Towards Better Carbohydrate Vaccines

Towards Better Carbohydrate Vaccines

Proceedings of a meeting organized by the World Health Organization, 9–11 October 1986, Geneva

Edited by

R. Bell and G. Torrigiani
Microbiology and Immunology,
World Health Organization,
Geneva, Switzerland

A Wiley Medical Publication

Published on behalf of the World Health Organization

JOHN WILEY & SONS
Chichester · New York · Brisbane · Toronto · Singapore

Library of Congress Cataloging in Publication Data:
Towards better carbohydrate vaccines.

(A Wiley medical publication)
'Published on behalf of the World Health Organization.'
Includes index.
1. Carbohydrates—Immunology—Congresses.
2. Vaccines—Congresses. I. Bell, R. II. Torrigiani, G. III. World Health Organization. IV. Series.
[DNLM: 1. Carbohydrates—immunology—congresses.
2. Immunotherapy—congresses. QU 75 T737 1986]
QR186.6.C37T68 1987 615'.372 87–10494

ISBN 0 471 91623 4

British Library Cataloguing in Publication Data:
Towards better carbohydrate vaccines:
proceedings of a meeting organized by the World Health Organization, 9–11 October 1986, Geneva.
1. Vaccines 2. Carbohydrates
I. Bell, Rosemary II. Torrigiani, G.
III. World Health Organization
615'.372 RM281

ISBN 0 471 91623 4

Typeset by Input Typesetting Ltd, London SW19 8DR
Printed and bound in Great Britain by Anchor Brendon Ltd, Colchester, Essex

Contents

V General Discussion

This book contains the view and statements
of an international group of scientists
meeting under the auspices of the
World Health Organization

Authors alone are responsible for views
expressed in signed papers

Towards Better Carbohydrate Vaccines
Edited by R. Bell and G. Torrigiani

Published by John Wiley & Sons Ltd

Carbohydrates and the immune system – an introduction

G. L. Ada
Department of Microbiology, John Curtin School of Medical Research, Australian National University, Canberra, ACT 2601, Australia

Three years ago, the World Health Organization (WHO) initiated a new Programme for Vaccine Development to complement other WHO programmes concerned with vaccines. Prior to the establishment of the new programme, a programme of research on the immunology of tuberculosis had been started and this was incorporated into the new programme. Four other diseases were chosen for which research leading to improved vaccines was considered to be of high priority. These were three diseases caused by viruses – dengue, hepatitis A and viruses involved in acute respiratory tract infections, principally respiratory syncytical virus and paramyxoviruses – and diseases caused by encapsulated bacteria, in which the evidence suggests that important epitopes are carbohydrate in nature. Initially, the programme on encapsulated bacteria was rather broad in its aim, but recently the Steering Committee operating this part of the programme reviewed their strategic plan and placed top priority on supporting research aimed at developing a vaccine to control meningococcal infections, though work on other related organisms may be supported if it has important conceptual or applied implications for the primary goal.

One of the main features of oligosaccharide antigenic determinants is that, generally, they react poorly with T cells and this is clearly shown during ontogeny. Vaccines featuring such epitopes may give adequate immune responses in adults, but lead to poor responses in children under 2 years of age. The reason for this poor response by T cells is not well understood, but advances in our general understanding of the requirements for T-cell responses to oligopeptide antigens and in other areas prompted the suggestion that now was an appropriate time to hold a meeting at which a number of features of carbohydrates could be discussed in relation to the immune system. All of these, in one way or another, may be related to future vaccine production, not only to control meningococcal infections but possibly diseases caused by other infectious agents, such as parasites.

We will hear at this meeting about the various disease agents, their distribution and disease patterns. The efficacy and shortcomings of current vaccines will be surveyed.

This will be followed by a session on the distribution of oligosaccharide epitopes and evidence regarding their importance as stimulators of the immune response will be discussed.

The next session is on molecular biology. Though short, it is potentially of great importance. One of the most exciting areas relevant to future vaccines is the use of recombinant or chimeric infectious agents as vectors for DNA coding for other antigens. If the genes coding for enzymes determining the antigenic specificity of carbohydrate epitopes of meningococcus could be transferred, for example, to *Neisseria lactamica* or *Salmonella typhimurium* Ty21a, this might be an effective means of immunization, not only for adults but possibly for young children. So this is potentially an important area.

In the next session, we have that great immunologist, Elvin Kabat, to give us of his wisdom, gained over many, many years, on the nature of carbohydrate epitopes and their reaction with antibodies. It is hard to conceive of a successful meeting on this topic without his participation. As part of this area of interest, two exciting prospects emerge. Antibodies recognize shapes; the work of Allen Edmundson [4] and others indicate that both the shapes involved – that of the epitope and that of the antibody, i.e. the antigen-combining site – demonstrate a degree of flexibility. The question arises – can the shape of an oligosaccharide epitope be sufficiently closely mimicked by other structures, e.g. oligopeptides, to deceive the immune system? That is, could one immunize with an oligopeptide and induce the formation of antibodies which will then bind with appropriate affinity to a carbohydrate determinant?

Evidence that this is theoretically possible has come from the study of anti-idiotypes. There are now reports [e.g. refs 5, 7] of the use of both idiotypes and anti-idiotypes to immunize against infection by bacteria where the epitope is oligosaccharide, and Dr Söderström will be telling us about findings in this area. The extension of this is – can an oligopeptide be synthesized *in vitro* and used as an immunogen to mount a protective antibody response to an encapsulated bacterium? This would represent a significant breakthrough indeed, and Mario Geysen will report on attempts to achieve this.

In the meantime, what can effectively be done about increasing the immunogenicity of carbohydrate epitopes? If this is essentially a matter of T-cell recognition, what can we learn about the structural requirements of epitopes in order for them to be recognized by T cells? There is now considerable evidence that oligopeptides recognized by T cells must have an amphipathic structure [3] and a programme is now available to identify such sites in proteins [6]. The precise reason for this is not absolutely clear. It seems that the hydrophilic portion of the epitope is recognized by the T-cell receptor and the hydrophobic portion of the molecule is at least in part to bind to the class II MHC antigen at the surface of the presenting cell. It may also play a role in attaching the epitope to the plasma membrane in the first place [1, 2, 8]. Can oligosaccharides *per se* adopt such a structure, or can they be modified, e.g. by attachment of a lipid tail, to have this structure? Work in the parasite area is teaching us some lessons in this respect, as will be mentioned by Emanuela Handman and André Capron. An alternative is to attach to the carbohydrate epitope a structure which is specially able to react with T cells, and the final speakers in the main part of the meeting will be discussing possibilities.

Provided our speakers adopt an adventurous attitude, this should be a very productive meeting and result in some important pointers for future vaccine development.

REFERENCES

1. Ashwell, J. D., and Schwartz, R. H. T cell recognition of antigens and the Ia molecule as a ternary complex. *Nature*, **320**, 176–8 (1986).
2. Babbitt, B. P., Allen, P. M., Matsueda, G., Haber, E., and Unanue, E. R. Binding of immunogenic peptides to Ia histocompatibility molecules. *Nature*, **317**, 359–61 (1985).
3. Delisi, C., and Berzofsky, J. A. T-cell antigenic sites tend to be amphipathic structures. *Proc. Natl. Acad. Sci. USA*, **82**, 7048–52 (1985).
4. Edmundson, A. B., and Ely, K. R. Binding of N-formylated chemotactic peptides in crystals of the Mcg light chain dimer: similarities with neutrophil receptors. *Mol. Immunol.*, **22**, 463–475 (1985).
5. McNamara, M. K., Ward, R. E. and Kohler, H. Monoclonal idiotype vaccine against *Streptococcus pneumoniae* infection. *Science*, **226**, 1325–6 (1984).
6. Sette, A., Doria, G., Adorini, L. A microcomputer programme for hydrophilicity and ampipathicity analysis of protein antigens. *Mol. Immunol.*, **23**, 807–10 (1986).
7. Stein, K., and Soderstrom, T. Neonatal administration of idiotype or antidiotype primer for protection against *Eschericia coli* K13 infection in mice. *J. exp. Med.*, 1984; **160**, 1001–11 (1984).
8. Watta, T. H., Gaub, H. E., and McConnell, H. M. T-cell mediated association

of peptide antigens and major histocompatibility complex protein detected by energy transfer in an evanescent wave-field. *Nature*, **320**, 179–81 (1986).

Part I: Occurrence of Carbohydrates on Various Cells

Towards Better Carbohydrate Vaccines
Edited by R. Bell and G. Torrigiani

Published by John Wiley & Sons Ltd

1

Carbohydrate antigens of mammalian cells

TEN FEIZI
Immunochemistry Research Group, MRC Clinical Research Centre, Watford Road, Harrow, Middlesex HA1 3UJ, UK

Carbohydrate chains of glycoproteins and glycolipids are prominent antigens of mammalian cells. These conclusions have been reached through studies of specificities of autoantibodies and hybridoma-derived monoclonal antibodies reactive with diverse cell types of man and mouse [2, 7]. Mono- and polyclonal antibodies to purified glycoproteins may also be directed against their carbohydrate moieties [3, 4]. Where there are homologies between carbohydrate structures of bacteria and those of host-cell membranes, as in the case of *Pneumococcus* type XIV [1, 8, 15] *Neisseria meningitides* Group B and *Escherichia coli* K1 [5, 6], it will be important to keep in mind the possibility that vaccination with the bacterial polysaccharides may elicit antibodies which react with the host-cell carbohydrates.

The carbohydrate structures of host-cell membranes serve as receptors for adhesion of several microbial agents and toxins [12]. In the case of infection with *Mycoplasma pneumoniae*, a pathogen of the human respiratory tract, autoantibodies are frequently elicited to the backbone of the host-cell carbohydrate receptor sequence [9, 10]. Thus the complexing of adhesive proteins of infective agents to specific saccharides of host-cell membranes may be a 'new' mechanism for eliciting autoantibodies.

There is a need for micro-scale immunoassays for monitoring antibody responses to specific oligosaccharide sequences. Such a procedure is well established for glycolipid oligosaccharides [11] but not for glycoprotein oligosaccharides. We have therefore designed a new micro-immunoassay procedure [13, 14] for analyses of the antigenicities of oligosaccharides released from glycoproteins. This procedure involves the conjugation of the oligosaccharides to a lipid (phosphatidyl ethanolamine diplomityl). The resulting neoglycolipids can be rendered multivalent by binding to plastic or silica plates, or they can be incorporated into liposomes and their antigenicities can be determined in low concentrations by binding or inhibition of binding assays. This approach has been successfully used with as little as 30 μg of starting glycoproteins (approx. 3 μg of carbohydrate material), and should be widely applicable for studies of antibody responses to carbohydrate moieties of glycoproteins.

REFERENCES

1. Feizi, T. The blood group Ii system: a carbohydrate antigen system defined by naturally monoclonal or oligoclonal autoantibodies of man. *Immunol. Commun.*, **10**, 127–56 (1981).
2. Feizi, T. Demonstration by monoclonal antibodies that carbohydrate structures of glycoproteins and glycolipids are onco-developmental antigens. *Nature*, **314**, 53–7 (1985).
3. Feizi, T., and Childs, R. A. Carbohydrate structures of glycoproteins and glycolipids as differentiation antigens, tumour-associated antigens and components of receptor systems. *Trends in Biochem. Sci.*, **10**, 24–9 (1985).
4. Feizi, T., and Childs, R. A. Carbohydrates as antigenic determinants of glycoproteins. *Biochem. J.*, in press.
5. Finne, J. Polysialic acid – a glycoprotein carbohydrate involved in neural adhesion and bacterial meningitis. *Trends in Biochem. Sci.*, **10**, 129–32 (1985).
6. Finne, J., Leinonen, M., and Makela, P. H. Antigenic similarities between brain components and bacteria causing meningitis. *Lancet*, **2**, 355–7 (1983).
7. Hakomori, S. Monoclonal antibodies directed to cell-surface carbohydrates. In *Monoclonal Antibodies and Functional Cell Lines* (ed. R. H. Kennet, K. B. Bechtol and T. J. McKearn), Plenum, New York, 1984, pp. 67–100.
8. Kabat, E. A. Contributions of quantitative immunochemistry to knowledge of blood group A, B, H, Le, I and i antigens. *Am. J. Clin. Pathol.*, **78**, 281–92 (1982).
9. Loomes, L. M., Uemura, K-I., Childs, R. A., Paulson, J. C., Rogers, G. N., Scudder, P. R. Michalski, J-C., Hounsell, E. F., Taylor-Robinson, D., and Feizi, T. Erythrocyte receptors for *Mycoplasma pneumoniae* are sialylated oligosaccharides of Ii antigen type. *Nature*, **307**, 560–3 (1984).
10. Loomes, L. M., Uemura, K-I., and Feizi, T. Interaction of *Mycoplasma pneumoniae* with erythrocyte glycolipids of I and i antigen types. *Infection and Immunity*, **47**, 15–20 (1985).
11. Magnani, J. L., Brockhaus, M., Smith, D. F., Ginsburg, V., Blaszczyk, M., Mitchell, K. F., Steplewski, Z., and Koprowski, H. A monosialoganglioside is a monoclonal antibody-defined antigen of colon carcinoma. *Science*, **212**, 55–6 (1981).
12. Mirelman, D. (ed.) *Microbial Lectins and Agglutinins*. John Wiley & Sons, New York, 1986.

13. Tang, P. W., and Feizi, T. Neoglycolipid micro-immunoassays applied to the oligosaccharides of human milk galactosyltransferase detect blood group related antigens on both O- and N-linked chains. *Carbohydr. Res.*, 161, 133–43 (1987).
14. Tang, P. W., Gooi, H. C., Hardy, M., Lee, Y. C., and Feizi, T. Novel approach to the study of the antigenicities and receptor functions of carbohydrate chains of glycoproteins. *Biochem Biophys Res Comm.*, **132**, 474–80 (1985).
15. Watkins, W. M. Biochemistry and genetics of the ABO, Lewis and P blood group systems. *Advances in Human Genetics* (ed. H. Harris and K. Hirschhorn), **10**, 1–136, 379–85 (1980).

DISCUSSION – Chaired by Dr J. B. Robbins

HANDMAN: One of the problems that we find, and so do my colleagues working on receptors on lymphocytes, is that the micro methods in carbohydrate chemistry are really macro methods as far as we are concerned. You are talking of 30 μg of protein. People working on growth factor receptors are talking about 700 receptors per cell; 30 μg of protein is really a huge amount that we cannot get. Is this your lowest limit, or is it possible to go down further?

FEIZI: Our assay procedure was designed with these problems in mind: 30 μg of galactosyltransferase contains only 3 μg of carbohydrate material, and this is sufficient for multiple assays using our procedure. Thus our procedure is substantially more sensitive than existing assay methods for glycoprotein oligosaccharides. We hope we shall render it even more microscale.

ROBBINS: In our laboratory Ronald Sekura has studied the bonding of pertussis toxin. Pertussis toxin recognizes that basic repeat structure in glycoproteins of galactose *N*-acetyl glucosamine both on serum proteins and on membrane proteins. This wide variety of activity might explain how the toxin is transported from the organism into the circulation and to various tissues.

Towards Better Carbohydrate Vaccines
Edited by R. Bell and G. Torrigiani

Published by John Wiley & Sons Ltd

2

A chemically modified Group B meningococcal polysaccharide vaccine*

HAROLD J. JENNINGS, ANDRZEJ GAMIAN, FRANCIS MICHON AND RENE ROY
Division of Biological Sciences, National Research Council of Canada, Ottawa, Ontario, Canada K1A 0R6
FRASER E. ASHTON
Bureau of Microbiology, Laboratory Center for Disease Control, Ottawa, Ontario, Canada K1A 0L2

ABSTRACT

In order to overcome the poor immunogenicity of the Group B meningococcal polysaccharide, chemical manipulation of its basic structure was attempted, on the premise that a structurally related synthetically derived artificial antigen might be capable of favourably modulating the immune response to the Group B meningococcal polysaccharide. One successful modification was to substitute *N*-propionyl groups for the *N*-acetyl groups in the polysaccharide. When conjugated to tetanus toxoid this immunogen successfully induced in mice much higher levels of cross-reactive Group B meningococcal-specific IgG antibodies than the similarly conjugated Group B meningococcal polysaccharide. In addition, only antisera produced in mice by the *N*-propionyl conjugate were bactericidal for Group B meningococcal organisms.

---

* This is NRCC Publication No. 27775.

INTRODUCTION

The poor immunogenicity of the Group B meningococcal polysaccharide (GBMP) and the structurally related *Escherichia coli* K1 capsular polysaccharide [16] preclude their use as human vaccines. With the exception of one report of the induction of high titre GBMP-specific antibodies by hyperimmunization of a horse [14] with Group B meningococcal (GBM) organisms, the latter organisms are usually only able to produce low levels of low-affinity GBMP-specific antibodies in humans and animals [12]. All of the above antibodies are exclusively of the IgM isotype and only recently was it reported [5] that GBMP-specific monoclonal antibodies of the IgG isotype could be produced by injecting a specialized strain of autoimmune NZB mice with GBM organisms.

The most probable reason for the poor immunogenicity of the GBMP is that it induces in humans and animals a state of immunological tolerance, due to the presence of cross-reactive tissue components. This hypothesis has been considerably strengthened by the identification of linear α-(2 → 8)-linked oligomers of sialic acid, similar to those associated with the structure of the GBMP [6], in the glycopeptides of human and rat foetal brain tissue [1, 2]. Furthermore, the oligosaccharide moieties of these glycopeptides were large enough, up to twelve sialic acid residues, to be able to generate the conformational determinant responsible for the immunological specificity of the GBMP [3, 6]. This is consistent with the fact that the polysialosylpeptides obtained from human and rat foetal brain bind to GBMP-specific equine polyclonal IgM antibodies and a GBMP-specific mouse monoclonal IgG_{2a} antibody [2].

Group B meningitis remains a major health problem in the world and the poor immunogenicity of the GBMP prevents the formulation of a comprehensive multivalent polysaccharide vaccine against meningococcal meningitis. Certainly experience would indicate that an immunogenic form of the GBMP would be a vaccine candidate worthy of serious consideration. One approach to produce an immunogenic form of the GBMP was to inject it in animals [4, 13] and humans [17] as a complex with meningococcal serotype outer membrane proteins. While enhancement of immunological responses was reported in some cases, the antibody levels were generally low, and the antibodies were exclusively of the IgM isotype.

MATERIALS AND METHODS

Materials

Neisseria meningitidis strain 608B was grown in a chemically defined medium and the GBMP isolated and purified as previously described [6, 8].

Methods

The GBMP was *N*-deacetylated by dissolving it in 2 M NaOH and heating the solution in a sealed tube for 6 hours at 105 °C [9, 10]. The *N*-deacetylated GBMP was *N*-propionylated using propionic anhydride [9, 10]. The GBMP–tetanus toxoid conjugate was made by a previously published procedure [8] and the *N*-propionylated GBMP–tetanus toxoid conjugate was made using the same procedure.

Female white (CFl) mice were immunized with the above polysaccharide conjugates in Freund's complete adjuvant and bled by procedures previously described [9]. The levels of GBMP-specific antibody were measured by a radioactive antigen binding assay using an extrinsically tritium-labelled GBMP antigen, and relative amounts of IgG and IgM GBMP-specific antibody were determined by ELISA [9].

RESULTS AND DISCUSSION

An alternative strategy to enhance the immunogenicity of the GBMP would be by means of its chemical manipulation. In this category is the covalent coupling of GBMP to a protein carrier, by which procedure many other polysaccharides [7] including the α-(2 → 9)-linked Group C meningococcal polysaccharide [8] have successfully induced high levels of polysaccharide-specific antibodies of the IgG isotype. However, when the GBMP was covalently linked to tetanus toxoid (TT) and the GBMP–TT conjugate was injected in rabbits, no GBMP-specific antibodies could be detected by immunodiffusion analysis [8]. However, recently, using more sensitive radioimmunoassay techniques [9], it has been possible to measure a distinct enhancement of GBMP-specific antibodies, including some of the IgG isotype, when mice were immunized with the same GBMP–TT conjugate vaccine (see later). Unfortunately, the antibody levels were low and this fact, together with the previous failure to detect bactericidal activity in animal post-immunization antisera [8], provides little encouragement for the use of this type of conjugate as a future human vaccine against GBM meningitis.

The relative failure of the direct coupling procedure prompted interest in the direct chemical modification of the GBMP itself. This was done with the idea of creating synthetic epitopes capable of modulating the immune system so as to produce enhanced levels of cross-reactive GBMP-specific antibodies. Although there is no precedent for this approach to succeed, serendipity played a role when it was demonstrated that a synthetic GBMP antigen could be made which was able to induce in mice high titres of cross-reactive GBMP-specific IgG antibodies [9, 10].

In selecting possible chemical modifications of the GBMP [9, 10], two

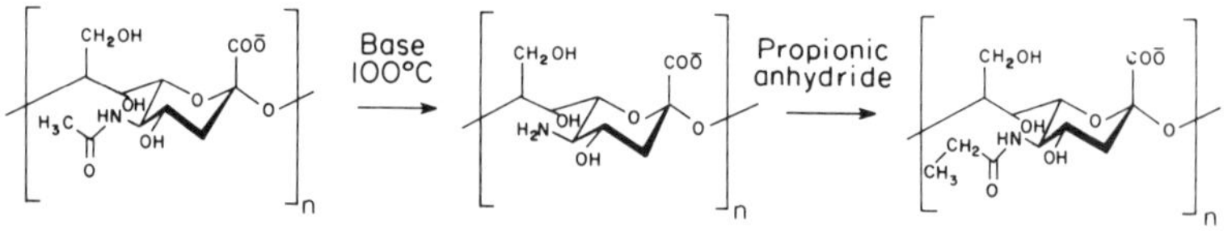

Figure 1. Reaction sequence leading to the formation of *N*-Pr–GBMP from *N*-Ac–GBMP

requirements had to be met. First, the modification had to be accomplished with ease and with minimal degradation of the polysaccharide. Secondly, in order to produce cross-reactivity, thc antigenicity of the modified polysaccharide to GBMP-specific antibodies had to be preserved. The carboxylate and amino groups of the sialic acid residues of the GBMP were obvious sites that could be modified with reasonable ease, and which satisfied the first requirement. However, in a number of modifications of both groups, only those involving the substitution of the *N*-acetyl (NAc) groups for other appropriate acyl groups, e.g. *N*-propionyl (NPr), satisfied the second requirement (Figure 1). Finally, the removal of NAc groups required that the GBMP be treated with strong base at 100 °C, conditions which depolymerize it considerably and render it non-immunogenic by virtue of its molecular size alone [9]. Therefore the NPr–GBMP was subsequently conjugated to TT using procedures previously described [8] for the formation of the NAc–GBMP–TT conjugate, thus yielding an artificial and virtually synthetic antigen.

The potential of the NPr–GBMP–TT conjugate to enhance the induction of GBMP-specific antibodies was first demonstrated by comparing the immune responses raised by the NPr–GBMP–TT- and NAc–GBMP–TT-conjugate vaccines in rabbits [10]. Serological analyses of these antisera indicated that the NPr conjugate not only elicited antibodies with homologous specificity but also raised higher levels of GBMP-specific antibodies than were induced by the NAc conjugate.

These observations made in the above preliminary experiments were amply verified by subsequent more comprehensive and statistically accurate experiments [9] in which the ability of the two conjugates to induce GBMP-specific antibodies in mice was compared. The results of this study are shown in Figure 2, and demonstrate that enhancement of the immune response to the GBMP was obtained from both conjugates. However, the NPr conjugate produced much higher levels of GBMP-specific antibodies than the homologous NAc conjugate, a booster effect being particularly pronounced following the second and third injections of the NPr conjugate. Interestingly, while the NAc conjugate also gave a noticeable but smaller booster effect after being injected three times in mice, it was much more effective following the priming of the mice with the NPr conjugate. In addition, following the priming of the mice with two injections of the NAc conjugate, a third immunization

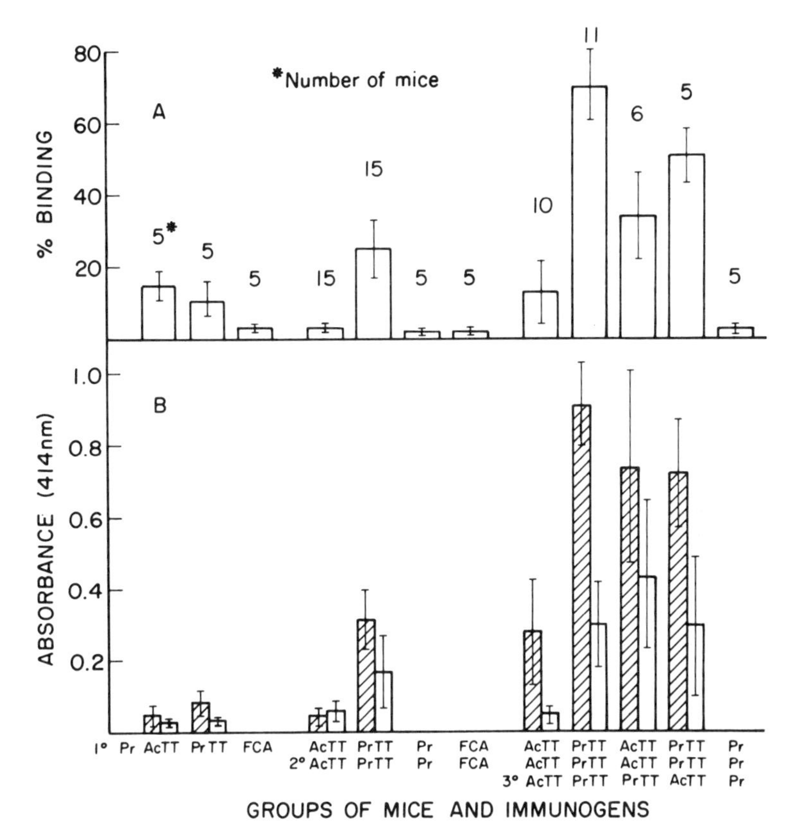

Figure 2. (A) Binding of GBMP to antibodies induced in groups of mice immunized with different antigens determined by radioactive antigen binding assay. Mean values ± standard deviation are shown. (B) Corresponding ratio of IgG (hatched bars) to IgM (open bars) antibodies in the antibody responses shown in A. The mice are grouped according to the antigen or antigens used, and the antigens are referred to by an abbreviated nomenclature; e.g. Pr, *N*-Pr–GBMP; PrTT, *N*-Pr–GBMP–TT; Actt, *N*-Ac–GBMP–TT

with the NPr conjugate also produced a pronounced booster effect. These booster effects are indicative of an anamnestic response based on the participation of T cells, which is also substantiated by the large proportion of IgG antibodies in all responses.

In comparative bactericidal assays, the pooled antisera produced by injecting the mice three times with the NPr conjugate proved to be highly bactericidal for a wide range of GBM organisms of different protein serotypes, whereas the equivalent NAc conjugate mouse antisera was inactive. The above bactericidal activity was also specific for GBM organisms [11].

Because the NPr–GBMP–TT conjugate is capable of inducing high titres of bactericidal GBMP-specific IgG antibodies in mice, it must be considered as a prototype vaccine against meningitis caused by Group B *N. meningitidis* and *E. Coli* K1. However, due to the structural and serological homology between the GBMP and the glycopeptides associated with foetal brain, it might be inferred that its success as a vaccine could only be achieved at the risk of breaking tolerance. Certainly the production of GBMP-specific IgG antibody in mice confirms that the NPr conjugate is capable of breaking tolerance. The consequences of this are unknown at present and, because of the importance of developing a viable GBM vaccine, the exploration of chemically modified GBMP vaccines needs to be actively pursued. Recent experiments [15] have been carried out which are encouraging to the pursuit of the above strategy. In these experiments it was found that while GBMP-specific IgG antibodies bind to foetal brain tissue *in vitro* there is evidence to suggest that these antibodies are incapable of crossing the blood–brain barrier. In addition it was also ascertained that the bactericidal antibodies induced in mice by the NPr–GBMP–TT conjugate did not bind to the GBMP [11].

REFERENCES

1. Finne, J., Finne, V., Deagostini-Bazin, H., and Goridis, C. Occurrence of a α-2 → 8-linked polysialosyl units in a neural cell adhesion molecule. *Biochim. Biophys. Acta*, **112**, 482–7 (1983).
2. Finne, J., Leinonen, M., and Mäkelä, P. H. Antigenic similarities between brain components and bacteria causing meningitis. *Lancet*, **ii**, 355–7 (1983).
3. Finne, J., and Mäkelä, P. H. Cleavage of the polysialosyl units of brain glycoproteins by a bacteriophage endosialidase. *J. Biol. Chem.*, **260**, 1265–70 (1985).
4. Frasch, C. E., Peppler, M. S., Cote, T. R., and Zahradnik, J. M. Immunogenicity and clinical evaluation of group B *Neisseria meningitidis* outer membrane protein vaccines. In *Seminars in Infectious Disease*, Vol. IV (ed. J. B. Robbins, J. C. Hill and J. C. Sadoff), Thieme-Stratton, New York, 1982, pp. 262–7.
5. Frosch, M., Görgen, I., Boulnois, G. J., Timmis, K. N., and Bitter-Süermann, D. NZB mouse system for production of monoclonal antibodies to weak bacterial antigens: isolation of an IgG antibody to the polysaccharide capsules of *Escherichia coli* K1 and group B meningococci. *Proc. Natl. Acad. Sci.*, **82**, 1194–8 (1985).
6. Jennings, H. J., Roy, R., and Michon, F. Determinant specificities of the groups B and C polysaccharides of *Neisseria meningitidis*. *J. Immunol.*, **134**, 2651–7 (1985).
7. Jennings, H. J. Polysaccharides and conjugated polysaccharides as human vaccines. In *New Developments in Industrial Polysaccharides* (ed. V. Crescenzi, I. C. M. Dea and S. S. Stivala), Gordon and Breach, New York, 1985, pp. 325–44.
8. Jennings, H. J., and Lugowski, C. Immunochemistry of groups A, B and C meningococcal polysaccharide-tetanus toxoid conjugates. *J. Immunol.*, **127**, 1011–18 (1981).

9. Jennings, H. J., Roy, R., Gamian, A. Induction of meningococcal group B polysaccharide-specific IgG antibodies in mice using an *N*-propionylated B polysaccharide–tetanus toxoid conjugate vaccine. *J. Immunol.*, **137**, 1708–13 (1986).
10. Jennings, H. J., and Roy, R. Enhancement of the immune response to the group B polysaccharide of *Neisseria meningitidis* by means of its chemical modification. In *The Pathogenic Neisseria* (ed. G. K. Schoolnik), American Microbiological Society, Washington DC, 1985, pp. 628–32.
11. Jennings, H. J., Gamian, A. and Ashton, F. E. N-propionylated group B meningococcal polysaccharide mimics a unique epitope on group B *Neisseria meningitidis*, J. exp. Med. **165**, 1207–11 (1987).
12. Mandrell, R. E., and Zollinger, W. D. Measurement of antibodies to meningococcal group B polysaccharide: low avidity binding and equilibrium constants. *J. Immunol.*, **129**, 2172–8 (1982).
13. Moreno, C., Esdaile, J., and Lifely, M. R. Thymic-dependence and immune memory in mice vaccinated with meningococcal polysaccharide group B complexed to outer membrane protein. *Immunology*, **57**, 425–30 (1986).
14. Orskov, F., Orskov, E., Sutton, A., Schneerson, R., Wenlii, L., Egan, W., Moff, G. E., and Robbins, J. B. Form variation in *Escherichia coli* K1: determined by *O*-acetylation of the capsular polysaccharide. *J. Exp. Med.*, **149**, 669–85 (1979).
15. Saukkonen, K., Haltia, M., Frosch, M., Bitter-Süermann, D., and Leinonen, M. Antibodies to the capsular polysaccharide of *Neisseria meningitidis* group B or *E. coli* K1 bind to the brains of infant rats *in vitro* but not *in vivo*. *Microbial Pathogenesis*, **1**, 101–5 (1986).
16. Wyle, F. A., Artenstein, M. S., Brandt, B. L., Tramont, D. L., Kasper, D. L., Altieri, P., Berman, S. L., and Lowenthal, J. P. Immunologic response of man to group B meningococcal polysaccharide antigens. *J. Infect. Dis.*, **126**, 514–22 (1972).
17. Zollinger, W. D., Mandrell, R. E., Griffiss, J. M., Altieri, P., and Berman, S. Complex of meningococcal group B polysaccharide and type 2 outer membrane protein immunogenic in man. *J. Clin. Invest.*, **63**, 836–48 (1979).

DISCUSSION – Chaired by Dr J. B. Robbins

CHAIRMAN: Dr Kabat would like to make some comments with some slides about a newly discovered human monoclonal antibody that reacts with the Group B meningococcus.

KABAT: I would first like as a matter of historical record, to call attention to the fact that, back in the Second World War, we had a contract with the Meningitis Commission of the US Army to study immunization against Group A meningococcus. In those days there was no radioimmunoassay and we immunized using the techniques that Michael Heidelberger had developed, and when we immunized with preparations that we had made in our own laboratory, as distinct from some of the other preparations which had been exposed to alkali, we got antibody levels of 9–18 μg of nitrogen per ml in 4 out of 30 individuals. Since Heidelberger got a much higher proportion of similar responses to the pneumococcal polysaccharides, this was not considered very promising at the time, but we did show that these antibodies were protective in animals (with C. P. Miller and A. Z. Foster), so that

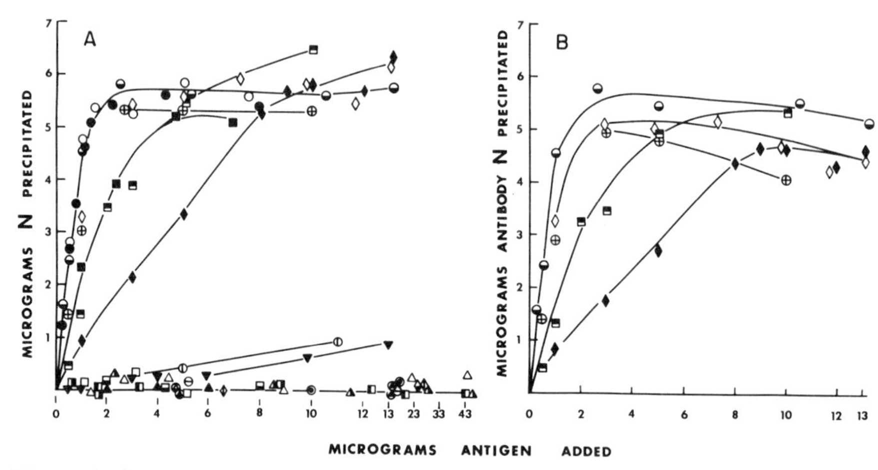

Figure 1. Quantitative precipitin curves for IgM^NOV with various polysaccharides, polynucleotides and DNA; 15 μl of a 1 : 10 dilution of IgM^NOV in a total volume of 200 μl. (A) Total nitrogen precipitated. (B) Antibody nitrogen precipitated. (○) Meningococcal CPS Group B; (○) *E. coli* K1 CPS LH *O*-acetyl-negative; (○) *E. coli* K1 CPS 016 *O*-acetyl-negative; (◇) poly (A); (○) poly (I); (■) *E. coli* K235 CPS *O*-acetyl-negative; (□) denatured DNA; (◆) poly(G); (○) colominic acid; (▽) bacto-agar, 20 °C, extracted; (□) *E. coli* K1 CPS LH *O*-acetyl-positive; (▲) *E. coli* K100 CPS; (△) *E. coli* K92 CPS N67; (△) *E. coli* K92 CPS MT1389; (□) meningococcal CPS Group C; (□) meningococcal CPS Group Y; (□) native DNA; (◇) chondroitin sulphate type A; (◇) chondroitin sulphate type B; (○) chondroitin sulphate type C; (○) *Klebsiella* K21; (○) *Klebsiella* K30; (○) polysialoglcoprotein. (From the *Journal of Experimental Medicine*, **164**, 642–4 (1986), by copyright permission of The Rockefeller University Press.)

actually we did demonstrate effective immunization back in 1945 against Group A meningococcus.

The first slide (Figure 1) will show you what is essentially an incredible finding because of its intrinsic low frequency. Elliot Osserman has been collecting proteins with monoclonal spikes and I have been testing them with my collection of polysaccharides, so we essentially make beautiful music together. We found quite a number of monoclonal spikes with various specificities, some of which Ten Feizi mentioned but, in this particular case, we found a very nice monoclonal antibody to poly-α-(2 → 8)-*N*-acetylneuraminic acid.

This is an individual of 81 years old, who is now 83, who gave a specific precipitive reaction with the Group B meningococcus polysaccharide and *E. coli* Kl. The first curve under A shows you two preparations of *E. coli* and two preparations of meningococcal polysaccharide in which about three quarters of a murogram gave maximum precipitation. These assays are done using 15 μg of a one-to-ten dilution of serum which calculates to 23 mg of antibody precipitated per ml anti-Group B, so that this individual is essen-

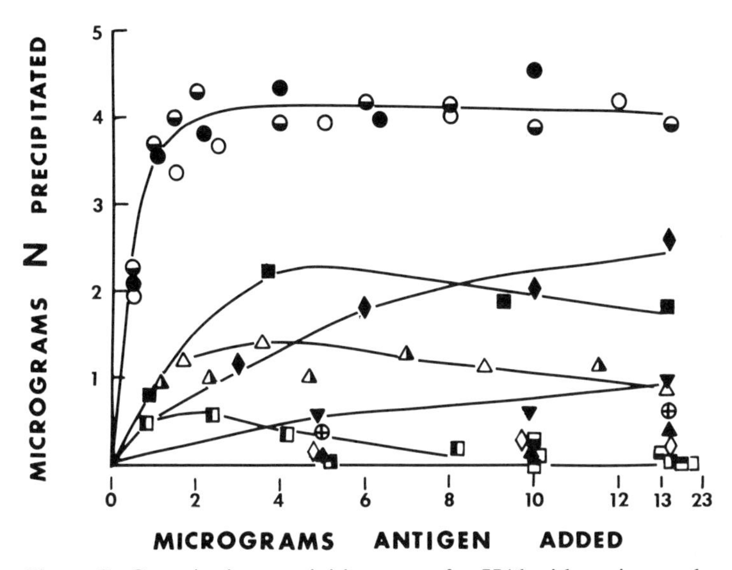

Figure 2. Quantitative precipitin curves for H46 with various polysaccharides, polynucleotides and DNA. Symbols as in Figure 1; 100 μl 1 : 5-diluted anti-horse 46, total volume 200 μl. (From the *Journal of Experimental Medicine*, **164**, 642–4 (1986), by copyright permission of The Rockefeller University Press.)

tially a potential walking factory for potent serum therapy of Group B meningitis or *E. coli* sepsis. Kathy Nickerson and Leonard Chess have been trying to get cell lines and make hybridomas so that one could preserve the antibody. We are, at the present time, doing amino acid sequencing of this antibody in case cell lines are not obtained. He has given us a plasmapheresis. We expect to be able to run a pilot clinical experiment in which alternate cases of Group B meningitis would be given, about 20 mg of this antibody with everybody getting the usual antibiotic therapy.

The same curve shows the four preparations of meningococcal Group B polysaccharides or *E. coli* (Carlos Moreno gave us one of his preparations). You can see their identity, but there is also on that initial curve a reaction with poly A and poly I, which per unit rate are equally good in precipitating the Group B polysaccharide. This is probably attributable to some oligomeric pattern in which the charged phosphates of poly A and poly I will occupy the same relative conformation as the carboxyls, and it is interesting that Michael Heidelberger, who is still working at the age of 98, showed a couple of years ago that, in two cross-reactions with type 8 and 19 polysaccharide, a phosphorylated mannose oligomeric pattern would function in cross-precipitating anti-carboxyl pattern, and *vice versa*. So there are several cases coming up of this type, and this is the basis for one group of what is called poly-specificity.

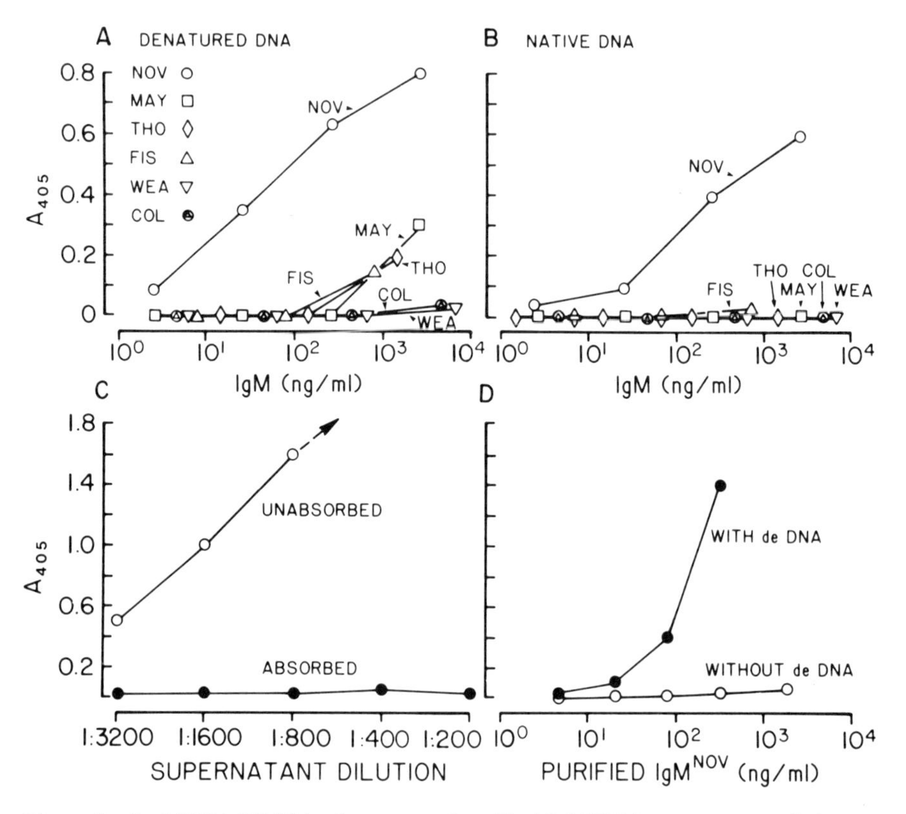

Figure 3. Anti-DNA ELISA of serum and purified IgM^NOV^ in nanograms of nitrogen per millitre. NOV serum and five other sera containing monoclonal IgM proteins tested against denatured (A), and native (B) DNA by ELISA. Serum dilutions have been converted to nanograms of IgM present per millitre, to adjust for the varying amounts of macroglobulin in each serum. Values represent mean of duplicate samples. (C) Anti-DNA ELISA of NOV serum before and after absorption with meningococcal polysaccharide. A 1 : 10 dilution of serum was added to 5.25 μg polysaccharide in a total volume of 200 μl. The dilutions shown are of the supernatants with and without polysaccharide. (D) Purified IgM^NOV^ with denatured (de) DNA as the substrate. Values shown are means of duplicates. Shaded circles indicate wells coated with DNA; open circles indicate control wells without DNA, (from the *Journal of Experimental Medicine*, **164**, 642–4 (1986), by copyright permission of The Rockefeller University Press.)

This (Figure 2) is John Robbins's standard anti-Group B meningococcal horse serum. Dr Robbins, Dr Schneerson and Dr Yang carried out studies on protective power in rats against *E. coli* Kl infection and, microgram for microgram, these are approximately as potent as our human anti-meningococcal antibody. With respect to the glycolipid reactions, Dr Laytor tested with GM3 and GD3 and did not find any particular cross-reaction.

Kathy Nickerson studied the reactions with DNA (Figure 3). This reacts in the precipitin reaction with denatured DNA. It takes about two or three times as much to give equal amounts of precipitation, and here are four other monoclonals which were studied as controls. You get a little bit of cross-reaction with native DNA by ELISA and probably one-thousandth as much reactivity to native DNA, and this could be due to frayed ends in the method of preparing the native DNA. Again, you can see that the antibody, unabsorbed, gives you very good reaction and if you absorb it either with meningococcal polysaccharide or with denatured DNA you do remove all of the antibody. This is essentially the picture and we are hoping to get some arrangements with the Bureau of Biologics at NIH whereby we can undertake to do this clinical study. As I say, we have a plasmapheresis from him. He is a very co-operative gentleman and it may be that we could carry out this experiment while we are trying to get cell lines and also to clone the genes and things like that.

ROBBINS: Dr Kabat, just in regard to your query about the safety involved in the use of such immunogens, does the fellow who has had a chronic malignancy removed, but does not seem to have any symptoms that could be related to the potential of this antibody, tend to react with nervous tissue?

KABAT: He is in perfectly good health. This condition goes under the name of benign monoclonal gammopathy. I have one myself, which we can date back to the appearance of a monoclonal spike to about 1970 since I had serum dating back to the 1950s. As far as I know it has never bothered me. It happens to be an antibody to a snail galactan. I must say that I would prefer to have the anti-meningococcal antibody.

JENNINGS: Do you think that the critical thing, though, would be the effect of putting the IgG into, say, pregnant women? You will get placental passage of the IgG and then interfere with the whole mechanism?

KABAT: You mean as a possible difficulty?

JENNINGS: Yes.

KABAT: I have no idea, but at the moment one would administer the IgM antibody in the treatment, of meningococcus meningitis intrathecally. I looked over the old literature from 1900 to 1930 on the use of horse anti-meningococcal serum and, believe it or not, they used to give 20 cc of horse antiserum intraspinally, three or four times a day for 4 days. We had a little meeting with the people from the Bureau of Biologics who were worried even about giving 1 ml of human serum intraspinally. They suggest that we actually purify the antibody before we use it, which of course is perfectly reasonable. But it shows you how far we have come since the 1900–30 period with respect to human therapy.

ROBBINS: Could I ask Dr Helena Mäkelä to comment about the potential immunopathogenic effects of having a foetus exposed to IgG antibody of this specificity?

MÄKELÄ, Helena: I do not think I have anything to say more than anybody else here, because we really do not know what happens. We know that this antigen is found in large quantities in the brain and also other tissues, at least close to birth. It disappears in a few weeks, as far as we can tell, but it also reappears after trauma for example. So it is not totally non-existent in adults either. Another consideration, of course, is that it might not be accessible to antibodies circulating in the serum and this is reasonable, but how can you be sure that small amounts of antibody would not leak into the sensitive sites anyway. I think that really is the crucial point.

The people in my laboratory did a very crude experiment in looking at binding of antibody injected in the blood of new-born rats and did not find any antibody in the brain, but I think this is a very insensitive assay. It is a starting-point that tells us that gross lesions do not occur, but one would really have to observe these animals for a very long time and to observe for undefined clinical symptoms, and I do not know how you can measure psychological changes in rats. I think it will be very difficult to find out what is happening. On the other hand, I do acknowledge that there is a great a need for this type of vaccine, because alternative attempts at finding vaccines to the Group B meningococcus, based mainly on the outer membrane proteins, are still indecisive. We do not know whether such antibodies work or whether one would need very high quantities of these antibodies of protection.

At least in experimental studies, it is sure that, when you cause an experimental infection with the encapsulated bacteria, they are very much more sensitive to antibodies directed to the capsule than antibodies directed to any components beneath the capsule. Definitely, many antibodies that bind to the outer membrane of non-capsulated bacteria, or non-capsulated mutants, do not bind, or are not bactericidal to the encapsulated form and are not protective in experimental studies. So I think there were many negative findings in respect of these other outer membrane components, consequently one must consider the capsular polysaccharide more seriously, but I am worried about the possible adverse effects and I do not know how to find out what happens if you induce antibodies to them in humans.

ROBBINS: Just a last comment, that those polysaccharide acid with the α-(2 → 8)-linked compounds that you find in foetal mammals were also found in fishes. Fish eggs, especially the salmon, have been well studied and those things are present in the eggs and disappear very quickly after hatching. It may be a general phenomenon of foetal development.

Towards Better Carbohydrate Vaccines
Edited by R. Bell and G. Torrigiani

Published by John Wiley & Sons Ltd

3

Schistosomes, a model for the study of parasite carbohydrate immunogens

A. Capron, C. Dissous, J. M. Grzych and M. Capron
Centre d'Immunologie et de Biologie parasitaire, Unité mixte, Institut national de la Santé et de la Recherche médicale 167 – Centre nationale de la Récherche scientifique 624, Institut Pasteur de Lille, France
J. Montreuil, G. Spik and P. M. Jacquinot
Unité associée, Centre national de la Recherche scientifique 217, Université des Sciences et Techniques de Lille I, France

The importance of carbohydrate antigens in trematode infections, and particularly in schistosomiasis, has been described by many authors. A glycoprotein antigen, called M antigen, specific for the *Schistosoma* genus and localized in the cell wall of adult worm gut, was found in a circulating form in serum and urine of animals and humans infected by *S. mansoni* [3, 4]. Biochemical studies revealed that M antigen contained an important carbohydrate moiety (63%) and the presence of *O*-glycosidic linkage allowed M antigen to be considered as a mucin or a mucus glycoprotein-like component [5]. Circulating anodic (CAA) and cathodic (CCA) antigens showing a large range of molecular weight (50–300 000) were purified from trichloracetic acid-soluble fraction of adult worms. These polysaccharide antigens were found to be gut-associated and present in excretory and secretory products of schistosomes, eliciting an immunological response in mouse, hamster and human infection [6]. During *S. mansoni* infection, antibodies were shown to be directed against a gut-associated proteoglycan (GASP) and a glycoprotein(s) of 90–130 000 molecular weight (PSAP) [19].

Monoclonal antibodies were produced against carbohydrate moieties of antigens from different developmental stages of *Schistosoma.* Weiss and Strand used different monoclonal antibodies to characterize a group of acidic *S. mansoni* egg glycoproteins that display heterogeneous molecular weight in SDS–PAGE. All of the epitopes were present in eggs, cercariae and adult worms. The reactivity of monoclonal antibodies with several glycosylated proteins in the different developmental stages and *Schistosoma* species, as well as the sensitivity of antigens to a mild periodate oxidation, suggested that epitopes involved carbohydrate structures [23]. These immunogenic carbohydrate epitopes were also recovered on glycolipids of each parasite stage [24].

The presence and the nature of carbohydrates exposed on the *S. mansoni* surface were determined by the binding of lectins with various sugar specificities [1, 18, 21]. Results also indicated significant modifications of the surface carbohydrate composition during *in vivo* maturation of the parasite [20]. Immunoprecipitation of surface-radioiodinated schistosomula by monoclonal antibodies allowed us to characterize a particular surface glycoconjugate of 38 000 molecular weight. The 38 kDa antigen was shown to be a potent immunogen in experimental [8] and human [11] infection and was precipitated by a rat monoclonal IgG_{2a} (IPLSml) [9] which induced eosinophil-mediated cytotoxicity *in vitro* and protected naïve rats by passive transfer [14]. The protective epitope was characterized on a 115 kDa molecule in adult metabolic products [7] and was also present on variable molecular weight components of cercariae [9] and miracidia [10] surfaces. These observations suggested that the protective epitope could involve carbohydrate chains linked to different protein or proteolipidic structures. Moreover, the sensitivity of the epitope to periodate treatment [7] and the inability of IPLSml to precipitate *in vitro* translation products from adult worm or schistosomulum mRNA, confirmed the hypothesis of a carbohydrate nature for the epitope. Additional results, indicating that a rat monoclonal antibody of IgG_{2c} subclass with similar antigenic specificity was able to block the protective activity of IPLSml [15], prompted us to attempt the production of anti-idiotype to IPLSml. In a recent series of experiments, we were indeed able to demonstrate that immunization of rats with monoclonal anti-idiotype antibodies (AB_2) against the protective AB_1 monoclonal led to the production of specific and highly cytotoxic antibodies and, more importantly, induced a high degree of protection to challenge infection in recipient animals [16].

Although encouraging, these results appeared of limited applicability for vaccination against human disease and encouraged further studies on the chemical characterization of the glycan epitope.

The original description in our laboratory some 20 years ago [2] of shared antigens between schistosomes and their intermediate hosts prompted us to study possible identity between characterized *S. mansoni* target antigens and

Biomphalaria glabrata components [10]. Antibodies against mollusc soluble extracts were produced in rabbits and used to immunoprecipitate surface-labelled antigens of miracidia and schistosomula. In both parasite stages these antibodies bound to surface molecules and the electrophoretic mobilities of the bound antigens were similar to those characterized with IPLSml. Evidence of binding to the same epitope was given by the ability of antibodies to *B. glabrata* to inhibit (by up to 80%) the recognition by IPLS ml of the 38 kDa schistosomulum antigen in a solid-phase competition assay. Confirming our previous observation on the glycan nature of the epitope, it was shown that rabbit antibodies produced against deglycosylated mollusc extracts failed to recognize surface-labelled parasite antigens and were not able to compete with IPLSml for binding to the 38 kDa molecule.

The identification of cross-reactive *B. glabrata* components was also confirmed by SDS–PAGE analysis of soluble mollusc extracts followed by Western blotting using the IPLSml antibody. Under these experimental conditions IPLSml was shown to bind preferentially to a 90 kDa *B. glabrata* component, and this band was not labelled when a deglycosylated *B. glabrata* extract was analysed.

The next question to be answered was whether this molecular mimicry was limited to the *S. mansoni–B. glabrata* host-parasite system. Whereas *B. glabrata* extracts strongly inhibited (up to 95%) the immunoprecipitation of labelled 38 kDa antigen by IPLSml, we observed that soluble extracts from *Bulinus truncatus* and *Lymnaea stagnalis*, which are respectively the intermediate hosts for *S. haematobium* and *Trichobilharzia ocellata*, were also both able to compete with the *S. mansoni* antigen showing respective inhibition of 80 and 65%. Moreover, a similar level of inhibition (75%) was observed with a non-schistosome host, *L. limosa*. Such results suggested that the presence of the protective epitope in molluscs was not restricted and would be found in a wide variety of snail species.

We next made a crucial observation which, in fact, was due more to serendipity than to a logical progression of experimental analysis. We showed, in the course of the immunization of rats with anti-idiotype antibodies conjugated to keyhole limpet haemocyanin (KLH), that sera collected from the control group of rats immunized with KLH alone could bind strongly to the schistosomulum surface and, more significantly, inhibit the binding of ^{125}I-labelled IPLSml to parasite antigen in exactly the same range of inhibition as serum from rats immunized with AB_2–KLH [13].

This preliminary observation suggesting the existence of a common epitope between the haemocyanin of *Megathura crenulata*, an ancestral marine mollusc, and the *S. mansoni* antigen was placed on a molecular basis by immunoprecipitation techniques. We showed that indeed sera from KLH-immunized rats were capable of binding to the 38 kDa schistosomulum surface antigen. The antigenic similarity between parasite antigen and KLH was also confirmed by the analysis of a purified fraction of KLH by SDS–PAGE and Western blotting. These experiments showed that molecules of about 150–200 kDa were recognized by IPLSml, and by sera from animals infected with *S. mansoni*.

The glycan nature of the parasite epitope, together with the documented existence of carbohydrate moieties in KLH, prompted us to study the potential importance of KLH oligosaccharides in this surprising cross-reactivity. Inhibition experiments were performed either with purified native KLH, KLH deglycosylated with TFMS (trifluoromethanesulphonic acid) or with sera collected from rats immunized with KLH or deglycosylated KLH. In such conditions it was shown that various concentrations of native KLH, but not of deglycosylated KLH, were able to inhibit strongly the binding of IPLSml to the 38 kDa antigen. Antibodies obtained from KLH-immunized rats induced the same level of inhibition as that observed for infected rat sera, IPLSml or purified KLH. We could also inhibit the binding of labelled IPLSml to KLH by various concentrations of sera from infected animals. In all these experiments deglycosylation of KLH ablated the effects of the native molecule. More recently, similar inhibition experiments performed with the purified carbohydrate moiety of KLH clearly confirmed the total identity between the glycan epitope of parasite and KLH oligosaccharides.

Moreover, using this approach, a total identity was demonstrated between KLH oligosaccharides and *Biomphalaria* allowing, therefore, the existence of a cross-reactive glycan epitope on schistosomula surface, on the intermediate host *B. glabrata* and in the ancestral marine snail *M. crenulata* to be ascertained.

It is also noteworthy that KLH almost totally inhibits the interaction between IPLSml and its anti-idiotype, thus confirming that the anti-idiotype which was produced against the MAb to the 38 kDa molecule was indeed the internal image of this antigen.

The essential role of anti-38 kDa antibodies in eosinophil-dependent cytotoxicity for schistosomula naturally led to the investigation of such cytotoxic antibodies in sera from KLH-immunized rats. Significant levels of cytotoxicity (46–94%) comparable to those obtained when using infected rat sera, were observed. The antibodies produced by immunizing rats with KLH were also found to be protective when passively transferred to recipient rats to a degree (48%) very close to that previously observed for the IPLSml protective antibody. In addition, KLH immunized rats were shown to be highly protected against a challenge infection.

Since it had been shown previously in human infected populations that antibodies to the 38 kDa parasite antigen could be detected in 97% of patients [11], we explored the possibility of using KLH for the detection of anti-schistosome antibodies in humans. Preliminary studies using a competition assay with human sera have indicated the potential use of KLH as a diagnostic reagent.

Work at present in progress now indicates the feasibility of defining the chemical structure of KLH oligosaccharides and their possible synthesis.

The sugar composition of commercially purified KLH (France Biochem., Meudon) has been determined by gas–liquid chromatography, and the identification of monosaccharides has been confirmed by mass spectrometry. Total sugars represent 5–5.25% of KLH and the molar ratios of monosaccharides in native KLH molecules are listed in Table I.

Table I. Molecular ratios[a] of monosaccharides in KLH

Monosaccharides	Native KLH	KLH glycopeptide (from pronase hydrolysis)	KLH oligosaccharides (from alkaline hydrolysis)
Mannose	3	3	3
Galactose	3–4	4–5	3.5–4
Fucose	2–3	1.6–3	2.5–3
Glucose	1.8–2.4	4	0.5–1
Xylose	0.5–1	0.5–1	0.5–0.8
N-acetylglucosamine	3–4	3.3–4.5	1.6–3
N-acetylglucosaminitol	—	—	1
N-acetylgalactosamine	1.7–2.3	2–2.5	0.8
N-acetylgalactosaminitol	—	—	1

[a] Calculated on the basis of three mannose residues.

The glucidic nature of the KLH epitope recognized by IPLSml was first confirmed by its sensitivity to mild periodate oxidation. Pronase hydrolysis of KLH (at 40 °C for 48 hours, pH 8.2) and gel-filtration chromatography on Biogel P2 of hydrolysis products have led to the obtention of a glycopeptide (bearing four to five amino-acid residues) exhibiting, in IPLSml-38 kDa binding competitive assay, the KLH inhibitory activity. The molar composition in monosaccharides of the glycopeptide was also shown to be very similar to that of native KLH (see Table I). More recently, alkaline hydrolysis was used to prepare oligosaccharidic fractions of KLH. Here, KLH was treated for 6 hours at 100 °C in NaOH 1 N in the presence of BH_4Na 1M and oligosaccharides were purified by chromatography on Biogel P2, then reacetylated by acetic anhydrid in the presence of $NaHCO_3$. The oligosaccharidic fraction kept the KLH inhibitory activity, and the molar composition of purified oligosaccharides was determined (Table I). The presence of both *N*-acetylglucosaminitol and *N*-acetylgalactosaminitol implicates the coexistence in KLH of *N*-glycosyl and *O*-glycosyl linkages (GlcNAc–Asn and GalNAc–Ser (Thr)).

Taken together, these observations appear to have several main consequences. They illustrate the expression on the surface of a human parasite of a major immunogen, not only present in its snail intermediate host, but of which the origins are found in a marine mollusc that has been in existence for the past several hundred million years. The evolutionary conservation of the structure and the similarities of the expression in a human parasite pose a fascinating problem of phylogeny and adaptation. It has been recently reported in various biological systems that membrane oligosaccharides play an important role in osmotic adaptation and osmolarity [17]. It is tempting to speculate that important changes affecting schistosomes in the osmolarity of their cellular environment during the rapid adaptation of the free larval forms to their vertebrate or invertebrate hosts might rely on this highly preserved structure [10].

The fact that almost all subjects infected by *S. mansoni* produce antibodies against the glycanic epitope of the 38 kDa antigen also present in KLH opens an entirely new path towards the development of a simple, easily standardized and cheap reagent for the sero-epidemiology of human schistosomiasis. The protective properties linked to this particular epitope might confer on KLH, and particularly on its glycanic moiety, an interesting potential in the vaccine strategy against schistosomes. Work presently in progress using mass-spectrometry analysis of purified KLH oligosaccharides makes feasible in the near future the access to a well-defined structure.

Finally, it will be certainly of interest to immunologists that have used KLH for 20 years as a carrier for human or animal immunization [12, 22] to know that such immunization can lead to the production of anti-*S. mansoni* antibodies.

CONCLUSION

Major progress has been recently made in the identification, purification and molecular characterization of an immunodominant carbohydrate epitope expressed on *S. mansoni* schistosomula surface.

The demonstration of an identical epitope in the snail intermediate host, *B. glabrata* and the ancestral marine snail *M. crenulata* (keyhole limpet) opens, besides its theoretical interest, new perspectives in the framework of a vaccine strategy against schistosomiasis.

It also appears that a precise knowledge of the structure of the oligosaccharide involved, together with the availability of monoclonal idiotypic and anti-idiotypic antibodies, will constitute the basis of a novel model for the understanding of carbohydrate immunogenicity.

ACKNOWLEDGEMENTS

This work was partially supported by a grant from the Edna McConnell Clark Foundation (EMCF No. 07585) and by the INSERM (U167) and by the CNRS (624).

REFERENCES

1. Bennett, J. L., and Seed, J. L. Characterization and isolation of concanavalin A binding sites from the epidermis of *S. mansoni*. *J. Parasitol.*, **63**, 250–8 (1977).
2. Capron, A., Biguet, J., Rose, F., and Vernes, A. Les antigènes de *Schistosoma mansoni*. II. Etude immunoélectrophorétique comparée de divers stades larvaires et des adultes des deux sexes. Aspects immunologiques des relations hôte–parasite de la cercaire et de l'adulte. *Ann. Inst. Past. Paris*, **109**, 798–810 (1965).
3. Carlier, Y., Bout, D., Bina, J. C., Camus, D., Figueiredo, J. F. M., and Capron, A. Immunological studies in human schistosomiasis. I. Parasitic antigen in urine. *Am. J. Trop. Med. Hyg.*, **24**, 949–54 (1975).
4. Carlier, Y., Bout, D., and Capron, A. Further studies on the circulating M antigen in human and experimental *Schistosoma mansoni* infections. *Ann. Immunol. (Inst. Past.)*, **129C**, 811–8 (1978).
5. Carlier, Y., Bout, D., Strecker, G., Debray, H., and Capron, A. Purification, immunochemical and biological characterization of the *Schistosoma* circulating M antigen. *J. Immunol.*, **124**, 2442–50 (1980).
6. Deelder, A. M., Kornelis, D., Van Marck, E. A. E., Eveleigh, P. C., and Van Egmond, J. G. *Schistosoma mansoni*: characterization of two circulating polysaccharide antigens and the immunological response to these antigens in mouse, hamster and human infections. *Exp. Parasitol.*, **50**, 16–32 (1980).
7. Dissous, C., and Capron, A. *Schistosoma mansoni*: antigenic community between schistosomula surface and adult worm incubation products as a support for concomitant immunity. *FEBS Lett.*, **162**, 355–9 (1983).
8. Dissous, C., Dissous, C., and Capron, A. Isolation and characterization of surface antigens from *Schistosoma mansoni* schistosomula. *Mol. Biochem. Parasitol.*, **3**, 215–225 (1981).
9. Dissous, C., Grzych, J. M., and Capron, A. *Schistosoma mansoni* surface antigen defined by a rat monoclonal IgG_{2a}. *J. Immunol.*, **129**, 2232–4 (1982).
10. Dissous, C., Grzych, J. M., and Capron, A. *Schistosoma mansoni* shares a protective oligosaccharide epitope with fresh water and marine snails. *Nature*, **323**, 443–5 (1986).
11. Dissous, C., Prata, A., and Capron, A. Human antibody response to *Schistosoma mansoni* surface antigens defined by protective monoclonal antibodies, *J. Inf. Dis.*, **149**, 227–33 (1984).
12. Dixon, F. J., Jacot-Guillormod, H., and McConahey, P. J. The antibody responses of rabbits and rats to hemocyanin. *J. Immunol.*, **97**, 350–5 (1966).
13. Grzych, J. M., Dissous, C., Capron, M., Lambert, P. H., and Capron, A. of *Schistosoma mansoni* shares with a protective carbohydrate epitope, Keyhole Limpet Hemocyanin (KLH) *J. exp. Med.*, **165**, 865–878 (1987).
14. Grzych, J. M., Capron, M., Bazin, H., and Capron, A. *In vitro* and *in vivo* effector function of rat IgG_{2a} monoclonal anti-*S. mansoni* antibodies. *J. Immunol.*, **129**, 2739–43 (1982).

15. Grzych, J. M., Capron, M., Dissous, C., and Capron, A. Blocking activity of rat monoclonal antibodies in experimental schistosomiasis. *J. Immunol.*, **133**, 998–1004 (1984).
16. Grzych, J. M., Capron, M., Lambert, P. H., Dissous, C., Torres, S., and Capron, A. An anti-idiotype vaccine against experimental schistosomiasis. *Nature*, **316**, 74–5 (1985).
17. Miller, K. J., Kennedy, E. P., and Reinhold, V. N. Osmotic adaptation by gram-negative bacteria: possible role for periplasmic oligosaccharides. *Science*, **231**, 48–51 (1986).
18. Murrell, K. D., Taylor, D. W., Vannier, W. E., and Dean, D. A. *Schistosoma mansoni*: analysis of surface membrane carbohydrates using lectins. *Exp. Parasitol.*, **46**, 247–55 (1978).
19. Nash, T., Lunde, M. N., and Cheever, A. W. Analysis and antigenic activity of a carbohydrate fraction derived from adult *Schistosoma mansoni. J. Immunol.*, **126**, 805–10 (1981).
20. Simpson, A. J. G., Correa-Oliveria, R., Smithers, S. R., and Sher, A. The exposed carbohydrates of schistosomula of *Schistosoma mansoni* and their modification during maturation *in vivo. Mol. Biochem. Parasitol.*, **8**, 191–205 (1983).
21. Simpson, A. J. G., and Smithers, S. R. Characterization of the exposed carbohydrates on the surface membrane of adult *S. mansoni* by analysis of lectin binding. *Parasitology*, **81**, 1–15 (1980).
22. Swanson, M. A., and Schwartz, R. S. Immunosuppressive therapy: the relation between clinical response and immunologic competence. *New Engl. J. Med.*, **277**, 163–70 (1967).
23. Weiss, J. B., and Strand, M. Characterization of developmentally regulated epitopes of *Schistosoma mansoni* egg glycoprotein antigens. *J. Immunol.*, **135**, 1421–9 (1985).
24. Weiss, J. B., Magnani, J. L., and Strand, M. Identification of *Schistosoma mansoni* glycolipids that share immunogenic carbohydrate epitopes with glycoproteins. *J. Immunol.*, **136**, 4275–82 (1986).

DISCUSSION – Chaired by Dr J. B. Robbins

GLAUDEMANS: This question may show my ignorance, but the use of anti-idiotypic antibodies to carbohydrates – specific antibodies – has anybody ever looked at that as a method of breaking tolerance as far as a vaccine is concerned? Because one would now have an immunogen which is a protein which would mimic the determinant on the polysaccharide.

CAPRON: This is a verv interesting question indeed. As I mentioned, one of the main drawbacks of using this particular oligosaccharide is that, at the same time, it can induce two different antibody isotypes in the rat, one is a IgG_{2a} protective, the other is IgG_{2c}, which is a blocking. The equivalent in man being an IgG and an IgM. I think you are right, in the sense that when we immunize rats with the purified molecule, if we can proceed into immunization we can produce blocking antibodies with KLH, which is not apparently the case with the anti-idiotype.

MORENO: In the process of inducing immunity to the schistosoma, wouldn't this immunization to KLH also be a phenomenal way of inducing allergy to molluscs as well?

CAPRON: You mean, could it be a possible molecular basis for the development of allergy and hypersensitivity reaction to snails? I have no answer to that.

MORENO: In particular, since you need IgE to protect.

ROBBINS: I hope it won't introduce immunity to lobsters!

GRIFFISS: In answer to the question about anti-idiotypes breaking tolerance. An anti-idiotype to the parotope that binds the Group A meningococcal capsular polysaccharide, which is mannosamine phosphate, does break tolerance in the mouse and induces high levels of antibody. This is work done by Dr Michael Apicella and supported by WHO.

FEIZI: I wonder if I could ask you whether you have looked for cross-reactions between *S. mansoni* antigens, KLH and mammalian cells. The reason I am asking is that you could be dealing with a common carbohydrate epitope shared by schistosomes, KLH, mammalian cells as well as antibodies. This could provide a very simple explanation for all these cross-reactions.

CAPRON: Yes. This is a very pertinent question and we, of course, have been anxious to answer it. The thing I would like to say is that our observation is consistent with what we know about the evolution of prosobranch snails and the freshwater Gasteropods. Interestingly enough, one of the very well-known snails, which you all know as the Burgundy snail (very famous in France), *Helix pomatia*, belongs to a different family. A likely result, if we were right in our hypothesis, is that this epitope wouldn't be expressed on this particular land snail. Indeed, oligosaccharide does not exist on *H. pomatia*. The haemocyanin oligosaccharide is different. Now, to answer the second part of your question, we have of course been looking for possible cross-reactivity with mammalian carbohydrate, and from Jean Montreuil's experience there is no evidence of such a structure in mammalian antigens.

FEIZI: Have you looked for reactivities with mammalian cells?

CAPRON: Yes, during our control experiments with anti-KLH antibodies.

FEIZI: Do they react?

CAPRON: No. We have so far observed no evidence for binding of our anti-KLH antibodies to any vertebrate cell, but we certainly need to extend these investigations.

FEIZI: Do lysates of mammalian cells (e.g. hamster cells) inhibit the antibodies, just as the lysates of the molluscs?

CAPRON: This has to be done.

ADA: Professor Capron, haemocyanin has been the most popular of all carriers used by immunologists, and if you were to ask most immunologists what it was about, it was a very large molecule, essentially composed of oligopeptides. I am curious to know whether you have thought of testing your deglycosylated haemocyanin to see whether it is any good as a carrier for other antigens.

CAPRON: Yes, we are in the process of using the protein of KLH as a carrier after deglycosylation.

ADA: Does it work?

CAPRON: I can't tell you. This is being done at the moment.

Towards Better Carbohydrate Vaccines
Edited by R. Bell and G. Torrigiani

Published by John Wiley & Sons Ltd

4

Towards a carbohydrate-based vaccine against leishmaniasis

E. HANDMAN, G. F. MITCHELL, M. J. MCCONVILLE AND H. MOLL
The Walter and Eliza Hall Institute of Medical Research, Melbourne, Victoria 3050, Australia

Leishmania are digenetic protozoa, alternating between the promastigote, a free-living flagellate in the gut of the vector sandfly, and the amastigote, the obligatory intracellular form which resides in phagolysosomes of mammalian macrophages. Infection with this organism begins with the recognition of the host macrophage by the promastigotes, attachment and uptake by 'facilitated phagocytosis' [1]. The basic lesion in leishmaniasis is the infected macrophage. The infected macrophage displays parasite antigens on its surface (reviewed in [9]) and there is no reason why these should not be recognized by T cells in an MHC restricted manner.

Leishmania major infection of mice produces a range of disease patterns, similar to the situation in man, depending on the strain of inbred mouse. However, hypothymic nude mice of both resistant and susceptible genotypes are highly susceptible, suggesting a role for T cell-dependent immunity in resistance to disease [3, 11].

In response to *L. major* infection, both delayed-type hypersensitivity (DTH) and antibodies are produced (reviewed in [11]). However, there appears to be no strict correlation between healing and development of cell-mediated immune responses, and progressive lesions may develop in the presence of DTH to crude antigen mixtures [11]. Animals of resistant genotypes recover from infection and are resistant to reinfection [9, 11]. Protection can be transferred with $L3T4^+$, $Ly2^-$ T cells to syngeneic recipients [11].

Vaccination against cutaneous leishmaniasis is feasible with crude antigens [reviewed in ref. 11]. The ideal vaccine would be a molecularly defined set of antigens, either involved in the induction of host-protective immune responses or critical to parasite uptake into the macrophage. We have focused on the characterization of the parasite molecules involved in recognition and uptake into host macrophages as potential vaccine candidates. Using the monoclonal antibody WIC-79.3, we have recently described an externally oriented, amphipathic membrane antigen of *L. major* which is shed into culture medium [5, 6]. This antigen had been shown previously to be part of a polymorphic family of carbohydrate antigens present in all *Leishmania*. Each antigen was shown to be species-specific and this has formed the basis for a serotyping system for the classification and diagnosis of leishmaniasis [17].

While the structure of this molecule in *L. major* is still unknown, and an area of considerable interest, it appears from our data that the molecule is anchored into the parasite membrane by covalently attached fatty acid. It contains sulphated and phosphated sugars, with galactose in a terminal position, accessible for recognition by ricin lectin and radiolabelled by [^{3}H] sodium borohydride following galactose oxidase treatment [6]. A similar molecule has been identified in *L. donovani* and partially characterized by Turco *et al.* [18]. Preliminary data indicate that it may be similar in structure to bacterial lipopolysaccharides (S. J. Turco, personal communication).

Our studies examining the biological function of this glycolipid, or lipopolysaccharide molecule, indicate that it binds specifically to macrophages *in vitro* [6]. In addition, antibodies to the carbohydrate moiety block attachment of promastigotes to macrophages. Taken together, our data suggest that the *L. major* glycolipid is involved in macrophage recognition and attachment, and that this interaction occurs *via* the carbohydrate part of the molecule. Interestingly, the presence of this molecule, or parts of it, on the surface of *infected macrophages* can be inferred from immunofluorescence studies using monoclonal antibodies [2, 4]. Consequently, this antigen is biologically important as a recognition molecule, and immunologically important because of its expression on the surface of the infected macrophage, available for T-cell recognition.

Mice immunized with the glycolipid antigen purified from detergent lysates of *L. major* promastigotes using the monoclonal antibody WIC-79.3 (i.e. L-LPS) are resistant to subsequent infection with *L. major* [7, 8]. When injected with L-LPS plus the adjuvant, killed *Corynebacterium parvum*, intraperitoneally, mice of healer phenotype (e.g. C3H/He, C57BL/6) may be totally resistant in terms of lesion development. Doses used have been in the range of 2–10 μg L-LPS and 100–200 μg *C. parvum*. Immunized mice of non-healer phenotype (BALB/c and BALB/c H-2 congenic mice) generally show a delayed appearance of lesions and/or lesions that remain small in size. As with crude antigen mixtures (including attenuated whole organisms), with or without adjuvants [7, 10, 12, 13], subcutaneous injections fail to induce resistance to disease in mice. The nature of this peculiar constraint imposed by route of injection remains unknown; it is also unknown whether it pertains to man.

No protective effect in mice has yet been demonstrated with the carbohydrate portion (CHO) of L-LPS prepared from promastigote culture supernatants and injected by any route, with any adjuvant or in any amount. In fact, CHO injected with Freund's complete adjuvant (FCA) will increase the duration of subsequent disease in C3H/He and C57BL/6 mice [8, 15] challenged with *L. major* promastigotes. Moreover, it can be shown readily be adoptive transfers in nude mice that BALB/c mice injected with CHO plus FCA have an increased frequency of disease-promoting ('suppressor') cells in their lymphoid organs [15]. Using *in vivo* titrations in BALB/c nu/nu mice, the frequency of disease-promoting cells (that from all other evidence in the cutaneous leishmaniasis–mouse system are likely to be $Ly2^-$ T cells) is increased by about 10. Other unpublished and preliminary data suggest that injections of FCA plus the CHO purified from *L. donovani* culture supernatants, by affinity chromatography on monoclonal antibody WIC-108.3 increase the susceptibility of C3H/He mice to *L. major*. Thus there may be a sharing of 'disease-promoting epitopes' between the carbohydrate moiety of the L-LPS of these two leishmania species.

We have proposed [14, 16] that $L3T4^+$ $Ly2^-$ T-cell recognition of L-LPS, oriented in the membrane of infected macrophages through its lipid component, results in the release of mediators of macrophage activation (such as INF-γ and others) with subsequent parasitostatic, if not parasitocidal, effects. In contrast, the CHO component of L-LPS should be oriented quite differently following binding to its receptor on the surface of macrophages. Both recognition of L-LPS and its CHO component should be class II MHC (Ia) restricted. Clearly, like L-LPS, any antigen recognized by appropriate T cells and present in appropriate amounts on the infected macrophage surface should serve as a target of aggressive T cell-mediated attack. If T-cell receptors stabilize associations between antigen and Ia molecules at the cell surface, then *amounts* of lipophilic antigen at the infected macrophage surface (in the absence of any real affinity of most antigens for Ia) will be the critical factor.

The nature of disease-promoting immunity remains unknown. Antibodies appear to play no role in either resistance or disease-promoting immunity. An hypothesis we favour at the moment is that CHO recognition by IFN-γ producing T cells at the surface of *uninfected* macrophages in lesions increases the expression of the macrophage receptors to which CHO binds in the process of 'facilitated phagocytosis' of leishmania. This increased display of receptors enables parasites released from destroyed macrophages to gain entry quickly and thereby facilitates spread of infection. Clearly, little more can be gained from speculation in the absence of (a) structural data on the L-LPS and its carbohydrate fragment(s) released by phospholipase treatment, (b) T-cell clones with specificity for these antigens and (c) clonal analyses of T-cell populations in immunized mice of various genotypes using defined antigens.

ACKNOWLEDGEMENTS

This work was supported by the National Health and Medical Research Council of Australia, the World Health Organization/IMMLEISH and The Rockefeller Foundation.

REFERENCES

1. Chang, K. P., and Fong, D. Cell biology of host–parasite membrane interactions in leishmaniasis. In *Cytopathology of Parasitic Disease*, Pitman Books, London, Ciba Foundation Symposium 99, (ed, D. Evered and G. M. Collins) 1983, pp. 113–37.
2. DeIbarra, A., Howard, J. G., and Snary, D. Monoclonal antibodies to *Leishmania tropica major*: specificities and antigen location. *Parasitol.*, **85**, 523–31 (1982).
3. Handman, E., Ceredig, R., and Mitchell, G. F. (1979). Murine cutaneous leishmaniasis: disease patterns in intact and nude mice of various genotypes and examination of differences between normal and infected macrophages. *Aust. J. Exp. Biol. Med. Sci.*, **57**, 9–29 (1979).
4. Handman, E., and Hocking, R. E. Stage-specific strain-specific, and cross-reactive antigens of *Leishmania* species identified by monoclonal antibodies. *Infect. Immun.*, **37**, 28–33 (1982).
5. Handman, E., Greenblatt, C. L., and Goding, J. W. An amphipathic sulphate glycoconjugate of *Leishmania*: characterization with monoclonal antibodies. *EMBO J.*, **3**, 2301–6 (1984).
6. Handman, E., and Goding, J. W. The Leishmania receptor for macrophages is a lipid-containing glycoconjugate. *EMBO J.*, **4**, 329–36 (1985).
7. Handman, E., and Mitchell, G. F. Immunization with Leishmania receptor for macrophages protects mice against cutaneous leishmaniasis. *Proc. Natl. Acad. Sci. USA.*, **82**, 5910–14 (1985).
8. Handman, E., and Mitchell, G. F. Leishmania–macrophage interaction: role of parasite molecules in infection and host protection. In *Molecular Strategies of Parasitic Invasion*, UCLA Symposia on Molecular and Cellular Biology, New Series, Vol. 42 (ed. N. Agabian, H. Goodman and N. Noguiera), Alan R. Liss, New York, 1987 (in press).
9. Handman, E. Leishmaniasis: antigens and host–parasite interactions. In Parasite Antigens: Toward New Strategies for Vaccines. (ed. T. W. Pearson), Marcel Dekker, New York and Basle, 1986, pp. 5–48.
10. Howard, J. G., Liew, F. Y., Hale, C., and Nicklin, S. Prophylactic immunization

against experimental leishmaniasis. II. Further characterization of the protective immunity against fatal *Leishmania tropica* infection induced by irradiated promastigotes. *J. Immunol.*, **132**, 450–5 (1984).
11. Howard, J. G. Immunological regulation and control of experimental leishmaniasis. *Int. Rev. Exp. Pathol.*, **28**, 80–113 (1986).
12. Mitchell, G. F., Handman, E., and Spithill, T. W. Vaccination against cutaneous leishmaniasis in mice using nonpathogenic cloned promastigotes of *Leishmania major* and importance of route of injection. *Aust. J. exp. Biol. Med. Sci.*, **62**, 145–53 (1984).
13. Mitchell, G. F., Handman, E., and Spithill, T. W. Examination of variables in the vaccination of mice against cutaneous leishmaniasis using living avirulent cloned lines and killed promastigotes of *Leishmania major*. *Int. J. Parasitol.*, **15**, 677–84 (1985).
14. Mitchell, G. F., and Handman, E. T-lymphocytes recognize Leishmania glycoconjugates. *Parasitology Today*, **1**, 61–3 (1985).
15. Mitchell, G. F., and Handman, E. The glycoconjugate derived from a *Leishmania major* receptor for macrophages is a suppressogenic, disease-promoting antigen in murine cutaneous leishmaniasis. *Parasite Immunol.*, **8**, 255–63 (1986).
16. Mitchell, G. F. Cellular and molecular aspects of host–parasite relationships. In Proceedings of the VI International Congress of Immunology, *Progress in Immunology* (VI) (ed. B. Cinader and R. G. Miller), Academic Press, Florida, 1987 (in press).
17. Schnur, L. F. The immunological identification and characterization of leishmanial stocks and strains, with special reference to excreted factor serotyping. In *Biochemical Characterization of Leishmania* (ed. M. L. Chance and B. C. Walton), UNDP/World Bank/WHO, Geneva, Switzerland, 1982, pp. 25–48.
18. Turco, S. J., Wilkerson, M. A., and Clawson, D. R. Expression of an unusual acidic glycoconjugate in *Leishmania donovani*. *J. Biol. Chem.*, **259**, 3883–9 (1984).

DISCUSSION – Chaired by Dr J. B. Robbins

HANDMAN: Our problems began, though, when we tried to induce the same type of protection using the water-soluble carbohydrate antigen alone. In this example we used genetically resistant mice which develop a lesion that will eventually heal so the uninjected mice or the ones injected with the adjuvant alone eventually heal. However, mice that were immunized or vaccinated with the carbohydrate in Freund's complete adjuvant, were not only not protected from disease but, in fact, the disease was exacerbated. I could put forward several hypotheses for what causes this peculiar type of immune response but I won't because we have no evidence for any of them and this is where I would like to get some feedback from you people who have worked with carbohydrate antigens for a long time. I think that it may be a matter of antigen presentation – that the glycolipid antigen is anchored in the membrane of the antigen-presenting cell in such a way that it can interact with the host-histocompatibility antigen in a way that will then induce a T-cell protective immune response, whereas the carbohydrate alone may interact with the initial ligand, the molecule it normally binds to, but then it probably doesn't interact with class II antigen in the same way that the glycolipid does. All of this though is speculation and we really don't understand it. What we do understand is that we will not rush into human vaccination trials until we know how to make a very stable preparation to ensure that we will induce the appropriate immune response.

ADA: If you immunize your mice with the soluble carbohydrates and then immunize with the lipid, what happens?

HANDMAN: We are doing these experiments now in both directions to see if the carbohydrate overrides protection or if the glycolipid overrides suppression.

ADA: One possibility might be that you are causing tolerance to suppressor-T cells, you are activating suppressor-T cells by giving the free carbohydrate. Now, if that were the case, if you gave the free carbohydrate, then treated with cyclophosphamide to get rid of those suppressor-T cells then your mice might become more responsive to the glycolipid. I would think that if you did those two sets of experiments you might get an indication whether that was what was happening.

HANDMAN: Well, Graham Mitchell is doing this experiment now and we should know soon.

HOOKE: Have you thought about incorporating the glycolipid into liposomes and looking at the immune response to that?

HANDMAN: Yes. In fact my very first experiment was to use a lipid adjuvant called Lipovant, sold by Accurate Biochemicals in the USA, which is egg lecitin and, in fact, I found that the adjuvant alone, or the liposomes alone, exacerbated the disease and we have not used them since, but we will try and prepare our own liposomes.

KABAT: I would like to say, I will say more about it this afternoon, that Charles Wood and Eric Lai in my laboratory have been quite successful in getting antibodies to the isomaltose oligosaccharides coupled to stearylamine, so that you could take your recovered carbohydrate, couple it to something like stearylamine and make another type of glycolipid which we found to be a very good antigen, which seems to be thymus independent.

MORENO: Just for clarification, did you follow the antibody titres in those animals immunized with soluble polysaccharide in complete Freund's adjuvant?

HANDMAN: Yes. I must stress though, that the antibodies are not believed to play a role in protection in cutaneous leishmaniasis, it is a T-cell mediated type of protection, but I did follow the antibody titres and the mice made no antibodies whatsoever, whereas they did make antibodies when immunized with the glycolipid.

MÄKELÄ, Helena: In one of your slides you had in parenthesis an indication that this glycolipid antigen would also be active as a virulence factor within

the macrophages. I wonder whether you have any evidence of the mechanism of this activity?
HANDMAN: We have been trying to produce parasite mutants that lack this molecule and we found one such parasite which is taken up by macrophages, probably by a different mechanism, and is killed inside macrophages very rapidly. There are two possibilities and I can't distinguish between them. One is that a parasite which has this glycolipid molecule on its surface will interact with a set of receptors on macrophages which will target it into a compartment in the macrophage where it can survive. The parasite that does not have this antigen on the surface will interact with a different set of ligands on the macrophage and will end up in a different compartment and be killed, let us say by lysosomal enzymes for example. The other possibility is that parasites with or without this coat will end up in the same compartment, but this glycolipid protects them from killing by lysosomal enzymes. I cannot, at the moment, distinguish between them, but when I took these mutant parasites and incorporated into their membrane the purified lipids from the wild-type parasite, they survived much better in macrophages. So I think that this molecule is also involved in survival, I am still not sure exactly at what level.
MÄKELÄ, Helena: We have made rather similar observations, still at a preliminary stage, with *Salmonella* bacteria, a bacterial parasite which, however, lives in the same compartment in the macrophages as does the *Leishmania*, and obeys very much the same rules. We have looked at mutants that are devoid of a glycolipid antigen called the enterobacterial common antigen; to our great surprise they were very much more sensitive to the intracellular compartment than the normal ones and we are at the moment in the process of finding out what the mechanism of that is.
HANDMAN: It would be intriguing if they were targeted to a different compartment. There was a time when we used to believe that a lysosome is a lysosome is a lysosome, now I think there is more and more evidence that there are various acidic compartments and they are not all the same.
SÖDERSTRÖM: Did you look at the presence of these receptors also in the Langerhans cells, in the skin?
HANDMAN: No, we have not yet.
SUTHERLAND: You mentioned a disaccharide repeating unit. Can you give us any indication of either the composition or the structure of this unit?
HANDMAN: Well these are not my own data. It is a preliminary personal communication from Sam Turco so I would like to be very careful. He thinks that, in the case of *Leishmania donovani* – the parasite causing visceral disease in man, it is a (mannose (β-1.4) galactose) disaccharide unit which is phosphodiester-linked. But I can't say any more.
ROTTA: I might have missed this, but I am wondering whether you looked in your immunized animals for cell-mediated immunity reactions?
HANDMAN: No, we have not looked at the mechanism which induces host

protection in mice vaccinated with the lipid. We know that T cells from these mice respond to the glycolipid *in vitro*. We are now in the process of making T-cell lines from these mice, but we haven't actually done any *in vivo* experiments yet.

Towards Better Carbohydrate Vaccines
Edited by R. Bell and G. Torrigiani

Published by John Wiley & Sons Ltd

5

Applications of synthetic complex oligosaccharides to areas of molecular biology

RAYMOND U. LEMIEUX
Department of Chemistry, University of Alberta, Edmonton, Alberta, Canada T6G 2G2

INTRODUCTION

An extremely wide range of complex carbohydrate structures occurs in the form of ligands, of molecular structures at the surface of mammalian cells, as components of microbial cell walls and in glycoproteins and glycolipids of widespread occurrence in biological fluids. It is well established that these structures play significant roles in the orchestration of biological activity as well as in providing a variety of the structural requirements for living organisms. The diversity of these structures is sufficiently great to specify species as well as organs and cells. Although this highly diverse range of substances which contain complex carbohydrates as building units has evolved for the maintenance and reproduction of living organisms, the quantities required, especially at cell surfaces, are extremely small and normally occur in highly complex mixtures from which they can be isolated only with great difficulty. Furthermore, not only are the purifications difficult but the amounts achieved are too small for other than research purposes. It is possible that such handicaps in terms of availability will be overcome in many instances through the emerging biotechnologies based on recombinant DNA. However, the physical and/or chemical properties of the complex carbohydrates obtained by way of such processes may not be those desired for specific health-care applications.

In certain instances, specific structural modifications of the natural substance have led to useful semisynthetic products. Such modifications may be accomplished by either biochemical (enzymatic) or chemical means (degradation or synthesis). A recent example is the enhancement of the immune response to the Group B meningococcal polysaccharide (GBM) by replacement of the *N*-acetyl groups of sialic acid residues by *N*-propionyl groups [11]. The *N*-propionylated GBM was conjugated to tetanus toxoid (TT) for the preparation of a semisynthetic antigen which induced higher levels of anti-GBM antibodies in rabbits. In addition, these antibodies bound the native GBM polysaccharide more strongly than did antibodies raised to the native GBM–TT conjugate. The possibilities for such applications of synthetic organic chemistry to improve the immunogenicity of natural antigens are numerous and have already received much attention. However, such transformations will not be considered in this presentation. Instead the chapter will deal with an overview of some of the achievements based on total chemical synthesis. Such syntheses normally employ commercially available mono- and disaccharides as starting materials.

The time available did not allow a comprehensive review of how synthetic chemistry has contributed to the field of immunology as it relates to carbohydrate antigens and their antigenicity. A brief review of contributions, largely from my own laboratory and those of collaborators, is presented in the hope that this will suffice to illustrate how and why synthetic carbohydrate chemistry has been and surely will be increasingly useful to medical science. The concentration on the human blood group related oligosaccharides in my laboratory was dictated by the great wealth of structural information which already existed [1]. Synthetic studies related to the antigenic determinants of bacterial polysaccharides began at about the same time in Sweden [6]. The great diversity and complexity of these substances can be appreciated from reviews by Lindberg [15, 31]. However, the contributions to molecular biology based on synthetic carbohydrate chemistry which have appeared in this and related areas are not the subject of this review. It must be noted, however, that numerous studies during the past decade have established that carbohydrate-binding proteins termed 'adhesins' are involved in the adherence of bacteria to tissues. Ofek and Perry [35] have provided evidence that these are carbohydrate–lectin types of interactions, involving carbohydrates on either the bacterial or the tissue surface or both. Artificial antigens prepared from αDGal(1 → 4)βDGalO$(CH_2)_8$COOMe and αDMan(1 → 2)αDManO$(CH_2)_8$COOMe were adsorbed on latex beads in order to study the receptor-binding specificities of strains of uropathogenic *Escherichia coli* by agglutination [38]. Similar studies involving the use of BSA-artificial antigen with αDGal(1 → 4)βDGalO$(CH_2)_2$S$(CH_2)_2$– as hapten were made by Lomberg *et al.* [33].

CHEMICAL METHODOLOGIES

The synthesis of complex carbohydrates of interest to immunochemical investigations has long been a goal for carbohydrate chemists [12]. This interest magnified as the structures of blood group determinants became established some 20 years ago [32, 53] and was amplified by the ever increasing knowledge of the structures of carbohydrate components of bacterial cell walls [31]. To do so became feasible about 15 years ago [16], particularly because the then available range of blocking and deblocking strategies was adequate to render feasible a large number of syntheses. Furthermore, methodologies for the establishment of a wide range of glycosidic linkages in the desired configurations were either in place or soon to become available. Most importantly, however, the physical methods required to monitor and register properly the synthesis of complex carbohydrate molecules had evolved. The availability of powerful means, based in chromatography, for isolation and purification of complex oligosaccharides both as such and a lipophilic derivatives was essential. The commercial availability of the necessary grades of adsorbents, especially silica gels for column and thin-layer chromatography and of gels and membranes for molecular sieving provided the road to success. However, the realization of success required the availability of the modern high-frequency Fourier-transform nuclear magnetic resonance spectrometers. All of these requirements began to be in place in about 1970 and reached the present levels of sophistication largely over the following decade. It is now possible to say that the achievement of virtually any complex neutral oligosaccharide up to the pentasaccharide level, in the hands of competent chemists, is simply a matter of the time and money. The achievement of still larger structures should also normally be possible, but acceptable reasons to do so may not always exist. In the case of acidic oligosaccharides, much progress has been reported but, for example, the attachment of a suitably protected sialosyl group will probably, under present circumstances, proceed in an unacceptable yield. For example, sialic acid is often found attached in 2 → 3 or 2 → 6 α-linkage to D-galactose, *N*-acetyl-D-glucosamine or *N*-acetyl-D-galactosamine. The best yields so far reported range from 34% when the glycosylation was at a primary position to yield a 2 → 6 sialoside [37] and from 6% [36] to 15.6% for 2 → 3 sialosides [40], where the attachments involve much less reactive secondary hydroxyl groups. A major complication is the formation in most cases of at least an equal yield of the thermodynamically more stable but unnatural β-isomer which can only be separated with difficulty. Although this situation will undoubtedly be improved through the continuing attention of the synthetic organic chemist, perhaps the best long-term solution to this and other similar problems for the achievement of synthetic oligosaccharides will be by way of biochemical rather than chemical methods. Thus, Barker and co-workers [44] accomplished enzymatic syntheses of oligosaccharides related to the human blood group determinants and Whitesides *et al.* [54] showed that *N*-acetyllactosamine could be prepared in gram quantities using immobilized enzymes. In the case of sialosides, Sabesan and Paulson [46] recently demonstrated that synthetic neutral oligosaccharides could be sialylated enzymatically using purified sialyltransferase. Both αDNeuAc(2 → 6) and (2 → 3)βDGal linkages could be formed to provide thirteen sialyloligosaccharides ranging from di- to hexasaccharides. There can be no doubt that such combined approaches for the achievement of complex oligosaccharides will find commercial application.

The publication in 1975 of the first chemical syntheses of human blood-group determinants at the trisaccharide level, namely the Lewis a (βDGal(1 → 3)-[αLFuc(1 → 4)]βDGlcNAcOR) [21, 23] and b (αLFuc(1 → 2)[αDGal(1 → 3)]βDGalOR) [22] was followed by a flood of activity in laboratories world-wide which has resulted in the chemical synthesis of the immunodominant portions of not only the known blood-group antigenic determinants, but also a wide range of their derivatives for structure–activity investigations. This chemical literature is only of specialist interest and will not be a subject of this review. Those interested probably are already aware of the many reviews that have appeared [16, 37, 39]. Instead, this presentation will focus on how these developments in synthetic carbohydrate chemistry have contributed to developments of interest to molecular biology as related to the health-care field. As was stated in 1978 [16]:

> The isolation of pure oligosaccharides with structures related to blood-group specificities from human milk and urine is possible. Nevertheless, the supplies are rather limited; the procedures are difficult and, at best, are amenable to the provision of only gram amounts of a limited range of structures. On the other hand, with the advent of appropriate synthetic methodologies, the supply of any given oligosaccharide would be limited only by the scale of operation. The foreseen range of products which are desirable and which can be made available in substantial amounts by synthesis is already large and will continue to grow.

Artificial antigens and immunoadsorbents

The main value of chemical synthesis in the provision of antigens is that the products are monospecific in terms of the carbohydrate antigenic determinants. The carrier molecule normally is not carbohydrate in nature and is antigenic in itself. In fact, the carbohydrate-free protein bovine serum albumin (BSA) is strongly immunogenic and most commonly used for the preparation of artificial antigens for the production of anti-carbohydrate antibodies in test animals. These preparations involve the haptenation of the amino groups of lysine units using a wide range of reagents. In my laboratory, we have focused on building the oligosaccharide in glycosidic union to 8-methoxycarbonyloctanol to provide haptens of type **1** [20, 21, 41]. The methyl ester grouping is readily converted under mild conditions by way of a hydra-

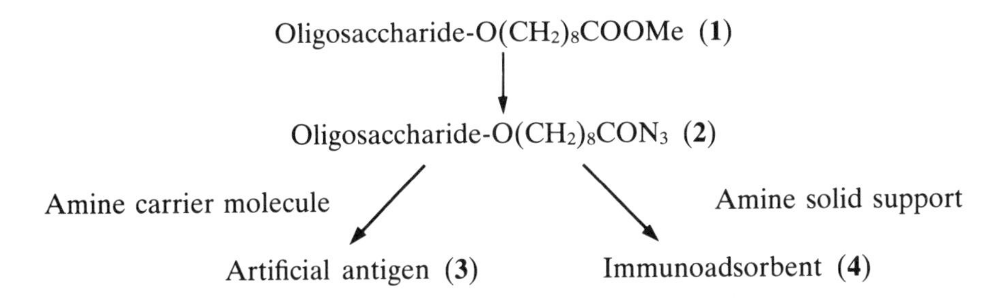

zide intermediate to the acyl azide (**2**) for the acylation of amino groups either to form a soluble artificial antigen (**3**) or an insoluble immunoadsorbent (**4**). This general technology has proved useful in a number of ways as will be illustrated by the following examples. It is noteworthy that, in addition to the acylation of proteins to form artificial antigens, the acylation of washed red blood cells has also proved useful for the immunization of animals [4, 21]. The adsorption of soluble artificial antigens on latex beads has provided a simulation of cells for the examination of agglutination [33]. Coated microtitre plates, prepared by adsorption of the artificial antigen, have proved highly effective in a solid-phase kinetic enzyme-linked immunoadsorbent assay (k-ELISA) for the detection of binding specificities [47, 49]. The procedure is especially useful at the cloning stage of the hybridoma technique for the production of monoclonal antibodies [4]. The immunoadsorbent prepared by haptenation of a calcined diatomaceous earth is most often used both for batch adsorptions [48] and the preparation of columns for affinity chromatography [20]. An increasingly large number of such immunoadsorbents, known by their product name Synsorb™, are available commercially (Chembiomed Ltd, University of Alberta, Canada).

A good example of the use of synthetic antigens and immunoadsorbents is provided by their application to the detection of Lewis determinants [20]. Artificial antigens of the type corresponding to **3** were synthesized using BSA as carrier molecule with the so-called Lewis a, b and blood-group determinants [54] as the carbohydrate antigenic structures.

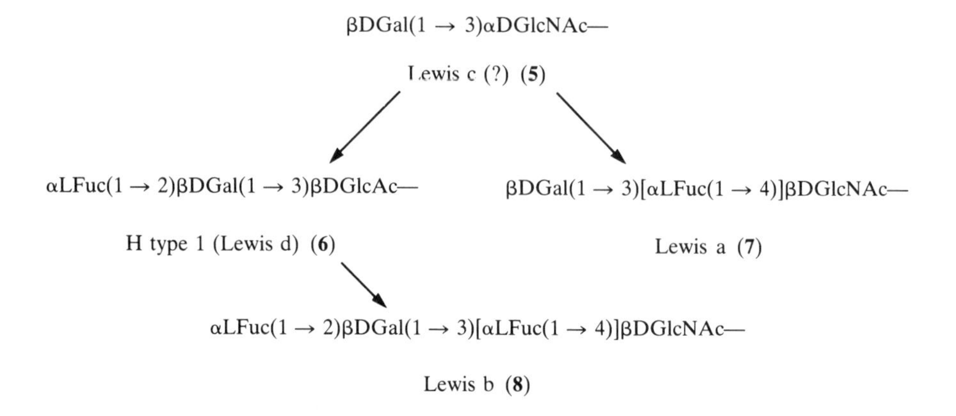

These antigens were used to raise antibodies in rabbits and the corresponding immunoadsorbent served to isolate those antibodies specific for the synthetic carbohydrate structure present in the antigen. A major asset was the availability of the other Lewis-type immunoadsorbents. Thus it was readily possible, for example, using the Lewis a and Lewis d immunoadsorbents, to remove any cross-reacting antibodies from the anti-Lewis b pool of antibodies. In this manner, refined anti-Lewis antibody reagents were obtained which proved thoroughly effective for the detection and location of Lewis antigens in stomach tissues [20]. This study demonstrated for the first time that sufficiently elaborated artificial antigens could be used in conjunction with the corresponding immunoadsorbents, for the preparation of reliable tissue-typing reagents. Also, the study confirmed that the so-called Lewis d activity arose from the H type 1 determinant and established the relationship of the H type 1 related fucosyl transferase to ABO secretor status. Synthetic haptens played the key role in the demonstration that at least two different H-blood-group-related βDGal-α-2-L-fucosyl transferases occur in human serum [27], as was recently confirmed by Betteridge Watkins [3].

As already mentioned, synthetic artificial antigens have proven highly useful for diagnostic and analytical purposes. The synthetic immunoadsorbents are also useful in these respects [5]. For example, the immunoadsorbent prepared from the Lewis c (?) type structure **5** absorbed the antibodies present in a so-called anti-Le[c] serum [29]. It was therefore expected that even the type 1 core structure βDGal(1 → 3)βDGlcNAc— (**5**) had a relationship to the Lewis blood group as an antigenic determinant. Indeed, very recently, Hanfland and co-worker [7] established strong inhibition by the well-characterized glycolipid (**9**) of the haemagglutination of the red cells of non-secretor OLe(a-b-) individuals by anti-Le[c] sera.

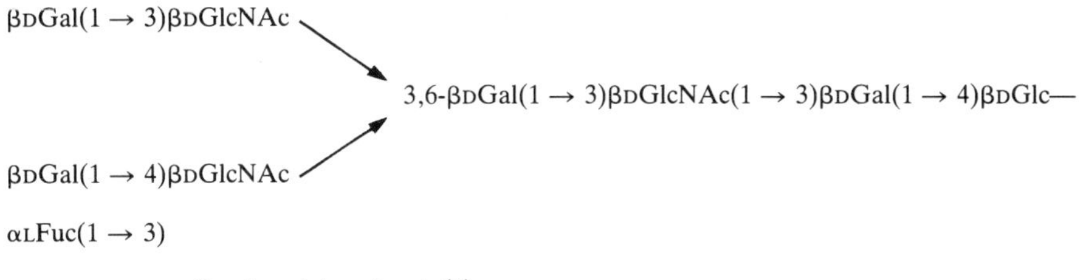

Lewis c determinant (**9**)

The βDGal(1 → 4)[αLFuc(1 → 3)]βDGlcNAc portion of (**9**) is known as the X blood group determinant. An immunoadsorbent of type **4** prepared from the X synthetic hapten was used (Lemieux and Parker, unpublished) to independently provide evidence for the binding of this structure by the SSEA-1 monoclonal antibody [10], supplied for this purpose by D. Solter and B. Knowles of the Wistar Institute Philadelphia, USA. Another example is the use of a synthetic H type 2 immunoadsorbent to establish the specificity of a hybridoma monoclonal antibody [14]. The procedure used in this laboratory involves incubation of a few mg of the immunoadsorbent with the biological fluid, followed by washing with buffer and treatment with base or acid to desorb any adsorbed protein which is detected by ultraviolet absorption and can serve as a simple technique for following the course of an immunization.

The most dramatic application of synthetic immunoadsorbents is for the selective removal of potentially offending antibodies from the plasma of an individual prior to the performance of an ABO-incompatible bone marrow transplantation. The procedure, which was introduced by Bensinger [2], at first involved blood separation into cellular and plasma components followed by passage of the plasma through a column of the required immunoadsorbent. The 'cleansed' plasma and cells were then recombined and returned to the patient. At present, the procedure allows the passage of whole blood through the column and will undoubtedly replace plasma exchange to lower the levels of incompatible antibodies prior to tissue transplantations. This approach may well be extended to the treatment of autoimmune diseases for which the structure of the antigenic determinant has become established. The chemical synthesis of an appropriate hapten will surely follow.

An option to the removal of offending antibodies from blood by adsorption with a specific immunoadsorbent is the neutralization of the antibody *in situ* by the administration of appropriate synthetic hapten. In fact, this approach was pioneered by Romano [42, 43] in studies of the therapeutic effect of a synthetic human blood group A trisaccharide in the haemolytic disease of the new-born due to A–O incompatibility. In the first three tests [42], the serum bilirubin levels of two of the infants fell to normal within 48 hours. Thus, grounds for a full evaluation of the *in vivo* use of synthetic haptens as neutralizing and therapeutic agents were established. In the case of a healthy O-blood-group adult, no trisaccharide was found in the urine. On the other hand, in the case of a blood-group A volunteer, the A trisaccharide was recovered in the urine collected in the first 8 hours after administration. Presumably, in the case of the O person, the A trisaccharide did not appear in the urine because it had been bound by the circulating A antibodies. Indeed, the administration of 100 mg of the trisaccharide produced a drop in the anti-A titre of three dilution tubes. These landmark experiments clearly suggest that synthetic oligosaccharides of lower molecular weight will be used in the future for the *in vivo* treatment of diseases related to the presence of offending antibodies of known specificity.

The artificial antigens have proved useful not only for the preparation of antisera specific for the synthetic hapten [19] but also for a variety of analytical purposes. The solid-phase radioimmunoassay developed by Oriol and co-workers [28, 30] employs immobilized antibodies or lectins and brings the carbohydrate structure to be assayed into competition with an appropriate ^{125}I-labelled artificial antigen. The method was successfully applied by Oriol and his associates in a wide range of investigations related to the occurrence, biosynthesis and distribution of ABO and Lewis antigens in man and lower animals [34]. The many ingenious studies of cell-surface carbohydrate structures using synthetic artificial antigens, immunoadsorbents and oligosaccharides that have been accomplished in that laboratory firmly established the advantages of methodologies based on monospecific, synthetic carbohydrate structures.

IMMUNOGENICHEMICAL SPECIFICITY

It has long been recognized [13] that the specificity of the binding of an oligosaccharide by an antibody may be appreciated by examination of its effect, through competition for the combining site, on the interaction between the antibody and the antigen used in the immunization. In this way, the relative potencies as inhibitors of the binding exhibited by different carbohydrate structures can be realized and a large immunochemical literature developed from such studies involving both antibodies and lectins [12]. However, until the advent of modern methods for the chemical synthesis of complex oligosaccharides, the information that could be gained was restricted to that provided by the commercially available mono- and disaccharides and simple derivatives and by glycoproteins, glycolipids or oligosaccharides isolated from various sources, but most importantly from milk. Chemical synthesis has now greatly increased the scope of such structure–activity studies, both in terms of range of structures and in the details for a given structure. About 5 years ago [17], I accepted the challenge of modifying, through total synthesis, selected human blood-group determinants in sufficient detail to allow an appraisal of how the oligosaccharides are recognized and bound by lectins or monoclonal antibodies. The synthetic programme in each case provided all of the monodeoxy derivatives of the oligosaccharides and included, for example, situations where a hydroxyl group was replaced by fluorine, chlorine or amine and either an acetyl, acetamido, methyl or hydroxymethyl group by hydrogen, etc. Furthermore, convincing evidence for their conformational preferences was obtained by detailed high-frequency ^{1}H-nuclear magnetic resonance studies [52]. The various derivatives were then used in inhibition studies involving the reaction of the protein with the appropriate artificial antigen under conditions of the solid-phase radioimmunoassay [28, 55]. These studies involved the binding of the H-type 2 (αLFuc(1 → 2)βDGal(1 → 4)βDGlcNAc) determinant by the lectin I of *Ulex europaeus* [8, 9], the B (αLFuc(1 → 2)[αDGal(1 → 3)]βDGal) determinant by two hybridoma monoclonal anti-B antibodies [25], the Lewis a (βDGal(1 → 3)[αLFuc(1 → 4)]βDGlcNAc) determinant by two hybridoma monoclonal anti-Le^a antibodies [24] and the Lewis b (αLFuc(1 → 2)βDGal(1 → 3)[αLFuc(1 → 4)]βDGlcNAc) determinant by the lectin IV of *Griffonia simplicifolia* [51] and a monoclonal anti-Le^b antibody [50]. In the case of the anti-IMa antibody [26], the inhibitions used a glycoprotein of natural origin in a precise microprecipitin assay in order to assess the effects on binding of structural changes in the trisaccharide βDGal(1 → 4)βDGlcNAc(1 → 6)βDGal and related compounds. These studies made it clearly apparent that the binding in each case involved the recognition of an amphiphilic surface comprising at one end a cluster of two or three hydroxyl groups, the integrity of which is required for substantial binding to occur. This grouping was termed the key polar grouping [18], since it appears to serve as a 'key' to 'open the gate', so to speak, to the combining site. Of major interest is the finding that, normally, the key polar grouping is provided by hydroxyl groups in different sugar units. It is not surprising, therefore, that, in these cases, simply glycosides of the individual sugars do not display appreciable inhibitory potencies. Obviously, this situation seriously limits the ability to gain information on binding specificities on the basis of the results obtained using simple carbohydrate structures as probes. It appears, therefore, that there will exist an interest to synthesize complex oligosaccharides simply because they are unknown and may well provide the 'key' to an important biological recognition.

The above-mentioned key polar groupings were found in each case to be adjacent to a much larger lipophilic surface consisting mainly of hydrocarbon groupings provided by the various sugar units [18]. It became clearly apparent that a high level of complementarity must exist between this essentially hydrophobic surface and the combining site for important binding to occur. The molecular surface area can, however, be curtailed with retention of activity, albeit reduced, should complementarity be retained. The evidence regarding the involvement of other hydroxyl groups in the binding reactions is inconclusive at present. Certainly, some appear to stay in contact with the aqueous phase, others may establish interactions with the complex that add more or less importantly, but not crucially, to the stability of the complex. Of major interest is the rather compelling circumstantial evidence that hydroxyl groups may form intramolecular hydrogen bonds in order to establish non-polar interactions within the complex. Although I am in favour of the view [18] that an important contribution to the stability of these complexes arises from thermodynamically favourable changes in dispersion forces of attraction, these are still open questions. It seems likely that answers will become available to at least some of the questions posed by this enormously complex system of interactions that involve a dominating contribution by the aqueous phase by comparing the crystal structures of the proteins with those of the complexes it forms with various oligosaccharides. We are attempting at present to gain such information in a collaboration with Dr L. T. J. Delbaere of the University of Saskatchewan, who has not only crystallized the lectin IV of *G. simplicifolia* but also its complex with the Lewis b tetrasaccharide and several of its derivatives. Certainly, our results to date indicate that the immunodominant surface of an oligosaccharide will tend to involve a key polar grouping that is contiguous to a large lipophilic surface [18, 45].

REFERENCES

1. Baker, D. A., Sugii, S., Kabat, E. A., Ratcliffe, R. M., Hermentin, P., and Lemieux, R. U. Immunochemical studies on the combining sites of Forssman hapten reactive hemagglutinins from *Dolichos biflorus*, *Helix pomatia* and *Wistaria floribunda*. *Biochem.*, **22**, 2741–50 (1983).
2. Bensinger, W. I. Plasma exchange and immunoadsorption for removal of antibodies prior to ABO incompatible bone marrow transplant. *Art. Organs*, **5**, 254–8 (1981).
3. Betteridge, A., and Watkins, W. M. Variant forms of α-2-L-fucosyltransferase in human submaxillary glands from blood group ABH 'secretor' and 'non-secretor' individuals. *Glycoconjugate*, **2**, 61–78 (1985).
4. Bundle, D. R., Gidneh, M. A. J., Kassam, N., and Rahman, A. F. R. Hybridomas specific for carbohydrates; synthetic human blood group antigens for the production, selection and characterisation of monoclonal typing reagens. *J. Immunol.*, **129**, 678–82 (1981).
5. Crawford, G., Adatia, A., Naylor, D. H., and Moore, B. P. L. Practical application of synthetic blood group immunoadsorbents. *Rev. Fr. Transfus. Immuno-Hematol.*, **24**, 281–8 (1981).
6. Ekborg, G., Garegg, P. J., and Gotthammar, B. Synthesis of *p*-isothiocyanatophenyl 3-*O*-(3,6-dideoxy-α-*D*-*arabino*-hexopyranosyl)-α-D-mannopyranoside. Synthetic tyvelosylmannose antigen. *Acta Chem. Scand. Ser. B.*, **29**, 765–71 (1975).

7. Hanfland, P., Kordowicz, M., Peter-Katalivic, J., Pfannschmidt, G., Crawford, R. J., Graham, H. A., and Egge, H. Immunochemistry of the Lewis blood-group system: isolation and structures of Lewis c active and related glycosphingolipids from the plasma of blood group Ole(a-b-) nonsecretors. *Arch. Biochem. Biophys.*, **246**, 655–72 (1986).
8. Hindsgaul, O., Khare, D. P., Bach, M., and Lemieux, R. U. Molecular recognition III. The binding of the H-type 2 human blood group determinant by the lectin I of *Ulex europaeus. Can. J. Chem.*, **63**, 2653–8 (1985).
9. Hindsgaul, O., Norberg, T., LePendu, J., and Lemieux, R. U. Synthesis of type 2 human blood group antigenic determinants. The H, X and Y haptens and variations of the H type 2 determinants as probes for the combining site of the lectin 1 of *Ulex europaeus. Carb. Res.*, **109**, 109–42 (1982).
10. Hounsell, E. F., Gooi, H. C., and Feizi, T. The monoclonal antibody anti-SSEA-1 discriminates between fucosylated type 1 and type 2 blood group chains. *FEBS Lett.*, **131**, 279–82 (1981).
11. Jennings, H. G., and Roy, R. Enhancement of the immune response to the group B polysaccharide of *Neisseria meningitidis* by means of its chemical modification. *Pathog. Neisseriae*, Proc. 4th Int. Symp. 628–32 (1984).
12. Kabat, E. A. *Structural Concepts in Immunology and Immunochemistry*, 2nd edn. Holt, Rinehart and Winston, New York, 1976.
13. Karush, F. The interaction of purified anti-β-lactoside antibody with haptens. *J. Am. Chem. Soc.*, **79**, 3380–4 (1957).
14. Knowles, R. W., Bai, Y., Daniels, G. L., and Watkins, W. Monoclonal anti-type 2 H: an antibody detecting a precursor of the A and B blood group antigens. *J. Immunogenetics*, **9**, 69–76 (1982).
15. Larm, O., and Lindberg, G. The pneumococcal polysaccharides: a re-examination. *Adv. Carbohydrate Chem. Biochem.*, **33**, 295–322 (1976).
16. Lemieux, R. U. Human blood groups and carbohydrate chemistry. *Chem. Soc. Rev.*, **7**, 423–52 (1978).
17. Lemieux, R. U. The binding of carbohydrate structures with antibodies and lectins. *Frontiers in Chemistry*, 3–26 (1982).
18. Lemieux, R. U. The hydrated polar-group 'gate' effect on the specificity and strength of the binding of oligosaccharides by protein receptor sites. *Proceedings of the VIIth International Symposium on Medicinal Chemistry*, 27–31 August 1984, Uppsala, Sweden, Vol. 1 pp. 329–51.
19. Lemieux, R. U., Baker, D. A., and Bundle, D. R. A methodology for the production of carbohydrate specific antibody. *Can. J. Biochem.*, **55**, 507–12 (1977).
20. Lemieux, R. U., Baker, D. A., Weinstein, W. M., and Switzer, C. M. Artificial antigens. Antibody preparations for the localization of Lewis determinants in tissues. *Biochemistry*, **20**, 199–205 (1981).
21. Lemieux, R. U., Bundle, D. R., and Baker, D. A. The properties of a 'synthetic' antigen related to the human blood-group Lewis a. *J. Am. Chem. Soc.*, **97**, 4076–83 (1975).
22. Lemieux, R. U., and Driguez, H. The chemical synthesis of 2-acetamido-2-deoxy-4-O-(α-L-fucopyranosyl)-3-O-(β-D-galactopyranosyl)-D-glucose. The Lewis a blood-group antigenic determinant. *J. Am. Chem. Soc.*, **97**, 4063–9 (1975).
23. Lemieux, R. U., and Driguez, H. The chemical synthesis of 2-O-(α-L-fucopyranosyl)-3-O-(β-D-galactopyranosyl)-D-galactose. The terminal structure of the blood-group B antigenic determinant. *J. Am. Chem. Soc.*, **97**, 4069–75 (1975).

24. Lemieux, R. U., Hindsgaul, O., Bird, P., Narasimhan, S., and Young, W. W. Jr Molecular recognition VI. The binding of the Lewis a human blood group determinant by two hybridoma monoclonal anti-Le^{a} antibodies. *Carbohydr. Res.*, in press.
25. Lemieux, R. U., Venot, A. P., Spohr, U., Bird, P., Mandal, G., Morishima, N., Hindsgaul, O., and Bundle, D. R. Molecular recognition V. The binding of the B human blood group determinant by hybridoma monoclonal antibodies. *Can. J. Chem.*, **63**, 2664–8 (1985).
26. Lemieux, R. U., Wong, T. C., Liao, J., and Kabat, E. A. The combining site of anti-I Ma (Group 1). *Mol. Immunol.*, **21**, 751–9 (1984).
27. LePendu, J., Cartron, J. P., Lemieux, R. U., and Oriol, R. The presence of at least two different H-blood group-related βDGal-α-2-L-fucosyl-transferases in human serum and the genetics of blood group H substances. *Am. J. Hum. Genet.*, **37**, 749–60 (1985).
28. LePendu, J., Lemieux, R. U., Lambert, F., Dalix, A.-M., and Oriol, R. Distribution of H type 1 and H type 2 antigenic determinants in human sera and saliva. *Am. J. Hum. Genet.*, **34**, 402–15 (1982).
29. LePendu, J., Lemieux, R. U., and Oriol, R. Purification of anti-Le-c antibodies with specificities for βDGal(1–3)βDglcNAc using a synthetic immunoadsorbent. *Vox. Sang.*, **43**, 188–95 (1982).
30. LePendu, J., Oriol, R., Lamberta, F., Dalix, A.-M., and Lemieux, R. U. Competition between ABO and Le gene specified enzymes. II. Quantitative analysis of A and B antigens in saliva of ABH nonsecretors. *Vox. Sang.*. **45**, 421–5. (1983).
31. Lindberg, B. Structural studies of polysaccharides. *Chem. Soc. Rev.*, **10**, 409–34 (1981).
32. Lloyd, K. O., Kabat, E. A., and Licerio, E. Immunochemical studies on blood groups. XXXVII. Structures and activities of oligosaccharides produced by alkaline degradation of blood-group Lewis a substance. Proposed structure of the carbohydrate chains of human blood-group A, B, H, Le-a, and Le-b substances. *Biochemistry*, **7**, 2976–90 (1978).
33. Lomberg, H., Cedergren, B., Leffler, H., Nilsson, B., Carlstrom, A.-S., and Svanborg-Eden, C. Influence of blood group on the availability of receptors for attachment of uropathogenic *Escherichia coli. Infection and Immunity*, **51**, 919–26 (1986).
34. Mollicone, R., Davies, D. R., Evans, B., Dalix, A.-M., and Oriol, R. Cellular expresion and genetic control of ABH antigens in primary sensory neurons of marmoset, baboon and man. *J. Neuroimmunol.*, **10**, 255–69 (1986).
35. Ofek, I., and Perry, A. Molecular basis of bacterial adherence to tissues. In *Molecular Basis of Oral Microbial Adhesion* (ed. S. E. Mergenhagen and B. Rosan), Soc. Chem. Microbiology, Washington, 1985, pp. 7–13.
36. Ogawa, T., and Sugimoto, M. Synthesis of β-Neu-5-Ac*p*-(2–3)-D-Gal and α-Neu-5-Ac*p*-(2–3)-β-D-Gal*p*-(1–4)-D-Glc. *Carbohydr. Res.*, **135**, C5–C9 (1985).
37. Ogawa, T., Yamamoto, H., Nukada, T., Kitaijima, T., and Sugimoto, M. Synthetic approach to glycan chains of glycoprotein and a protoglycan. *Pure Appl. Chem.*, **56**, 779–95 (1984).
38. O'Hanley, P., Low, D., Romero, I., Lark, D., Vosti, K., Falkow, S., and Schoolnik, G. Gal-Gal binding and hemolysin phenotypes and genotypes associated with uropathogenic *Escherichia coli. New. Eng. J. Med.*, **313**, 414–20 (1985).
39. Paulsen, H. Advances in selective chemical syntheses of complex oligosaccharides. *Angew. Chemie. Int. Ed. Engl.*, **21**, 155–73 (1982), and Synthesis of

complex oligosaccharide chains of glycoproteins. *Chem. Soc. Rev.*, **13**, 15–45 (1984).
40. Paulsen, H., and von Deesen, U. Glycosidsynthese von *N*-Acetylneuraminsaure mit sekundaren Hydroxylgruppen. *Carbohydr. Res.*, **146**, 147–53 (1986).
41. Ratcliffe, R. M., Baker, D. A., and Lemieux, R. U. Synthesis of the T-antigenic determinant in a form useful for the preparation of an effective artificial antigen and the corresponding immunoadsorbent. *Carb. Res.*, **93**, 35–41 (1981).
42. Romano, E. L., Soyano, A., and Linares, J. Preliminary therapeutic study in humans of a synthetic blood group A trisaccharide. *Abstract, 27th Meeting of the Am. Soc. Hematology*, 4 September, 1985; *Blood*, November Supplement, 1985.
43. Romano, E. L., Zabner-Oziel, P., Soyano, A., and Linares, J. Studies on the binding of IgG and F(ab) anti-A to adult and newborn group A red cells. *Vox. Sang.*, **45**, 378–83 (1983).
44. Rosevear, P. R., Nunez, H. A., and Barker, R. Synthesis and solution conformation of the type 2 blood group oligosaccharide αLFuc(1–2)βDGal(1–4)βDGlcNAc. *Biochemistry*, **21**, 1421–31 (1982).
45. Sabesan, S., and Lemieux, R. U. Synthesis of tri- and tetra-saccharide haptens related to the *Asialo*-forms of the gangliosides G_{M2} and G_{M1}. *Can. J. Chem.*, **62**, 644–54 (1983).
46. Sabesan, S., and Paulson, J. C. Combined chemical enzymatic synthesis of sialyloligosaccharides and characterization by 500–Mhz ^{1}H and ^{13}C-NMR spectroscopy. *J. Am. Chem. Soc.*, **108**, 2068–80 (1986).
47. Spitalnik, S., Cowles, J., Cox, M. T., Baker, D., Holt, J., and Blumberg, N. A new technique in quantitative immunohematology: solid-phase kinetic ELISA. *Vox. Sang.*, **45**, 440–8 (1983).
48. Spitalnik, S. L., Cowles, J. W., Cox, M. T., and Blumberg, N. Neutralization of Lewis blood group antibodies synthetic immunoadsorbents. *Am. J. Clin. Path.*, **80**, 63–5 (1983).
49. Spitalnik, S., Pfaff, W., Cowles, J., Ireland, J. E., Scornik, J. C., and Blumberg, N. Correlation of humoral immunity to Lewis blood group antigens with renal transplant rejection. *Transplantation*, **37**, 265–8 (1984).
50. Spohr, U., Morishima, N., Hindsgaul, O., and Lemieux, R. U. Molecular recognition IV. The binding of the Lewis b human blood group determinant by a hybridoma monoclonal antibody. *Can. J. Chem.*, **63**, 2659–63 (1985).
51. Spohr, U., Hindsgaul, O., and Lemieux, R. U. Molecular recognition II. The binding of the Lewis b and Y human blood group determinants by the lectin IV of *Griffonia simplicifolia. Can. J. Chem.*, **63**, 2644–52 (1985).
52. Thøgersen, H., Lemieux, R. U., Bock, K., and Meyer, B. Further justification for the *exo*-anomeric effect. Conformational analysis based in nuclear magnetic resonance spectroscopy of the B human blood group determinant. *Can. J. Chem.*, **60**, 44–57 (1982).
53. Watkins, W. M. Biochemistry and genetics of the ABO, Lewis and P blood group systems. *Adv. Hum. Genet.*, **10**, 1–136 (1980).
54. Wong, C. H., Haynie, S. L., and Whitesides, G. W. Enzyme-catalyzed synthesis of N-acetyllactosamine with *in situ* regeneration of uridine 5′-diphosphate glucose and uridine t′-diphosphate galactose. *J. Org. Chem.*, **47**, 5416–18 (1982).
55. Young, W. W., Johnson, H. S., Tamura, Y., Karlsson, K. A., Larson, G., Parker, J. M. R., Khare, D. P., Spohr, U., Baker, D. A., Hindsgaul, O., and Lemieux, R. U. Characterization of monoclonal antibodies specific for the Lewis a human blood group determinant. *J. Biol. Chem.*, **258**, 4890–4 (1983).

DISCUSSION – Chaired by Professor E. A. Kabat

ROBBINS: Some carbohydrates which are important virulence and protective antigens for bacteria are phosphorylated polysaccharides. Have you had any experience with trying to control the synthesis of a repeating unit that had a phosphate diester and then can you take the repeating unit and perhaps make block synthesis for longer materials?

LEMIEUX: I don't have any experience. In fact, I had just started work in that direction when I reached retirement age a year ago. I decided to cut my group down and that's one of the things that peeled off. It can be done, all the chemistry's there, there's no problem, it's just a matter of time and money.

GLAUDEMANS: It might be interesting in relation to a remark about different determinants. Dr Lee, of Johns Hopkins University, has an idea that he is testing now; that antibodies may form against different saccharidic parts of glycopeptides sitting next to each other on a membrane. In other words, have strands of glycoproteins, and obtain an antibody recognizing the ends of several *separated* chains of oligosaccharides. I wonder if anybody's ever seen any evidence of that, or knows anything about a similar occurrence?

LEMIEUX: Well I would venture the thought that perhaps some of the work that Dr Jennings talked about this morning is somehow connected with these ideas an that this happens because the chain of seventeen sialic acid residues that is involved is folding back in some sort of way.

KABAT: The other problem that arises is that, if you have an antibody which is directed towards the inside of a chain, as you go up in the size of the unit, let's say it is as big as six, as we have in the dextran, you then introduce multiple ways of combining and so you can get additional binding energy, so to speak, by the fact that you have multiple choices for reacting, whereas with only six you have the limit of what is filling the site. If you get up to nine, you can fill the site in many ways and that gives you a competitive advantage, but the conformational change is also important.

JENNINGS: We don't fully understand the minimum requirement for ten sialic acid residues to form the Group B polysaccharide epitope. However, we do have preliminary evidence that there is a conformational difference between the ends of the decasaccharide and the middle residues. Therefore, the oligosaccharide needs to be large before it starts to look like the polysaccharide.

KABAT: How much difference is there between the end of the chain, how many units are involved in your structure?

JENNINGS: The analysis of the NMR spectrum of the decasaccharide indicates that its two terminal disaccharide units are completely different from its internal hexasaccharide unit. Incidentally, the size of the latter is fairly

consistent with the maximum size that you originally proposed for the linear dextran epitope.
KABAT: So you are essentially implying that you are dealing with a sort of groove-type site because the four at the ends are sort of making knobs which are non-reactive and the six are then forming the usual type of determinants and then, as you go up further – how big have you got them? What is the longest oligosaccharide?
JENNINGS: The biggest we have is eighteen.
KABAT: Does it precipitate?
JENNINGS: No.
KABAT: You might have some high solubility in it. Maybe one could get it to . . .
GLAUDEMANS: What I meant that Dr Lee is doing is that he actually has one antibody-combining site reacting with several molecules that are in proximity to one another on the cell surface. That could have tremendous implications for cell-surface recognition, which is different from causing an oligosaccharide to have a tertiary structure like a polypeptide does. That's the point I was trying to make.
GEYSEN: I'd just like to make a couple of comments which might put it into perspective. At the moment, a question which is fundamental to some of the work we are doing is: are antibodies to polysaccharide antigens different fundamentally from antibodies to protein epitopes? It was quite interesting to see your data. In the first instance, if I could make any generalization at all with the epitopes that we have studied, to single-residue resolution which number between 50 and 60 to date, in terms of protein epitopes, all of them show at least one, what we call 'hydrophilic' residue, adjacent to one or two hydrophobic residues. Now that is a generalization I can make. So that's reasonably consistent, I think, with what you find, and maybe suggests that antibodies to polysaccharide epitopes are no different fundamentally from those against protein epitopes. The second thing I would like to say is, again as a generalization, that all the epitopes that we have located, for which we have a structure of the antigen itself, show evidence of conformational change. By that I am not necessarily implying that the alpha carbon of the main chain – I am talking here about protein epitopes, of course – is significantly altered. But what we do see is that side chains that are completely buried, i.e. have no surface exposure whatsoever, turn up as contact residues and they are invariably hydrophobic residues. Now, again, it is an interesting thing that, if there is no fundamental difference between polysaccharide epitopes and protein epitopes, then it seems to me that it is distinctly possible that you can get significant conformational change in your carbohydrate epitopes as well, in the same day as we see conformational change in protein epitopes.
ADA: There is great interest at the present time in synthetic vaccines and

interest particularly in making oligopeptide vaccines. I don't know what the cost of making say, a six-amino acid peptide, is. If you make it by the traditional methods, it may cost so many dollars; if you make some by enzymatic methods, it may cost a fraction of that cost. The question I wanted to ask is, if you wanted to make an epitope out of a pentamer oligosaccharide, how much would it cost to make that? Is it feasible to think that you could make it on a large scale very, very cheaply or not?

KABAT: Well it depends on whether you want to sell a kilo or a microgram.

ADA: If you were selling a kilo, what would it cost? You talk of vaccines costing maybe sixty cents per dose. Is it conceivable at all to think of making an oligosaccharide molecule for that sort of cost?

KABAT: I don't have any idea of the cost, but I can't afford it.

ROBBINS: It's not a commonly appreciated fact, but most of the cost in vaccine is putting it in the bottles, putting labels on, storing and testing. The production of the vaccine itself is only a fraction of its cost. Even if it were an expensive material, if it could be considered as a useful material, engineers and chemists would get together and make it cheap enough. Now that's never a factor. The major cost of making meningococcus vaccine is freeze-drying it.

LEMIEUX: Chemistry can provide you molecularly well-defined structures. You know what the structure is, this is a useful contribution, but it does not necessarily provide a low-cost vaccine.

ROBBINS: We should have a little time for hallucinating, that's what meetings like this are for. It seems to me that there's some suggestions now that you can make a better antigen by synthetic methods than occurs in nature. This seems to be unpublished but what we've seen are good data that an interesting polypeptide, 13- or 14-amino-acid peptide, which is called a heat-stable toxin and one of the exotoxins of enteropathogenic *E. coli*, can be improved in its immunogenicity by altering the residues. Unfortunately, one of the companies that is doing this is loath to give out the material, but they have shown the data and the data look good.

Now we have Dr Jennings showing us that you can do this with a material that's fully immunogenic by changing its structure. I'm not so sure the syntheses should be worried about making things that bacteria make, because commercially they can be made by fermentation probably cheaper, but try to see if, by chemistry, you can improve upon nature and make materials that are more effective immunogens by trying to take a look at the nature of the antigen–antibody combination itself.

LEMIEUX: In our work in modifying these haptens for inhibition studies, we have found that certain changes can give you much more potent inhibitors, up to a factor of 18 for example. So if you have a factor of 18, then for diagnostic purposes that could become quite important. It's another way that maybe we could contribute.

KABAT: I'd like to point out that quite a number of years ago when the National Research Council was interested in polypeptide plasma expanders that Paul Maurer made several of them and they turned out to be extremely potent in inducing delayed-type hypersensitivity reactions in humans which were very severe. So one has to worry about synthetic antigens of a polypeptide nature and I think that should be borne in mind.
ASSAAD: The price of any vaccine (as we have seen in all vaccines), drops steadily once it is on the market; the good manufacturers continue with research on more and more efficient production processes. The WHO Expanded Programme on Immunization (EPI) is acquiring poliomyelitis vaccine for approximately three cents per dose. One manufacturer in a developing country finds it more expensive to obtain poliomyelitis vaccine in bulk, buy the phials, dilute, mix the three poliomyelitis vaccine types and put in bottles, simply because the bottles *per se* are more expensive than the vaccine already on the market. It is really fascinating. There is a lot of know-how in vaccine production. For instance, in poliomyelitis, when the late Dr Frank Perkins put the vaccine of one manufacturer in bottles of another manufacturer, the titres were different from the original vaccine; the manufacturer calculates how much of the virus adheres to the bottle walls.
KABAT: On the other hand, with polysaccharide vaccines, the antibody protective levels stays up for many years from the earlier studies of Heidelberger. We found the same thing.
ASSAAD: Dr Griffiss knows very well that the studies carried out by CDC in West Africa, have shown that immunity wanes within 2–3 years, as it does in Egypt.
GRIFFISS: The problem is that there is a great deal of difference between a vaccine in a field trial that is carefully controlled, and the public health use of the vaccine somewhere in the world. In fact, Group A meningococcal vaccine, which is highly protective in all field trials, is a disaster as a public health vaccine because, 3 years after immunization, the target population no longer has protection, not antibody, but protection. Whether or not you can boost those people, because the data with polysachaarides in young adults are that, when you boost, they do not respond. It is possible that memory has been lost in these individuals and you are, in a sense, immunizing someone all over again and they would respond again. But, none the less, countries that have spent lots of money, not so much on the vaccine, but on the delivery of that vaccine, and diverted all their health-care resources to delivery.
MÄKELÄ, Helena: I would like to add something about the possibility of giving a booster dose of these polysaccharide vaccines. We have some experience in Finland of two such polysaccharides. One is the *Haemophilus influenzae* polysaccharide which we gave 3½ years after the first injection. The children were anywhere in the range between 3 months and 5 years when they got

their vaccine for the first time and, in each case, the response to the second dose was similar to the response in naïve children of the same age. So that, in each case, one did not get a booster response, but one did not get any impaired responses either. The second experience is in giving meningococcal Group A vaccine to young adults who had received the Group A vaccine about 8 years previously, at an age of between 5 and 15. Again, the responses were typical for that age without previous vaccination. So these experiences would show that it is possible to give new doses of vaccine but, obviously, it is a problem in the developing countries if you have to go back and give the vaccine every 3 years.

ROBBINS: Dr Assaad, I do not mean to be combative, but I would like to say that scientists have little enough control of their own budget, they should not be worried about national health budgets. No one gave us the budget of a country to spend and I do not think that should enter our considerations – what we should deal with is scientific principles. If we make products that are useful and countries wish to use them, or they have to use them, somehow they find a way of doing it and I do not think we should deal with that because we have no control over it.

ASSAAD: I am sorry, but I insist that price should not come in at all. I am not talking price at all. I am talking about the feasibility of getting to children, once, twice and three times. It is the operative part and not the cost.

ROBBINS: But if the money was available for the vaccine and the support of personnel, could this problem be solved?

ASSAAD: Not necessarily. This is not money, it is infrastructure.

ROBBINS: I know, that is right, but that is not our control.

ASSAAD: But can we get a better vaccine? That is the point.

ROBBINS: That is another issue.

KABAT: These things make for very serious problems, besides the scientific issues, and it is obvious that we are not equipped to deal with them.

Towards Better Carbohydrate Vaccines
Edited by R. Bell and G. Torrigiani

Published by John Wiley & Sons Ltd

6

Microbial polysaccharide antigens – biosynthesis, genes and gene products

IAN W. SUTHERLAND
Department of Microbiology, Edinburgh University, West Mains Road, Edinburgh EH9 3JG, UK

SUMMARY

Most microbial polysaccharides likely to be of antigenic importance are essentially polymers formed of repeating units of regular structure. These units vary in size from 2 to 8 monosaccharides and frequently carry *O*-acetyl and pyruvate ketal substituents. Few bacteria have been the subject of systematic studies on large numbers of serotypes, but there is now detailed information on the structures of exopolysaccharides from many *Klebsiella* serotypes, and a number of *Escherichia coli*, *Neisseria* and *Haemophilus* strains as well as several *Streptococcus pneumoniae* serotypes. These provide an indication of what may be expected in other micro-organisms. Very few genetic studies on exopolysaccharide-synthesizing bacteria have been reported. Such studies as do exist indicate the possibility of either chromosomal or plasmid control of polysaccharide synthesis. The genes and gene products form several groups – precursors common to other polysaccharides synthesized by the cell, sugar nucleotide glycosyl donors specific to the exopolysaccharide product, and the enzymes essential for exopolysaccharide synthesis. The regulatory systems identified so far, vary considerably in their complexity.

INTRODUCTION

The number of polysaccharide antigens produced by any microbial cell depends on the type of micro-organism. Because of the limited information available on many of these systems, this chapter will discuss primarily gram-negative bacteria. These yield two types of carbohydrate-containing antigens – lipopolysaccharides (LPS) which form part of the outer membrane wall complex of the bacteria, and extracellular polysaccharides found either as material attached to the bacterial cell or, alternatively, secreted into the extracellular environment.

Microbial exopolysaccharides (EPS) vary in their structure and composition. Many are constructed from a limited range of hexoses, 6-deoxyhexoses and uronic acids to form repeating units containing 2–8 monosaccharides [30]. Others contain *N*-acetylamino sugars and phosphate groups. In some genera, such as *Klebsiella*, and to a lesser extent in *E. coli*, most serotypes are formed from similar structures and a relatively limited range of common monosaccharides [1] (Figure 1). In addition. *O*-acetyl groups and ketal-linked pyruvate groups are present. In other genera, *N*-acetylamino sugars may be present, including the relatively rare *N*-acetylaminouronic acids, and also phosphorylated sugars in structures closely resembling the teichoic acid components of gram-positive bacterial walls [7]. Thus, a range of mechanisms of genetic control and of gene products can perhaps be anticipated, together with a range of different regulatory systems. Information obtained directly from genetic studies on EPS antigen systems is relatively limited and must frequently be extrapolated from other bacteria.

→4)-α-D-Glc*p*A(1→3)-α-L-Fuc*p*(1→3)β-D-Glc*p*(1→
                                                    ↑4
                                                    |
                                                   1|
                                               β-D Glc*p*

Acyl substituents : 0 acetate
½ acetate (alternate fucose residues)
1 acetate (all fucose residues)

Figure 1. The *Enterobacter aerogenes* K54 polysaccharides

GENE PRODUCTS

Biosynthesis of EPS is a complex process involving considerable numbers of enzymes. These enzymes can be regarded as belonging to three distinct groups. Group 1, are enzymes which synthesize precursors common to the production of EPS antigens and other cell components, including not only

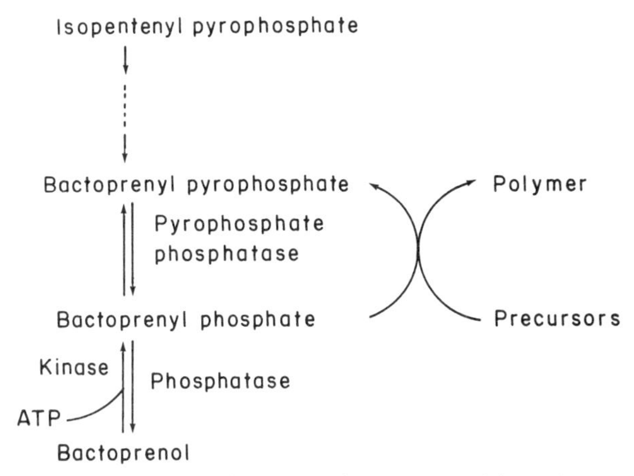

Figure 2. The involvement of bactoprenol in polysaccharide synthesis (polymer = exopolysaccharide, lipopolysaccharide or peptidoglycan)

polysaccharides but other polymers and intracellular constituents. While most are concerned with anabolic processes of the cell, a few are also involved in bacterial catabolism. Thus such enzymes include those yielding the isoprenoid lipids (bactoprenol or, in eukaryotes, dolichol) which are essential for the synthesis of repeating unit-containing EPS antigens. These enzymes are *essential* for the viability of the microbial cell. Their absence would lead to failure to produce a cell wall and consequent lysis and death. The only way in which mutations in such enzymes can be studied, therefore, is through the isolation and examination of conditional mutants. Also essential for the metabolic processes of all cells are the enzymes yielding acetyl CoA and phosphoenolpyruvate (PEP). This group of enzymes and products is relatively large and can be expected to form segments of the chromosome clearly separated from those *directly* involved in regulation of EPS antigens. Some of the enzymes involved in isoprenoid alcohol biosynthesis and utilization have been identified in gram-positive bacteria and in at least one gram-negative species [18, 29]. It is *possible* that the group of enzymes responsible for the phosphorylation of bactoprenol and dephosphorylation of bactoprenyl pyrophosphate (Figure 2) could be involved in the regulation of polysaccharide antigen synthesis, as was suggested initially by Goldman and Strominger [14] Neither *O*-acetyl groups nor pyruvate ketals are essential features of EPS, and examples are known, such as *Klebsiella* type 2 [33], in which both acylated and non-acylated versions of this polymer are synthesized. A mutant of *E. coli* producing non-acetylated colanic acid has also been isolated [12], while other bacterial strains can, under certain physiological conditions, synthesize non-acylated polymers [5]. A pyruvate-less extracellular polysaccharide has also been obtained from one mutant bacterial strain [39]. However, both acyl

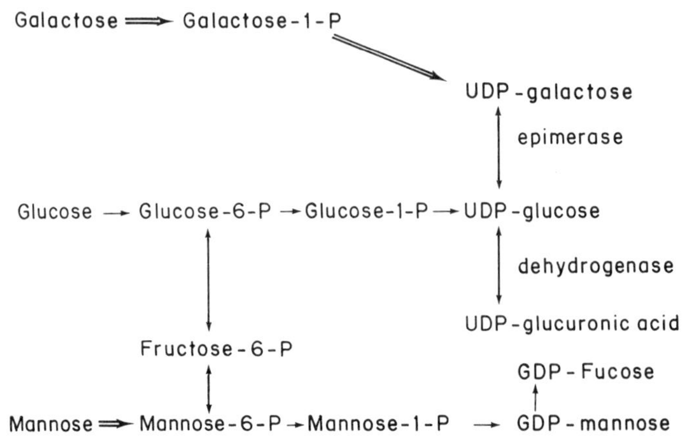

Figure 3. Interconversion of sugars and sugar nucleotides involved in polysaccharide synthesis (⇨ = catabolic systems used on specific substrates)

donors are required for the synthesis UDP-*N*-acetylmuramic acid, essential as a precursor of peptidoglycan in prokaryotes.

Group 2 gene products form the sugar nucleotides which are the activated glycosyl precursors for all polysaccharides synthesized within microbial cells. This group of gene products can be subdivided into those sugar nucleotides which are common to EPS and other polysaccharides such as LPS or teichoic acid, and those which are required for the EPS only. It has frequently been shown that, in both eukaryotic and prokaryotic cells, three sugar nucleotides – UDP-D-glucose, GPD-D-mannose and UDP-*N*-acetyl-D-glucosamine – are important both as direct precursors of these three sugars when present in polysaccharides and as key intermediates in the synthesis of other sugars such as D-galactose and D-glucuronic acid, *N*-acetyl-D-galactosamine and L-fucose respectively. The mechanisms of interconversion of some of these sugar nucleotides are illustrated in Figure 3.

Although these sugar nucleotides are essential for EPS synthesis, and mutants unable to form them do not produce EPS, they are not essential for cell viability. The synthesis of some of the sugar nucleotides has been examined and the key roles of enzymes such as GDP-mannose pyrophosphorylase has been demonstrated [22]. In particular, feedback control permitted the bacteria studied to regulate independently the rate of synthesis of GDP-mannose and GDP-fucose, when these acted as glycosyl donors for polysaccharide synthesis. Similar regulation has been suggested for UDP-glucose dehydrogenase in the control of the synthesis of the glucuronic acid-containing K27 EPS antigen of *E. coli* [27]. However, this is clearly not the sole regulatory mechanism in the synthesis of the EPS colanic acid by *E. coli*. Non-EPS-synthesizing mutants accumulated relatively large amounts of

UDP-glucuronic acid [23]. Two specific precursors of colanic acid, UDP-glucuronic acid and GDP-fucose, are produced by the enzymes UDP-glucose dehydrogenase and GDP-fucose synthase respectively. The two sugar nucleotides were detectable in bacteria in which colanic acid synthesis was repressed, but the levels of the sugar nucleotides and of the enzymes responsible for their synthesis, were increased in derepressed strains [17]. Thus it appeared that there existed one or more operons containing genes for key enzymes in colanic acid synthesis. Those sugar nucleotides, which were precursors common to LPS and colanic acid, were found at essentially the same levels in bacteria in which colanic acid had been repressed as in derepressed cells. This was also reflected in the levels of UDP-glucose pyropophorylase and UDP-galactose-4-epimerase.

In serotypes 1 and 8 *K. aerogenes*, enzymes assumed to be involved in the synthesis of sugar nucleotides specific to the capsular and other polysaccharide antigens had high specific activities, whereas those solely involved in capsular synthesis were present at lower levels [26]. Mutants in which there was loss of EPS-synthezising capacity had similar specific activities of the enzymes tested to wild type bacteria. These results strongly suggest that enzymes and their products belonging to Group 1 are controlled constitutively, while those forming Group 2 can be repressed under certain conditions. It should, however, be remembered that it is possible to control synthesis of many antigenic polysaccharides, and presumbly the enzymes and precursors necessary for their formation, through variations in the physiological conditions under which the bacteria are grown [35].

The third group of gene products are those controlling enzymes exclusively concerned with the biosynthesis of the repeating units of the polysaccharide antigens. The number of these will obviously depend on the complexity of the macromolecule. Relatively few EPS-synthesizing systems have been studied in sufficient detail to identify the enzymes catalysing repeating unit assembly and polysaccharide secretion. However, from the elegant studies of Troy *et al.*]37] using a *K. aerogenes* strain, it was clear that each sugar in the sequence required a distinct sugar transferase (or, in the initial reaction, a sugar-1-phosphate transferase). Similar results from another *K. aerogenes* strain of serotype 8 [34] confirmed the enzyme pattern (Figure 4). More recently, studies on *Xanthomonas campestris* have revealed a similar enzymic sequence and have, in addition, confirmed the predicted requirement of specific transferases for *O*-acetyl groups from acetyl CoA and pyruvate from PEP [3, 20, 21] (Figure 5). All these gene products are membrane-bound enzymes, two of which in *K. aerogenes* type 8, were extractable with acid butanol [24] and thus likely to be lipoproteins. It is probable that they must reside in correct spatial relationships with one another, and with the enzymes supplying or regulating isoprenoid lipid availability, if polysaccharide is to be synthesized. Most of the studies indicated above were performed on

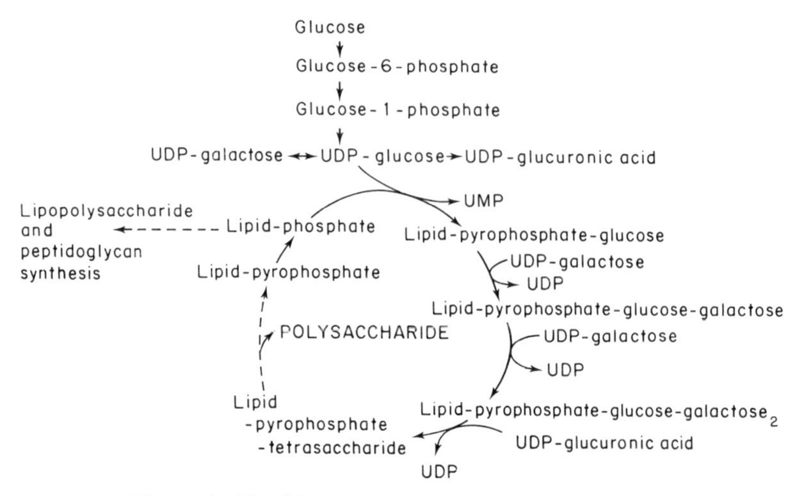

Figure 4. The biosynthesis of an exopolysaccharide

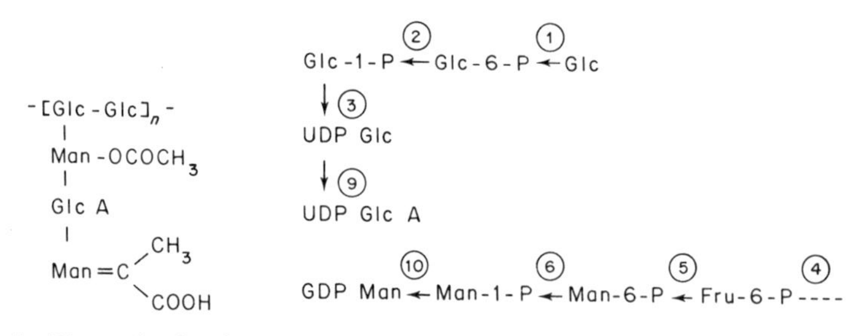

Figure 5. Biosynthesis of xanthan.

Enzymes required (a) for other systems: (1) hexokinase; (2) phosphoglucomutase; (3) UDP-glucose pyrophosphorylase; (4) phosphoglucose isomerase; (5) Phosphomannomutase; (7) Pyruvate kinase; (8) enzymes for acetyl CoA and isoprenoid lipid syntheses.

(b) For specific precursors: (9) UDP-glucose dehydrogenase; (10) GDP-mannose pyrophorylase.

(c) For polymer synthesis: (11) glucose-1-phosphate transferase; (12) glucosyl transferase; (13) mannosyl transferase; (14) mannose acetylase; (15) glucuronosyl transferase; (16) mannosyl transferase II; (17) ketal transferase; (18) ligases, polymerases

membrane fragments of varying size, or using bacterial cells which had been rendered permeable to the sugar nucleotide substrates of the enzymes by treatment with toluene or other organic solvents.

The later stages of EPS synthesis and excretion are poorly understood. The possible role of outer membrane proteins in gram-negative bacteria has been postulated. One such protein, designated protein K, has been observed in a number of different capsulate *E. coli* strains, although it was absent from most non-capsulate strains [28]. Protein K is a porin with effective pore diameter 1.2 nm and it is conceivable that it could function in EPS export, although the dimensions suggest that this is unlikely [32, 40]. Another protein, the precursor of outer membrane protein *a* was a product of the *lon* gene [13]. It is clear, therefore, that gene products involved in EPS synthesis may, in gram-negative bacteria, include outer membrane proteins. although whether or not these have a *direct* role in polysaccharide production remains to be elucidated. The different categories of gene product associated with polysaccharide antigen synthesis are summarized in Table I.

Table I. Gene products associated with polysaccharide antigen synthesis

Group 1	Products not specifically associated with the antigens
	Sugar phosphates
	Some sugar nucleotides
	Isoprenoid lipids
	Acetyl CoA
	Phosphenolpyruvate
Group 2	Specific precursors
	e.g. UDP-glucuronic acid
	GDP-fucose, etc.
Group 3	Specific enzymes and proteins
	Monosaccharide transferases
	Acetyl and ketal transferases
	Polymerase(s)
	Ligase(s)
	Export system?
	Outer membrane protein

GENES

As the individual enzymes involved in the final stage of synthesis cannot be isolated and assayed, relatively little information on their genetic regulation is available. It seems highly likely that they form single linkage groups under co-ordinated control. Two models for this exist. In *E. coli*, synthesis of colanic acid (Figure 6) a polysaccharide of relatively complex structure (hexasaccharide repeat unit carrying acetyl and ketal groups), formed by various enterobacterial strains [16], has been the subject of numerous studies by Markovitz and his colleagues [25]. This polysaccharide is, unlike many EPS antigens, not produced normally in large amounts by those bacteria capable of its synthesis, the exception being *Enterobacter cloacae*. Its synthesis is greatly increased by mutations at a number of different loci, one of which has been designated *lon* [25]. This gene is responsible for other

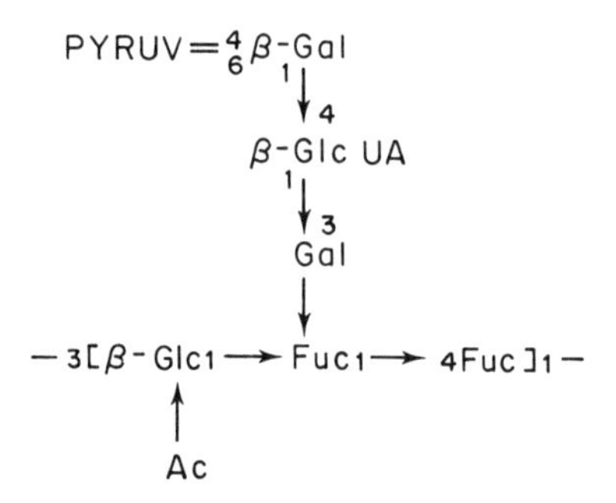

Figure 6. Synthesis of colanic acid

properties in addition to colanic acid synthesis. A set of at least five genes required for colanic acid synthesis show negative transcriptional regulation by the *lon* gene product [36], and the number of enzymes involved in polysaccharide synthesis under such control may amount to ten; however, the *lon* regulatory system does not regulate all the genes necessary for colanic acid biosynthesis. Notable exceptions are the enzymes of the gal operon, one of which at least is essential for polysaccharide synthesis.

Further studies revealed the regulation of colanic acid to be even more complex than at first thought. Control was exerted by at least two positive regulators of capsule synthesis – rcsA and rcsB at 43 and 47 minutes respectively on the *E. coli* map, and rcsC a negative regulator located close to rcsB [15]. It has also been possible to clone a 2 megadalton DNA fragment in *E. coli* which controls cell division, capsular polysaccharide synthesis and enzymes involved in EPS synthesis [2]. More recently, an 8.2 megadalton fragment was cloned and one of its products, a 94 kilodalton polypeptide, identified as the *lon* gene product [31, 41]. The 94K protein was an ATP-dependent protease, capable of binding to DNA. It is possible, but not yet proved, that such regulation may also include some of the genes common to LPS synthesis, such as those required for sugar nucleotide production. Studies on *lon* mutants in *Salmonella typhimurium*, showed them to be similar to those in *E. coli* [6]. The product, the ATP-dependent protease La, normally functions to degrade protein products of the *sulA* gene, but probably has regulatory roles in addition to a role in the SOS response.

The alternative to the very complicated regulatory mechanisms reported from *E. coli* is probably of more widespread occurrence. Certainly, a tight clustering of several genetic loci associated with EPS synthesis in *Pseudomonas aeruginosa* has been reported [4]. The biosynthetic system for this polymer is likely to be much simpler than that for colanic acid, but *P. aeruginosa* is a further example in which polysaccharide synthesis is normally repressed. Mutation in a regulator gene close to the origin causes derepression and polysaccharide synthesis [10]. Genetic mapping indicates that at least two regions of the chromosome in the strain studied are involved in repression of polysaccharide synthesis [11]. Even in a relatively simple repeating unit structure of four sugars, as is found in many *K. aerogenes* strains, this would still involve regulation of perhaps eight structural genes. In more complex structures this number would be much higher.

In *H. influenzae*, the cap-b region of the chromosome consists of two large repeated DNA segments [19], but only one functional copy is required for expression of the capsular serotype [8]. This feature may be relatively common, as other EPS-synthesizing bacteria have also been found to contain sufficient DNA to account for multiple copies of their chromosomes [11].

Control of polysaccharide antigen synthesis through plasmids has been demonstrated in some bacteria such as *E. coli* and other enteric species [25] and in *Rhizobium meliloti*. In this last bacterium, a megaplasmid of several megadaltons includes four loci involved in EPS synthesis [9], although other genes responsible for EPS synthesis were chromosomally located. The cellulose-producing bacterium *Acetobacter xylinum* also contains a number of plasmids, and evidence for their involvement in polysaccharide synthesis has been presented [38]. It is clear that, while many of the genes and gene products necessary for polysaccharide antigen synthesis can be predicted, extrapolation of results between species is probably seldom possible. Various mechanisms for genetic regulation have been identified in the few polysaccharide-producing bacteria which have been extensively studied. These can probably be separated into the relatively simple systems likely to be involved in micro-organisms where a single capsular polysaccharide is produced (e.g. *K. aerogenes*, *S. pneumoniae*, etc.) and the much more complex systems found when polysaccharide production is normally repressed (*E. coli*, *P. aeruginosa*). Some bacteria are capable of multiple polysaccharide production and these may include a number of polymers of antigenic importance. In these bacteria, even more complex regulatory systems can be expected, to ensure supply of appropriate precursors and enzymes to the different biosynthetic complexes.

REFERENCES

1. Atkins, E. D. T., Isaac, D., and Elloway, H. F. Conformations of microbial extracellular polysaccharides by x-ray diffraction: Progress on the Klebsiella serotypes. In *Polysaccharides and Polysaccharases* (ed. R. C. W. Berkeley, G. W. Gooday and D. C. Ellwood), Academic Press, London and San Francisco, 1969, pp. 161–89.
2. Berg, P. E., Gayda, R., Avni, H., Zehnbauer, B., and Markovitz, A. Cloning of *Escherichia coli* DNA that controls cell division and capsular polysaccharide synthesis. *Proc. Natn. Acad. Sci., USA,* **73**, 697–701 (1976).
3. Couso, R. O., Ielpi, L., Garcia, R. C., and Dankert, M. Biosynthesis of polysac-

charides in *Acetobacter xylinium*. Sequential synthesis of a *hepta*saccharide diphosphate isoprenol. *Europ. J. Biochem.*, **123**, 617–27 (1982).
4. Darzins, A., Wnag, S.-K., Vanags, R. I., and Chakrabarty, A. M. Clustering of mutations affecting alginic acid biosynthesis in mucoid *Pseudomonas aeruginosa*. *J. Bacteriol.*, **164**, 516–24 (1985).
5. Davidson, I. W. Production of polysaccharide by *Xanthomas campestris* in continuous culture. *FEMS Microbiol. Letts.*, **3**, 347–9 (1978).
6. Downs, D., Waxman, L., Goldberg, A. L., and Roth, J. Isolation and characterization of lon mutants in *Salmonella typhimurium*. *J. Bacteriol.*, **165**, 193–7 (1986).
7. Duckworth, M. Teichoic acids. In *Surface Carbohydrates of the Prokaryotic Cell* (ed. I. W. Sutherland), Academic Press, London and San Francisco, 1977, pp. 177–208.
8. Ely, S., Tippett, J., Kroll, J. S., and Moxon, E. R. Mutations affecting expression and maintenance of genes encoding the serotype b capsule of *Haemophilus influenzae*. *J. Bacteriol.*, **167**, 44–8 (1986).
9. Finan, T. M., Kinkel, B., de Vos, G. F., and Signer, E. R. Second symbiotic megaplasmid in *Rhizolium melilati* carrying exopolysaccharide and thiamine synthesis genes. *J. Bacteriol.*, **167**, 66–72 (1986).
10. Fyfe, J. A. M., and Govan, J. R. W. Alginate synthesis in mucoid *Pseudomonas aeruginosa*: a chromosomal locus involved in control. *J. Gen. Microbiol.*, **119**, 443–50 (1980).
11. Fyfe, J. A. M., and Govan, J. R. W. Synthesis, regulation and biological function of bacterial alginate. *Progr. Ind. Microbiol.*, **18**, 45–83 (1983).
12. Garegg, P. J., Lindberg, B., Onn, T., and Holme, T. Comparative structural studies on the M-antigen from *Salmonella typhimurium*, *Escherichia coli* and *Aerobacter cloacae*. *Acta Chem. Scand*, **25**, 1185–94 (1971).
13. Gayda, R. C., Avni, H., Berg, P. E., and Markovitz, A. Outer membrane proteins and other polypeptides regulate capsular polysaccharide synthesis in *E. coli* K-12. *Molec. Gen. Genet.*, **175**, 325–32 (1979).
14. Goldman, R., and Strominger, J. L. Purification and properties of C55-isophenylpyrophosphate phosphatase from micrococcus lysodeikticus. *J. Biol. Chem.*, **247**, 5116–22 (1972).
15. Gottesman, S., Trisler, P., and Torres-Cabassa, A. Regulation of capsular polysaccharide synthesis in *Escherichia coli* K-12: characterization of three regulatory genes. *J. Bacteriol.*, **162**, 1111–19 (1985).
16. Grant, W. D., Sutherland, I. W., and Wilkinson, J. F. Exopolysaccharide colanic acid and its occurrence in the enterobacteriaceae. *J. Bacteriol.*, **100**, 1187–93 (1969).
17. Grant, W. D., Sutherland, I. W., and Wilkinson, J. R. Control of clonic acid synthesis. *J. Bacteriol.*, **103**, 89–96 (1970).
18. Higashi, Y., Siewert, G., and Strominger, J. L. Biosynthesis of the peptiologlycan of bacterial cell walls. *J. Biol. Chem.*, **245**, 3683–90 (1970).
19. Hoiseth, S. K., Moxon, E. R., and Silver, R. P. Genes involved in *Haemophilus influenzae* type b capsule expression are part of a 18-kilobase tandem duplication. *Proc. Natn. Acad. Sci., USA*, **83**, 1106–10 (1986).
20. Ielpi, L., Couso, R., and Dankert, M. Pyruvic acid acetal residues are transferred from phosphoenolpyruvate to the pentasaccharide-P-P lipid. *Biochem. Biophys. Res. Commun.*, **102**, 1400–8 (1981).
21. Ielpi, L., Couso, R., and Dankert, M. Xanthanygum biosynthesis: acetylation occurs at the prenyl-phosphate sugar stage. *Biochem. Intern.*, **6**, 323–33 (1983).

22. Kornfeld, R. H., and Ginsburg, L. Control of synthesis of guanosine 5′-diphosphate D-mannose and guenosine 5′-diphosphate L-fucose in bacteria. *Biochim. Biophys. Acta*, **117**, 79–87 (1966).
23. Lieberman, M. M., Shaparis, A., and Markovitz, A. Control of uridine diphosphate-glucose dehydrogenase synthesis and uridine diphosphate-glucuronic acid accumulation by a regulator gene mutation in *Escherichia coli* K-12. *J. Bacteriol.*, **101**, 959–64 (1970).
24. Lomax, J. A., Poxton, I. R., and Sutherland, I. W. Butanol-soluble glycoryl transferases in *Klebsiella aerogenes. FEBS Letts*, **34**, 232–3 (1973).
25. Markovitz, A. Genetics and regulation of bacterial capsular polysaccharide synthesis and radiation sensitivity. In *Surface Carbohydrates of the Procaryotic Cell* [ed. I. W. Sutherland), Academic Press, London and San Francisco, 1977, pp. 415–62.
26. Norval, M., and Sutherland, I. W. The production of enzymes involved in exopolysaccharide synthesis in *Klebsiella. Europ. J. Biochem.*, **35**, 209–315 (1973).
27. Olson, A. C., Schmidt, G., and Jann, K. Biochemistry of the K antigens of *Escherichia coli*. Formation of the nucleoside diphosphate sugar precursors of the K27 antigen of *E. coli*, 08: K27(A):H-. *Europ. J. Biochem.*, **11**, 376–85 (1969).
28. Paakanen, J., Gotschlich, E. C., and Mäkelä, P. H. Protein K: a new major outer membrane protein found in encapsulated *Escherichia coli. J. Bacteriol.*, **139**, 835–41 (1979).
29. Poxton, I. R., Lomax, J. A., and Sutherland, I. W. Isoprenoid alcohol kinase – a third butanol-soluble enzyme in *Klebsiella aerogenes* membranes. *J. Gen. Microbiol.*, **84**, 231–3 (1974).
30. Sandford, P. A. Exocellular, microbial polysaccharides. *Adv. Carb. Chem. Biochem.*, **36**, 265–313 (1979).
31. Schoemaker, J. M., and Markovitz, A. Identification of the gene on (cap R) product as a 94-kilodalton polypeptide by cloning and selection analyses. *J. Bacteriol.*, **147**, 46–56 (1981).
32. Sutcliffe, J., Blumenthal, R., Walter, A., and Foulds, J. *Escherichia coli* outer membrane protein K is a porin. *J. Bacteriol.*, **156**, 867–72 (1983).
33. Sutherland, I. W. The exopolysaccharides of *Klebsiella* serotype 2 strains as substrates for phage-induced polysaccharide depolymerases. *J. Gen. Microbiol.*, **70**, 331–8 (1971).
34. Sutherland, I. W., and Norval, M. The synthesis of exopolysaccharide by *Klebsiella aerogenes* membrane preparations and the involvement of lipid intermediates. *Biochem. J.*, **120**, 567–76 (1970).
35. Tait, M. I., Sutherland, I. W., and Clarke-Sturmen, A. J. Effect of growth conditions on the production, composition and viscosity of *anthomonas campestris* exopolysaccharide. *J. Gen. Microbiol.*, **132**, 1483–92 (1986).
36. Trisler, P., and Gottesman, S. Lon transcriptional regulation of genes necessary for capsular polysaccharide synthesis in *Escherichia coli* K-K. *J. Bacteriol.*, **160**, 184–91 (1984).
37. Troy, F. A., Frerman, F. E., and Heath, E. C. The biosynthesis of capsular polysaccharide in *Aerobacter aerogenes. J. Biol. Chem.*, **246**, 118–33 (1971).
38. Valla, S., Coucheron, D. H., and Kjosbakken, J. A new extracellular polysaccharide from *Acetobacter xylinum. Arch. Microbiol.*, **134**, 9–11 (1983).
39. Wernau, W. C. UK Patent 2008 600A (1979).
40. Whitfield, C., Hancock, R. E. W., and Costerton, J. W. Outer membrane protein

K of *Escherichia coli*: purification and pore-forming properties in lipid bilayer membranes. *J. Bacteriol.*, **156**, 873–9 (1983).
41. Zehnbauer, B. A. and Markovitz, A. Cloning of gene lon (cap R) of *Escherichia coli* K-12 and identification of polypeptides specified by the cloned deoxyribonucleic acid fragment. *J. Bacteriol.*, **143**, 852–63 (1980).

DISCUSSION – Chaired by Professor E. A. Kabat

KABAT: I would like to point that we have had some monoclonal antibodies to *Klebsiella* K30 and *Klebsiella* 21 polysaccharides, which are specific for the 3,4- or 4,6-pyruvylated galactoses and that these monoclonals will also be quite useful. An anti-idiotype to a monoclonal anti-lupus, made in Bob Schwartz's laboratory, reacts with these anti-*Klebsiella* human monoclonals and the reaction is inhibited by *Klebsiella* polysaccharide.

ROBBINS: There are some instances among capsular polysaccharides of bacteria that caused disease in which acetyl does have some effect on the immunogenicity. The first was shown in the early 1930s with the degree of acetylation of pneumococcus type 1, another example is meningococcus Group C. Of the isolates, 90% have the variant that is *o*-acetyl positive (i.e. the material that is used as the vaccine) and 10% are not *o*-acetylated. In experiments in children and adults, the variant that appeared the least frequently (not *o*-acetylated) seems to have a slightly better immunogenicity than the one that caused disease more frequently (*o*-acetyl positive). Unfortunately, this difference disappeared when the *o*-acetyl variant vaccines were tried on infants. I wonder if that degree of acetylation could reflect a selective pressure on allowing the variant that was least immunogenic to cause more disease.

Just one other thing, Dr Sutherland, do you have any idea of how the bacterium determines the chain length of the capsule? What does it do to shut it off and excrete it?

SUTHERLAND: Yes, we have been actually quite interested in this aspect, how does the bacterium first of all control excretion and, secondly, the stage at which it controls chain length.

Basically, the control is, as far as we can tell, a very rigid one. In other words, under any given set of physiological conditions, the chain length appears to be pretty tight. The size of the molecules is not very variable. On the other hand, we can change that by two techniques. First of all we can alter the physiological conditions and, for example, we can get a much shorter chain. Alternatively, we can select mutants which have lost the ability to shut off at the earlier chain length and produce a much larger chain. We can show this in sequence, i.e. we can take one lot of mutants, we can then mutate them again, get a double mutant, which makes an even longer chain, and so on. We have never been able to get it the other way around. There we have problems because, although we have a very nice selective procedure for getting the increase in length, we do not have good selective procedures for getting the decreased chain length. It does seem to be built into the biosynthetic mechanism, but we still do not know how it operates.

KABAT: I would also like to mention in connection with Dr Robbins's statement that, with our monoclonal human anti-meningococcus Group B, the acetylated compounds are less reactive than the unacetylated.

MORENO: With reference to chain length of the polysaccharides, we have established that the requirements for molecular weight of polysaccharides, for instance meningococcal saccharides, have nothing to do with the actual chain length of the molecule itself. Being molecules that have lipids at the reducing end, the results of gel filtration usually indicate apparent molecular weights above a million, where the chain length is only 60–70 residues long. That difference is important because the aggregate is immunogenic.

SUTHERLAND: Yes, this is true where you have the possibility of aggregation, and I think one should remember that there are various ways in which this can be achieved, not just with lipids. One can also achieve it with some polymers in the presence of multivalent cations. For example, we can see almost cross-linking effects with aluminium or with chromium, but the polysaccharides that I was specifically referring to in answer to Dr Robbins's query are polysaccharides totally free of lipid or of protein, where we do know that they are a true measure of molecular weight.

KABAT: Actually, the use of glycolipids in inhibition reactions can give spurious results due to aggregation, with the fatty acid material giving micelles compared to what you would get with the same oligosaccharides without the fatty acid.

ADA: You said that the control of oligosaccharide can be plasmid controlled. If so, can you transfect another cell type with that plasmid and what is produced when you do this? Do you get production of the unique oligosaccharide?

SUTHERLAND: This is not work that we have done, but people have been working in this field. The control mechanisms can in fact be transfected from one species, for example from *Klebsiella* into *E. coli*. The product in this particular example that I know of was actually the *E. coli* product. In other words, the *E. coli* product was repressed in the mutant; it was derepressed in the transfected mutants. I am not aware of anything equivalent to the binary capsulation story in pneumococcus occurring in gram negatives yet. I think it may be possible that it may yet be developed, but I do not think anyone has looked at that particular type of system.

Part II: Carbohydrates as Antigens

Towards Better Carbohydrate Vaccines
Edited by R. Bell and G. Torrigiani

Published by John Wiley & Sons Ltd

7

Carbohydrates as antigens and immunogens: size, shape and nature of carbohydrate epitopes and idiotopes polysaccharide vaccines

ELVIN A. KABAT
Department of Microbiology, Genetics and Development and Neurology, Columbia University, New York, NY 10032 and the National Institute of Allergy and Infectious Diseases Bethesda, MD 20892, USA

The history of immunization with bacterial polysaccharides begins with the observations of Schiemann and Casper [89] and of Francis and Tillett [27] that the capsular polysaccharides of the pneumococcus would induce an immune response in mice and in humans respectively. These findings led to intensive efforts to study their efficacy in the 1930s to 1950s, culminating in the demonstration by MacLeod *et al.* [69] in a large-scale field trial that immunization with purified pneumococcal capsular polysaccharides offered substantial protection against pneumococcal infection of the four types used, as compared with two control types. Other efforts to use various bacterial polysaccharides as vaccines [4] were also being carried out. During the Second World War, my laboratory was involved in trying to immunize medical student volunteers with the type I (now Group A) meningococcal polysaccharide [55, 56]. By quantitative precipitin assays using 4.0 ml of serum per test (as employed by Michael Heidelberger) to assay the immune response to pneumococcal polysaccharides, we found 4 of 38 individuals who developed significant and sustained responses of 9–18 μg Ab/ml to the three

Group A preparations of polysaccharide made in the laboratory. The antibodies were found to be protective in Dr Philip Miller's laboratory at the University of Chicago, USA [55]. Addition of antigen to these sera removed the protective power. At the time, more sensitive methods of measuring the antibody response were not available and these findings were not considered sufficiently promising. DeVoe [19] has misinterpreted our findings as indicating that the study 'failed, probably, because of the small molecular weight of their preparations (<50 000 daltons) which failed to stimulate antibody'. Subsequent investigations have employed radioimmunoassay which was hundreds of times more sensitive. Employing such a technique, we would most probably have detected antibodies in many of the other individuals who had received the Group A polysaccharide.

Subsequent studies [32], which took care to avoid depolymerization of the meningococcal polysaccharides in preparing the vaccine and utilized the more sensitive radioimmunoassays, established the effectiveness of immunization in humans with Groups A and C meningococcal polysaccharides. The successes with pneumococcal and with Groups A and C meningococcal vaccines led to extensive efforts to develop vaccines using other polysaccharides including *Haemophilus influenzae* types, Group B beta haemolytic streptococci, *Klebsiella pneumoniae*, *Escherichia coli* K antigens, etc. Of these, *H. influenzae* type b is the only licensed vaccine (for references see Austrian [4]).

Despite these successes, difficulties and problems were recognized which necessitated extensive study. Certain capsular polysaccharides, most notably those of the Group B meningococcus and of *E. coli* K1, did not induce a sufficient immune response. Moreover, the effectiveness of different polysaccharides in young children was much poorer and the age at which satisfactory immune responses occurred varied from 3 months with the type 3 pneumococcus and with Group A meningococcus, which requires a second injection 3 months later, to 18 months for *H. influenzae* type b and to over 4 years for type 6 pneumococcal polysaccharide (see Austrian [4] for references).

The meningococcal Group B and *E. coli* K1 polysaccharides, both of identical structure and composed of poly-$\alpha(2 \rightarrow 8)$ *N*-acetylneuraminic acid (NeuNAc) [22, 61], have been found to be poor antigens even in adults, and a satisfactory polysaccharide vaccine is not available. Thus it was surprising when, in the course of screening individuals having elevated serum immunoglobulins with our collection of specific polysaccharides, to discover [57] a person with a benign monoclonal gammopathy with 23 mg/ml of IgM anti-poly-$\alpha(2 \rightarrow 8)$NeuNAc (IgM^{NOV}). On a weight basis, the protective power of IgM^{NOV} in infant rats against infection with *E. coli* K1 was similar to that of a horse anti-Group B meningococcal serum.

This unique finding offers promise, if cell lines producing antibody can be obtained from this individual [57], of the use of these antibodies as an adjunct to antibiotic therapy of Group B meningococcal meningitis and of *E. coli* K1 sepsis. The mortality and morbidity from these diseases, despite the best available therapy, is considerable, and in a significant proportion of the cases of Group B meningococcal meningitis, the patient becomes deaf. Other neurological difficulties also occur. Treatment of meningococcal meningitis in the first four decades of this century by intraspinal administration of polyvalent horse anti-meningococcal serum, using doses of 20 ml or more several times a day for 4 days, was considered to be effective in reducing mortality, despite the absence of knowledge of meningococcal groups and of methods of standardization of the antisera [7, 31]. We have obtained IgM^{NOV} serum by plasmapheresis to conduct initial studies to determine its value in a clinical trial in which alternate cases are treated with the antiserum, all patients being given the standard antibiotic therapy.

The question naturally arises as to how this extraordinary response was generated, in view of the generally unsatisfactory immune responses to the Group B meningococcal and *E. coli* K1 capsular polysaccharides [72, 108]. As far as it is known, Mr Nov did not have Group B meningococcal meningitis or *E. coli* K1 sepsis. A possible origin [16, 87] of these antibodies is a response to non-symptomatic carriage of these organisms at some point in Mr Nov's life, followed by expansion of a single clone by stimulation of a memory cell.

These inferences are largely those of classical immunology. However, in the last 4 or 5 years, extensive studies have been carried out on anti-idiotypic and anti-anti-idiotypic responses to various antigens including polysaccharide antigens. These provide a mechanism for the production of antibodies specifically reacting with a given antigen in animals which have never been deliberately stimulated with the antigen. The role of prior contact with the antigen or with some structurally related cross-reacting antigen can, of course, not be evaluated.

I shall attempt, therefore, to summarize our current knowledge of the sizes, shapes and structures of antibody combining sites to polysaccharide antigens with a view to localizing idiotypic determinants in relation to the complementarity-determining regions (CDRs) [49, 59, 107], i.e. those portions of the variable regions of the light and heavy chains which make contact with the antigenic determinant (epitope).

Dextran [38, 94] has served as a model antigen [52, 53, 71] for these studies, since it is a high-molecular-weight polymer composed of a single sugar (glucose) with predominantly $\alpha(1 \rightarrow 6)$linkages which may have many structures depending upon the proportions of $\alpha(1 \rightarrow 2)$, $\alpha(1 \rightarrow 3)$ and $\alpha(1 \rightarrow 4)$linkages and their distribution in relation to the $\alpha(1 \rightarrow 6)$linkages [38]. The most important findings about antigenic determinants and antibody-combining sites have been made with dextran of the B512 strain of *Leuconostoc mesenteroides* with 96% of $\alpha(1 \rightarrow 6)$ and 4% of $\alpha(1 \rightarrow 3)$linkages which serve as branch points. Most of the $\alpha(1 \rightarrow 3)$ branches are one or two sugars long [67] and a small proportion join longer branches of α(1 → 6)-linked glucoses [15].

Although dextran had been known to cross-react with types 2, 12 and 20 antipneumococcal horse serum [33, 74, 99], it became of major immunological interest during the Korean War when it was found that a highly branched dextran, used as a plasma expander for the treatment of shock, produced a high frequency (*circa* 50%) of severe allergic reactions in humans [58], whereas the B512 strain produced far fewer allergic reactions. Antibodies precipitating with dextran occur in many normal individuals, the antibody probably being formed to dextran-producing micro-organisms in the gastrointestinal tract, to dextran in commercial sucrose or with cross-reacting antigens of other micro-organisms. Native B512 dextran, as well as other native dextrans, were found to induce precipitating antibody and wheal and erythema-type skin sensitivity on injection into humans [52, 53, 71].

In a field trial with US Air Force volunteers [58], it was established that the incidence of allergic reactions to infusion correlated with pre-existing skin sensitivity of the wheal and erythema type to dextran, and with pre-existing precipitating antibody to dextran, that the incidence of such pre-existing skin sensitivity was higher to the more highly branched dextrans and that the lowest incidence of these skin reactions was to the B512 dextran.

Assays of the antigenicity of B512 dextran fractions of graded molecular weight prepared by controlled acid hydrolysis showed that fractions with average molecular weights of 51,300 or below had a substantially reduced capacity to elicit formation of antidextran [54]. Moreover, skin reactions to intracutaneous injection of 10–20 μg of the dextran fractions required a level of circulating precipitins of about 7 μg AbN/ml or more, whereas native B512 dextran elicited skin reactions in individuals with circulating precipitin levels as low as 3 μg AbN/ml.

The finding of precipitin reactions to dextran [52, 53], and the isolation and purification of the isomaltose series α(1 → 6)-linked oligosaccharides [39, 102] from isomaltose (IM2) to isomaltohexaose (IM6) and isomaltoheptaose (IM7), provided a system which could serve as a molecular ruler for probing the sizes [45–47] and later the shapes [13, 14, 64, 75, 92] of antidextran combining sites. The principle used was essentially based on the findings of Landsteiner [66] with azoproteins and their antibodies, that a low-molecular-weight hapten representing a portion of an antigenic determinant would enter the combining site and inhibit the antigen–antibody reaction. Measurements of the amount of precipitate in the presence of the inhibitor, as compared with the quantity of antigen–antibody precipitate in the absence of inhibitor, were made by a micro modification of the quantitative precipitin methods of the Heidelberger school [36]. In recent years, radioimmunoassay and ELISA have come into widespread use because of their high sensitivity.

Results are generally plotted in terms of per cent inhibition *versus* micro- or nanomoles of inhibitor added.

With the sera of humans immunized with dextran, it could be shown that, as the oligosaccharide length from the di- to the hexa- and heptasaccharide increased, the degree of inhibition increased, but the incremental increase became less and generally reached an upper limit with oligosaccharides composed of six or seven glucoses [45–47]. This limit was taken to be the size or extent of the complementary area of the antibody-combining site [14, 46, 47]. The lower limit in size of an antibody-combining site was found to be between one and two glucose units [3]. These values have generally held for antibody-combining sites, not only to polysaccharides but to all types of antigenic determinants [48].

A practical consequence of the inhibition studies was the development by Richter and Hedin [81] of a 150 mg/ml oligosaccharide solution (Promit, Pharmacia) which, when administered prior to the B512 dextran to be infused or added to the dextran before administration, caused substantially reduced anaphylactic reactions.

With monoclonal mouse myeloma and later with hybridoma anti-α(1 → 6)dextrans, antibody-combining sites were found to be complementary to four, five, six or seven α(1 → 6)-linked glucoses [13, 14, 64, 75, 92, 93]. However, using synthetic glycolipid antigens prepared by coupling the various oligosaccharides to stearylamine [105, 106], it was found that the combining sites of nine hybridoma mouse antibodies to stearylisomaltotetraose, composed of three intact glucose rings plus an open chain linked to the stearyl moiety, were in all instances complementary to six and seven glucoses [64]. Only one hybridoma, from a mouse immunized with stearylisomaltopentaose with four intact glucose rings plus an open chain linked to the stearyl group, had a combining site of a size compatible with that of the immunizing antigen, namely to four glucoses [64]. These findings indicate that the stearyl-isomaltosyl oligosaccharide had induced proliferation of pre-existing clones with sites complementary to oligosaccharides larger than those present in the immunizing antigen. This strongly resembles the concept of 'original antigenic sin' put forward by Davenport *et al.* [17] and by Fazekas de St Groth [25]. It may well provide a serious limitation to our ability to obtain hybridoma antibodies of a desired specificity.

It should also be emphasized that these studies on monoclonal anti-α(1 → 6)dextrans have been carried out with T-independent antigens [65]. Stein *et al.* [98] have immunized mice with T-dependent antigens, IM6 and IM3 coupled to KLH; IM3–BSA and IM6–BSA had previously been used in rabbits to study the immune response with respect to the cross-reactivity of the antibodies with α(1 → 6)dextran [3]. The IM3–KLH and IM6–KLH induced anti-α(1 → 6)dextran in CBA, but only the IM6–KLH induced anti-α(1 → 6)dextran in C75/BL6 mice. CBA antidextrans cross-reacted with

IM3 and IM6 coupled to BSA, but C57BL antibodies bound IM3–BSA very poorly. Study of hybridomas of anti-α(1 → 6)specificity produced to these T-dependent antigens should substantially augment our information about the repertoire and perhaps further elucidate the role of somatic mutation in T-dependent *versus* T-independent antigens.

The chemical synthesis of long, strictly linear chains [85] of 200 or more α(1 → 6)-linked glucoses permitted further analysis of antibody–combining sites of anti-α(1 → 6)dextrans. With two mouse monoclonal myeloma antidextrans W3129 and W3434, it was found that the synthetic linear dextran inhibited on a molar basis as if five glucoses from the terminal non-reducing end saturated the combining site [14]. It was thus complementary to the non-reducing end of the sugar chain; competitive equilibrium dialysis using the IM2 oligosaccharides had indicated that most of the binding energy of these sites was specific for methyl α-glucoside or IM2 which had over 50% of the total binding energy of the saturating isomaltopentaose. These findings indicated that the combining sites of W3129 and W3434 were directed towards the non-reducing ends of chains and that the non-reducing terminal one or two sugars made more contacts with the antibody-combining sites, perhaps as if they were held in a tridimensional cavity, and we have loosely termed these cavity-type sites.

A third monoclonal mouse myeloma protein and 38 mouse hybridomas [13, 14, 64, 75, 92, 93] showed an entirely different behaviour with synthetic linear dextran. Rather than being specific for the terminal non-reducing ends of the linear dextrans, D3 and LD7 [83], these proteins actually precipitated with the linear dextran [14], whereas with myelomas W3129 and W3434 the linear dextrans were monovalent and inhibited dextran–antidextran precipitation. With the others, the linear dextran was multivalent and multiple segments of six or seven glucose units were reacting with the combining sites. This was consistent with earlier findings by equilibrium dialysis that methyl α-glucoside and IM2 only contributed less than 5% of the total binding energy [14]. Such findings would suggest a groove-type site, perhaps resembling the lysozyme site [78], except that antibody-combining sites are formed by two chains.

It is of interest that the rabbit responded to the isomaltosyl glycolipids by synthesis of sites predominantly specific for terminal non-reducing ends of chains [105, 106], e.g. cavity-type sites; these were not monoclonal responses. Thus the differences between the antibodies produced by the rabbit and the hybridoma antibodies produced by the mouse to the isomaltosyl glycolipids re-emphasized the problems of elucidating the repertoire of antibody-combining sites.

These two kinds of sites had been established for myelomas W3129 and QUPC52 by equilibrium dialysis [14], and by fluorescence quenching [6, 14]. Studies in the myeloma anti-β(1 → 6)galactan system with myeloma protein

J539 have also shown the presence of a groove-type site complementary to four β(1 → 6)-linked galactoses [6].

The antibody-combining site to the type 3 capsular polysaccharide of the pneumococcus has also been shown [70] to be complementary to six sugars consisting of alternating glucuronic acid and glucose. These results are consistent with model-building studies [18] in which a myeloma protein McPC603 with a cavity-type site which bound phosphorylcholine was converted to a groove-type site specific for the type 3 pneumococcal polysaccharide by replacing the CDRs of McPC603 with those of a type 3 rabbit antipneumococcal antibody.

A recent high-resolution x-ray crystallographic study [2] of a crystalline complex of lysozyme with a monoclonal antilysozyme shows that contacts between lysozyme and antibody occur on a rather flat surface with the interactions largely due to protuberances and depressions formed by the amino-acid side-chains, producing a tightly packed region of interaction. The lysozyme determinant involves two non-contiguous stretches, residues 18–27 and 116–119 of its polypeptide chain. All six CDRs of the antibody and two residues outside the CDRs but adjacent to the CDRs, Tyr 49 in V_L and Thr 30 in V_H, make contact with the lysozyme. Ten of the seventeen contacting residues are in V_H. Four of the ten contacting V_H residues and three of the seven contacting residues in V_L are in the corresponding CDR3s. These findings – if and to the extent applicable to anti-carbohydrate sites with respect to interactions of side chains on essentially flat surface – could have substantial implications for our understanding of these antigen–antibody and idiotype–anti-idiotype interactions. However, the J539 site would appear to be some type of groove complementary to a tetrasaccharide [30]. Unfortunately, so far the crystal form has not allowed the ligand to enter the site [100].

It will be extremely important to obtain crystals suitable for high-resolution x-ray studies to establish the differences between those antibodies specific for terminal ends of chains and those reacting with the linear internal portions of carbohydrate chains.

Cloning and sequencing cDNA of hybridoma anti-α(1 → 6)dextrans

We have cloned and sequenced cDNA from about fourteen of our anti-α(1 → 6)dextran hybridomas, so that we may correlate our immunochemical site-mapping data on the sizes, shapes, binding constants and idiotypic specificities of the sites with amino acid sequences [1, 95]. An important finding, using two T-independent antigens, α(1 → 6)dextran itself [39] and the IM2 oligosaccharides coupled to stearylamine [64], is that the repertoire of antibody-combining sites formed by each antigen differs sharply, even though their specificities are very similar. This clearly emphasizes the necessity of evaluating the repertoire with as many parameters and conditions as possible and from different species.

Also very unusual is the finding that the antibodies are almost entirely of IgM and IgA [64, 75, 91], only one IgG_3* [13] hybridoma having been found. These results which are unlike those with other polysaccharides, in which the response is mostly IgG. Indeed in the anti-2-phenyloxazolone system, which uses the same germ-line V_k gene, almost all of the reported antibodies are IgG; only a single IgM has been found [5, 34, 43, 44].

Even with the limited sampling of the potential repertoire, the very unusual finding is that the set of anti-$\alpha(1 \rightarrow 6)$dextrans having similar sizes and shapes and with only relatively small differences in Ka relative to the wide ranges found in other antigen–antibody systems, use several very different germ-line genes in both V_k and V_H. The nineteen V_k genes with groove-type combining sites complementary to six and seven $\alpha(1 \rightarrow 6)$-linked glucoses employ at least three different major families [1, 79]. One of these is the V Ox–1 gene for antibodies to 2-phenyloxazolone which was used in both BALB/c and C57BL/6 mice immunized with dextran. Another in C57BL/6 belongs to a very different germ-line family of five members from one fusion, all having six additional amino acids in CDR1, 27 A, B, C, D, E and 28 and extensive framework differences throughout the V-region. One C57BL/6 hybridoma, 10.11.3.9.2.3, belongs to a third germ-line family; it lacks the six additional residues in CDR3 and has extensive framework and CDR differences from V_k Ox–1 and has an additional residue in CDR3 ascribable to V_k–J_k joining. One C57BL hybridoma, 58.2C.10.3 anti-$\alpha(1 \rightarrow 6)$dextran, with a smaller size site complementary to four $\alpha(1 \rightarrow 6)$-linked glucoses [64] has six amino-acid substitutions, one in CDR1, three in CDR3 before the V_k–J_k junction, and one each in FR2 and FR3; one of the three in CDR3 involves a two-base change. Thus it might be a member of a germ-line subfamily of V_k Ox–1 or possibly may be a consequence of somatic mutation. The fourteen chains use three J_k minigenes, J1, J2 and J5; J2 is used most often.

The findings with 10α and 6μ V_H chains are essentially similar, the chains belonging to three of the major germ-line families reported by Dildrop [21] and by Brodeur and Riblet [10], J558, J606 and 36–60. The J558 germ-line family includes six BALB/c and two C57BL/6 mice immunized with $\alpha(1 \rightarrow 6)$dextran; they fall into two subfamilies, one containing five BALB/c and one C57BL/6, and the second containing one BALB/c and one C57BL. The J606 family is represented by a hybridoma from a C57BL/6 mouse immunized with stearylisomaltopentaose; and of the two members of the 36–60 family,

* A second IgG_3 has recently been obtained.

one, 37.1.1, was from a BALB/c mouse immunized with dextran and the other, 42.7C.11.2, from a C57BL/6 immunized with stearylisomaltotetraose.

Members of the J558 germ-line family have residues 100A and 100B which are lacking in the J606 family and the two members of the 36–60 family not only lack these residues, but one, 37.1.1, has a deletion of residue 100 and in the other, 42.7C.11.2, residues 97, 98 and 99 are also deleted. There are extensive framework as well as CDR differences between the two J558 subfamilies. The two members of the 36–60 also differ extensively and the J606 family is also very unlike others in nucleotide and amino acid identities [1]. Thus, as with the V_k chains, these very similar sites can be formed by the very different sequences of three germ-line families.

Among the six members of one of the J558 subfamilies, amino-acid substitutions are relatively sparse, there being two in FR1, one in CDR1, none in FR2, five in CDR2, five in FR3 and three in CDR3; all six chains use J3.

Among the 42. series of six hybridomas from a single fusion, all use J2 and there is but one amino-acid difference in CDR1 and one each in FR2 and FR3. CDR3 is extremely short, consisting of only four amino acids.

These findings that sets of similar sites can be formed by very different families of V_k, V_H and by different J and D minigenes have important implications. Thus, the question arises as to whether additional germ-line V_L and V_H families and subfamilies might not also be found using different conditions of inducing the antibody response, of selecting the hybridomas etc. Indeed, they seriously pose the problem that the repertoire of combining sites, even to a single antigenic determinant such as the chain of six or seven $\alpha(1 \rightarrow 6)$-linked glucoses, may never be fully elucidated. It is important to emphasize that these findings could not have been made without the extensive immunochemical mapping which was provided for the $\alpha(1 \rightarrow 6)$dextran–anti-dextran system.

Since there are now several instances in which idiotypic or even antibody specificity may be altered or abolished by single amino acid substitutions [11, 20, 42], it will obviously be necessary to do chain recombinations between V_L and V_H chains of the hybridomas with one another and with members of other germ-line families and with the anti-2-phenyloxazolone V_k chains to delineate further the structural basis of antibody complementarity.

Multi- or polyspecificity

Most immunological reactions studied since the beginnings of immunology have tended to show a high degree of specificity and, as chemical structures of various polysaccharides, proteins, nucleotides, etc., were elucidated, these could be correlated with immunological similarities or three-dimensional resemblances in structure. The concept of cross-reactions being due to such chemical or structural identities or resemblances among antigenic determinants has been deeply ingrained in the literature.

However, in the last 15 years a series of observations has been accumulating which suggests that many of these involved unusual cross-reactions. Some of these are still controversial [50, 80], but it is important for the present discussion in consider a number of instances in which the unusual specificities involved cross-reactions between charged groups, notably those containing phosphate, sulphate and carboxyl groups.

Among the earliest observations of multispecificity were those of Cameron and Erlanger [12], who found that three anti-AMP globulin fractions separated by isoelectric focusing behaved differently, relative to AMP, with respect to binding structurally unrelated ligands. Kahana and Erlanger [60], using poly(A) coupled to bovine serum albumin as an antigen, found cross-reactions with various polynucleotides and with polyribose phosphate, a major component of the capsule of *H. influenzae* type b.

Subsequently, Heidelberger [37] showed an unusual cross-reaction between type 8 and 19 pneumococcal polysaccharides and their antisera, which he interpreted as indicating that the cross-reactivity was ascribable to the negatively charged phosphoryl-βDManNAc of type 19 being able to enter the type 8 site specific for cellobiuronic acid with its COO^- and *vice versa*. One of our IgM anti-*Klebsiella* K monoclonals specific for K30 polysaccharide reacted with poly(G), another with poly(G), poly(I) and single-stranded DNA. The reaction with polynucleotides was specifically inhibited by K30 polysaccharide [7]. A monoclonal lupus anti-DNA 16/6 reacted weakly with K30 and K21. Four of six monoclonals specific for 3,4-pyruvylated-D-galactose shared an idiotypic determinant with the 16/6 anti-DNA, and this idiotype-anti-idiotype reaction was also inhibitable by *Klebsiella* polysaccharide [73]. Cross reactions have also been noted between DNA and phospholipids and ascribed to phosphodiester groups with a given spacing [63]. High-resolution X-ray crystallographic studies of phosphorylcholine binding myeloma protein McPC603 in 42% ammonium sulphate have shown that a sulphate ion at the bottom of the combining site displaces the phosphate of phosphorylcholine from the site [77].

The concept of multispecificity involving sites specifically reacting with different charged groups derives much support from the findings with IgM^{NOV} [57]. IgM^{NOV} does not react with poly-α(2 → 9)NeuNAc or with a polysaccharide composed of alternating poly-α(2 → 8)α(2 → 9)NeuNAc, thereby showing substantial specificity almost certainly for an oligomer of α(2 → 8)NeuNAc; nevertheless, per unit weight it, reacts just as well with poly(A) and poly(I) as with poly-α(2 → 8)NeuNAc; denatured DNA and poly(G) cross-react to a somewhat lesser degree. These data are most readily interpretable on the basis of a similarity in oligomeric patterns of poly-α(2 → 8)NeuNAc, poly(A) and poly(I), permitting the phosphate ions of DNA and the ionized carboxyls of poly-α(2 → 8)NeuNAc to be recognized by the IgM^{NOV} combining site. We shall attempt modelling studies of poly-α(2 → 8) NeuNAc, poly(A), poly(I), etc., to see whether these findings can be more precisely interpreted in terms of three-dimensional structure. It is of interest that the horse 46, an antimeningococcal Group B antiserum, did not react with poly(A), poly(I), poly(G) or with native or denatured DNA. There is no evidence that the IgM^{NOV} is in any way adversely affecting Mr Nov, who is now 83 years old.

Idiotypic vaccines and three-dimensional structure of antibody-combining sites

The concept is based on the Jerne network theory [40] that anti-idiotypic antibody (Ab2) formed on immunization with antibody (Ab1) to a given antigen may in some instances show properties of original antigenic determinants (Ab2β) [41] and that immunization with such Ab2 may elicit the formation of antibodies (Ab3) which will react with the original antigen as does Ab1 [103].

Since the pioneering study of Sege and Peterson [90], there have been a growing number of such studies [23, 24, 83], especially with hormones, showing that some Ab2 can compete with hormone for interaction with the receptor for the hormone, thus having an antigenic determinant resembling the hormone, often termed 'idiotypic mimicry'. The power of the method is greatly enhanced when hybridomas are used. The potential importance of such studies for immunization against infectious agents [76, 82] is that they open the possibility of inducing immunity in an animal which has not deliberately been given the antigen. A number of such studies have now been carried out [62, 86, 101, 104], indicating that the method is quite promising.

As applied to potential vaccines and to bacterial polysaccharides, a variety of interesting questions develop of both a regulatory and a structural nature. Thus, many bacterial polysaccharide antigens to which individuals are naturally exposed have already induced low levels of antibody and perhaps auto-anti-idiotype (Ab2) [29, 86]. Immunization with Ab1 either deliberately, generally with a foreign species of antibody, or by an autoimmune response or by antigen, dextran [26] or levan [9], could induce anti-idiotype (Ab2). A further formulation of successive stages is that of Urbain *et al.* [103]. Immunization with Ab2 induces anti-anti-idiotype (Ab3) which may be of several types: Ab3α, which recognizes idiotopes of Ab2; Ab3β, antibodies which do not bind antigen but have idiotopes similar to those of Ab1 – Jerne [40] has termed this the 'parallel set'; Ab3γ antibodies share idiotopes of

Ab1 and also bind antigen – animals containing Ab3γ produce large amounts of Ab1′, many of which share cross-reacting idiotypic determinants with Ab1; Ab4, anti-anti-anti-idiotypic antibodies obtained by immunization with Ab3. Many Ab4 antibodies react with Ab1 and Ab1′.

That some Ab2 react with Ab1 and thus possess properties of the original antigen is widely spoken of as 'internal image' antibodies [41] also called 'related epitopes' [35] and homobodies [68]. What requires further analysis is what such an 'antigenic determinant' would look like in relation to the original antigenic determinant [96]. This may not be a problem when the original antigenic determinant is a protein, since there could be similar cross-reacting or identical structures making up the determinants in the two instances. However, there is much to be learned as to how an immunoglobulin possessing an 'internal image' antigenic determinant which is a polysaccharide, or a steroid, etc., can look like the antigen [96]. Some of these interactions might be explainable by multispecificity if various charged groups are present in both. It seems to be more difficult to visualize such 'internal image antigenic determinants' in the case of a linear chain of $\alpha(1 \rightarrow 6)$-linked glucoses as in dextran. The crystallographic and immunochemical site-mapping studies on the anti-$\alpha(1 \rightarrow 6)$ galactan, J539, suggest the antigenic determinant to be as large as a tetrasaccharide fitting into a groove-type combining site [30, 100].

Regulatory aspects related to immunization to bacterial polysaccharides are based on findings [84] that the idiotype of ABPC48, a myeloma antilevan, or anti-idiotype can prime for an antibody response to bacterial levan administered subsequently. Moreover, data have been obtained that the idiotype itself may prime new-borns to respond to subsequent injection of antigen and so may overcome the failure of infants to respond to bacterial polysaccharides. This is thought to involve priming of idiotype-specific T-helper cells [84]. Further studies have demonstrated a similar effect of priming with an IgM monoclonal idiotype or anti-idiotype to *E. coli* K13 to protect against *E. coli* K1 infection [97].

It is not always easy to sort out whether a given antibody is an internal image type or a regulatory type (see [8, 28, 76, 82, 88]. Nisonoff and Lamoyi [76] propose that an Ab2β should react with Ab1 that is specific for the same antigenic determinant from different species, that the reaction be inhibitable by antigen and that the Ab2β injected into various species should induce a response similar to that of the original antigenic determinant. These developments offer important new approaches to immunization against infectious diseases caused by bacteria with polysaccharide capsules which determine virulence. For studies on the location of idiotopes with amino acid sequence and correlations see reference [51].

ACKNOWLEDGEMENTS

This research was supported by grants from the National Science Foundation (PCM 81-02321) and the National Institute of Allergy and infectious Diseases (1R01AI-19042) to E.A.K.; by a programme project grant to Elliott F. Osserman (CA-21112) and by a Cancer Center Grant to Columbia University.

The author thanks Drs B. F. Erlanger, Rose G. Mage, J. B. Robbins, R. Schneerson and K. E. Stein for helpful suggestions and Mr Darryl J. Guinyard for typing the manuscript.

REFERENCES

1. Akolkar, P. N., Sikder, S. K., Bhattacharya, S. B., Liao, J., Gruezo, F., Morrison, S. L., and Kabat, E. A. BALB/c and C57BL/6 hybridoma antibodies to $\alpha(1 \rightarrow 6)$dextrans use different V_L and V_H germline genes to produce similar combining sites (*J. Immunol.* in press).
2. Amit, A. G., Mariuzza, R. A., Phillips, S. E. V., and Poljak, R. J. Three-dimensional structure of an antigen–antibody complex at 28 A resolution. *Science*, **233**, 747–53 (1986).
3. Arakatsu, Y., Ashwell, G., and Kabat, E. A. Immunochemical studies on dextrans. V. Specificity and cross-reactivity with dextrans of the antibodies formed in rabbits to isomaltonic and isomaltotrionic acids coupled to bovine serum albumin. *J. Immunol.*, **97**, 858–866 (1966).
4. Austrian, R. Polysaccharide vaccines. *Ann. Inst. Pasteur/Microbiol.*, **1368**, 295–307 (1985).
5. Berek, C., Griffiths, G. M., and Milstein, C. Molecular events during maturation of the immune response to oxazolone. *Nature*, **316**, 412–18 (1985).
6. Bhattacharjee, A. K., Das, M. K., Roy, A., and Glaudemans, C. P. J. The binding sites of the two monoclonal immunoglobulin as J539 and W3129. Thermodynamic mapping of a groove- and a cavity-type immunoglobulin both having antipolysaccharide specificity. *Mol. Immunol.*, **18**, 277–80 (1981).
7. Blackfan, K. D. The treatment of meningococcus meningitis. *Medicine*, **1**, 140–212 (1922).
8. Bona, C. A., and Pernis, B. Idiotypic networks. In *Fundamental Immunology* (ed. W. E. Paul), Raven Press, New York, 1986, pp. 577–92.
9. Bona, C., Lieberman, R., Chien, C. C., Mond, J., House, S., Green, I., and Paul, W. E. Immune response to levan. I. Kinetics and ontogeny of anti-levan and anti-inulin antibody response and of expression of cross-reactive idiotype. *J. Immunol.*, **120**, 1436–42 (1978).
10. Brodeur, P. H., and Riblet, R. The immunoglobulin heavy chain variable region (Igh-V) locus in the mouse. I. One hundred Igh-V genes comprise seven families of homologous genes. *Eur. J. Immunol.*, **14**, 922–30 (1984).
11. Bruggemann, M., Muller, H.-J., Burger, C., and Rajewsky, K. Idiotypic selection of an antibody mutant with changed hapten binding specificity resulting from a point mutation in position 50 of the heavy chain. *EMBO. J.*, **5**, 1561–6 (1986).

12. Cameron, D. J., and Erlanger, B. F. Evidence for multispecificity of antibody molecules. *Nature*, **286**, 763–5 (1977).
13. Chen, H.-T., Makover, S. D., and Kabat, E. A. Immunochemical studies on monoclonal antibodies to stearylisomaltotetraose from C58/J and a C57BL/10 nude mouse. *Molec. Immunol.* **24**, 333–8.
14. Cisar, J., Kabat, E. A., Dorner, M. M., and Liao, J. Binding properties of immunoglobulin combining sites specific for terminal or nonterminal antigenic determinants in dextran. *J. Exp. Med.*, **142**, 435–59 (1975).
15. Covacevich, M. T., Richards, G. N. Frequency and distribution of branching in a dextran: an enzymatic method. *Carbohy. Res.*, **54**, 311–15 (1977).
16. Craven, D. E., Frasch, C. E., Mocca, L. F., Rose, F. B., and Gonzalez, R. Rapid serogroup identification of *Neisseria meningitidis* using antiserum agar: prevalence of serotypes in a disease free military population. *J. Clin. Microbiology*, **10**, 302–7 (1979).
17. Davenport, F. M., Hennessy, A. V., Francis, T. Jr Epidemiological and immunologic significance of age distribution of antibody to antigenic variants of influenza virus. *J. Exp. Med.*, **98**, 641–56 (1953).
18. Davies, D. R., and Padlan, E. A. Correlations between antigen binding specificity and the three-dimensional structure of antibody combining site. In *Antibodies in Human Diagnosis and Therapy* (ed. E. Haber and R. M. Krause), Raven Press, New York, 1976, pp. 119–32.
19. DeVoe, I. W. The meningococcus and mechanisms of pathogenicity. *Microbiological Rev.*, **46**, 162–90 (1982).
20. Diamond, B., Scharff, M. D. Somatic mutation of the T15 heavy chain gives rise to an antibody with autoantibody specificity. *Proc. Nat. Acad. Sci. USA*, **81**, 5841–4 (1984).
21. Dildrop, R. New classification of mouse V_H sequences. *Immunol. Today*, **5**, 85–93 (1984).
22. Egan, W. Structure of the capsular polysaccharide antigens from *Haemophilus influenzae* and *Neisseria meningitidis*. by ^{13}C NMR spectroscopy. *Magnetic Resonance in Biol.*, **1**, 197–258 (1980).
23. Erlanger, B. F. Anti-idiotypic antibodies: what do they recognize? *Immunol. Today*, **6**, 10–11 (1985).
24. Erlanger, B. F., Cleveland, W. L., Wassermann, N. H., Hill, B. L., Penn, A. S., Ku, H. H., and Sarangarajan, R. Anti-receptor antibodies by the auto-anti-idiotypic route. In *Investigation and Exploitation of Antibody Combining Sites* (ed. Eric Reid, G. M. W. Cook and D. J. Morre), Plenum, New York, 1985, pp. 91–107.
25. Fazekas de St Groth, S., and Webster, R. G. Disquisitions on original antigenic sin. I. Evidence in Man; II. Proof in lower vertebrates. *J. Exp. Med.*, **124**, 331–45; 347–61 (1966).
26. Fernandez, C., and Moller, G. Primary immune response to dextran B512 followed by a period of antigen-specific immunosuppression caused by autoanti-idiotypic antibodies *Scand. J. Immunol.*, **11**, 53–62 (1980).
27. Francis, T. J. Jr, and Tillett, W. S. Cutaneous reactions in pneumonia. The development of antibodies following the intradermal injection of type-specific polysaccharides. *J. Exp. Med.*, **52**, 573–85 (1930).
28. Gaulton, G. N., and Greene, M. I. Idiotypic mimicry of biological receptors. *Ann. Rev. Immunol.*, **4**, 253–80 (1986).
29. Geha, R. S. Presence of autoantiidiotypic antibody during the normal human immune response to tetanus toxoid antigen. *J. Immunol.*, **129**, 139–44 (1982).

30. Glaudemans, C. P. J., Bhattacharjee, A. K., and Manjula, B. N. Monoclonal anti-galactan IgA J 539 binds intercatenarily to its polysaccharide antigen. Observations on the binding of antibody to a macromolecular antigen. *Molec. Immunol.*, **23**, 655–60 (1986).
31. Gold, R. Prevention of bacterial meningitis by immunological means. In *Bacterial Meningitis* (ed. M. A. Sande, A. L. Smith and R. K. Root), Churchill-Livingstone, London, 1985, pp. 105–22.
32. Gold, R., and Lepow, M. L. Present status of polyvalent vaccines in the prevention of meningococcal diseases. *Advanc. Pediat.*, **23**, 71–93 (1976).
33. Goodman, J. W., Kabat, E. A. Immunochemical studies on cross reactions of antipneumoccocal sera. I. Cross reactions of types II and XX antipneumococcal sera with dextrans and of type II antipneumococcal serum with glycogen and Friedlander type B polysaccharide. *J. Immunol.*, **84**, 333–46 (1960).
34. Griffiths, G. M., Kaartinen, B. M., and Milstein, C. Somatic utation and the maturation of immune response to 2-phenyloxazlone. *Nature*, **312**, 271–5 (1984).
35. Gurish, M. F., Ben-Porat, T., and Nisonoff, A. The use of antiidiotypic antibodies as vaccines. In *Primary Immunodeficiency Diseases* (ed. M. M. Eibl and F. S. Rosen), Elsevier Science Publishers, 1986, pp. 217–27.
36. Heidelberger, M. *Lectures in Immunochemistry*. Academic Press, New York, 1956.
37. Heidelberger, M. Precipitating cross-reactions among pneumococcal types. *Infect. and Immun.*, **41**, 1234–44 (1983).
38. Jeanes, A., Haynes, W. C., Wilham, C. A., Rankin, J. C., Melvin, E. H., Austin, M. J., Cluskey, B. E., Fisher, H. M., Tsuchiya, H. M., and Rist, C. E. Characterization and classification of dextrans from ninety-six strains of bacteria. *J. Am. Chem. Soc.*, **76**, 5041–52 (1954).
39. Jeanes, A., Wilham, C. A., Jones, W., Tsuchiya, H. M., and Rist, C. E. Isomaltose and isomaltotriose from enzymatic hydrolysates of dextran. *J. Am. Chem. Soc.*, **75**, 5911–15 (1953).
40. Jerne, N. K. Towards a network theory of the immune system. *Ann Immunol. (Inst. Pasteur)*, **125**, 373–89 (1974).
41. Jerne, N. K., Roland, J., and Cazenave, P.-A. Recurrent idiotopes and internal images. *EMBO Journal*, **1**, 243–7 (1982).
42. Jeske, D. J., Jarvis, J., Milstein, C., and Capra, J. D. Junctional diversity is essential to antibody activity. *J. Immunol.*, **133**, 1090–2 (1984).
43. Kaartinen, M., Griffiths, G. M., Hamlyn, P. H., Markham, A. F., Karljalainen, K., Pelkonen, J. L. T., Makela, O., and Milstein, C. Anti-oxazolone hybridomas and the structure of the oxazolone idiotype. *J. Immunol.*, **130**, 937–45 (1983).
44. Kaartinen, M., Griffiths, G. M., Markham, A. F., and Milstein, C. mRNA sequences define an unusually restricted IgG response to 2-phenyloxazolone and its early diversification. *Nature*, **304**, 320–4 (1983).
45. Kabat, E. A. Some configurational requirements and dimensions of the combining site on an antibody to a naturally occurring antigen. *J. Am. Chem. Soc.*, **76**, 3709–13 (1954).
46. Kabat, E. A. Heterogeneity in extent of the combining regions of human antidextran. *J. Immunol.*, **77**, 377–85 (1956).
47. Kabat, E. A. Size and heterogeneity of the combining sites on an antibody molecule *J. Cell. Comp. Physiol.*, **50** (Supplement 1), 79–102 (1957).
48. Kabat, E. A. *Structural Concepts in Immunology and Immunochemistry*. Holt, Rinehart and Winston, New York, 1976.
49. Kabat, E. A. The structural basis of antibody specificity. In *27th Mosbacher*

Colloquium (ed. F. Melchers and K. Rajewsky), Springer-Verlag, Berlin, Heidelberg, 1976, pp. 1–18.
50. Kabat, E. A. The structural basis of antibody complementarity. In *Advances in Protein Chemistry*, Academic Press, New York, 1978 pp. 1–75.
51. Kabat, E. A. Idiotypic determinants minigenes and the antibody combining site. In *The Biology of Idiotypes* (ed. M. I. Greene and A. Nisonoff), Plenum, New York, 1984, pp. 3–17.
52. Kabat, E. A., and Berg, D. Production of precipitin and cutaneous sensitivity in man by injections of small amounts of dextran. *Ann. N.Y. Acad. Sci.*, **55**, 471–6 (1952).
53. Kabat, E. A., and Berg, D. Dextran – an antigen in man. *J. Immunol.*, **70**, 514–32 (1953).
54. Kabat, E. A., and Bezer, A. E. The effect of variation in molecular weight on the antigenicity of dextran in man. *Arch. Biochem. Biophys.*, **78**, 306–18 (1958).
55. Kabat, E. A., Kaiser, H., and Sikorski, H. Preparation of the type-specific polysaccharide of the type I meningococcus and a study of its effectiveness as an antigen in human beings. *J. Exp. Med.*, **80**, 299–307 (1944).
56. Kabat, E. A., Miller, C. P., Kaiser, H., and Foster, A. Z. Chemical studies on bacterial agglutination. VII. A quantitative study of the type specific and group-specific antibodies in antimeningococcal sera of various species and their relation to mouse protection. *J. Exp. Med.*, **81**, 1–8 (1945).
57. Kabat, E. A., Nickerson, K. G., Liao, J., Grossbard, L., Osserman, E. F., Glickman, E., Chess, L., Robbins, J. B., Schneerson, R., and Yang, Y. A human monoclonal macroglobulin with specificity for α(2 → 8)-linked poly-*N*-acetylneuraminic acid the capsular polysaccharide of group B meningococci and *Escherichia coli* K1 which crossreacts with polynucleotides and with denatured DNA. *J. Exp. Med.*, **164**, 642–54 (1986).
58. Kabat, E. A., Turino, G. M., Tarrow, A. B., and Maurer, P. H. Studies on the immunochemical basis of allergic reactions to dextran in man. *J. Clin. Invest.*, **37**, 1160–70 (1957).
59. Kabat, E. A., and Wu, T. T. Attempts to locate complementarity-determining residues in the variable positions of light and heavy chains. *Ann. N.Y. Acad. Sci.*, **190**, 382–93 (1972).
60. Kahana, Z. E., and Erlanger, B. F. Immunochemical study of the structure of poly(adenylic acid). *Biochem.*, **2**, 320–4 (1980).
61. Kasper, D. L., Winkelhake, J., Zollinger, W. D., Brandt, B. L., and Artenstein, M. S. Immunochemical similarity between polysaccharide antigens of *Escherichia coli* 07 : K1(L) : NM and group B *Neisseria meningitidis. J. Immunol.*, **110**, 262–8 (1973).
62. Koprowski, H., Herlyn, D., Lubeck, M., Defreitas, E., and Sears, H. F. Human anti-idiotype antibodies in cancer patients: is the modulation of the immune response beneficial for the patient? *Proc. Natl. Acad. Sci. USA*, **81**, 216–19 (1984).
63. Lafer, E. M., Rauch, J., Andrzejewski, C., Mudd, D., Furie, B., Schwartz, R. S., and Stollar, B. D. Polyspecific monoclonal lupus autoantibodies reactive with both polynucleotides and phospholipids. *J. Exp. Med.*, **153**, 897–909 (1981).
64. Lai, E., and Kabat, E. A. Immunochemical studies of conjugates of isomaltosyl oligosaccharides to lipid: production and characterization of mouse hybridoma antibodies specific for stearyl-isomaltosyl oligosaccharides. *Molec. Immunol.*, **22**, 1021–37 (1985).
65. Lai, E., Kabat, E. A., and Mobraaten, L. Genetic and nongenetic control of

the immune response of mice to a synthetic glycolipid stearylisomaltotetraose. *Cellular Immunol.*, **92**, 172–83 (1985).
66. Landsteiner, K. *The Specificity of Serological Reactions*, rev. edn. Harvard University Press, Cambridge, Massachusetts, 1945.
67. Larm, O., Lindberg, B., and Svensson, S. Studies on the length of the side chains of the dextran elaborated by *Leuconostoc mesenteroides* NRRL B-512. *Carbohy. Res.*, **20**, 39–48 (1971).
68. Lindemann, J. Homobodies: do they exist? *Ann. Immunol. (Paris)*, **130**, 311–19 (1979).
69. MacLeod, C. M., Hodges, R. G., Heidelberger, M., and Bernhard, W. G. Prevention of pneumococcal pneumonia by immunization with specific capsular polysaccharides. *J. Exp. Med.*, **82**, 445–65 (1945).
70. Mage, R. G., and Kabat, E. A. The combining regions of the type III pneumococcus polysaccharide and homologous antibody. *Biochem.*, **2**, 1278–88 (1963).
71. Maurer, P. H. Dextran an antigen in man. *Proc. Soc. Exp. Biol. Med.*, **83**, 879–84 (1953).
72. Moreno, C., Lifely, M. R., and Esdaile, J. Immunity and protection of mice against *Neisseria meningitidis* group B by vaccination using polysaccharide complexed with outer membrane proteins: a comparison with purified B polysaccharide. *Infect. Immun.*, **47**, 527–33 (1985).
73. Naparstek, Y., Duggan, D., Schattner, A., Madaio, M. P., Goni, F., Frangione, B., Stollar, B. D., Kabat, E. A., and Schwartz, R. S. Immunochemical similarities between monoclonal antibacterial Waldenstrom's macroglobulins and monoclonal anti-DNA lupus autoantibodies. *J. Exp. Med.*, **161**, 1525–38 (1985).
74. Neill, J. M., Sugg, J. Y., Hehre, E. J., and Jaffe, E. *Proc. Soc. Exp. Biol. Med.*, **47**, 339–44 (1941).
75. Newman, B., and Kabat, E. A. An immunochemical study of the combining site specificities of C57BL/6J monoclonal antibodies to $\alpha(1 \rightarrow 6)$-linked dextran B512. *J. Immunol.*, **135**, 1220–31 (1985).
76. Nisonoff, A., and Lamoyi, E. Implications to the presence of an internal image of the antigen in anti-idiotypic antibodies: possible application to vaccine production. *Clin. Immunol. Immunopathol.*, **21**, 397–406 (1981).
77. Padlan, E. A., Segal, D. M., Spande, T. F., Davies, D. R., Rudikoff, S., and Potter, M. Structure at 45 A resolution of a phosphorylcholine-binding Fab. *Nature (Lond). New Biol.*, **145**, 164–7 (1973).
78. Phillips, D. C. The three dimensional structure of an enzyme molecule. *Scientific American*, **215** (11), 78–90 (1966).
79. Potter, M., Newell, J. B., Rudikoff, S., and Haber, E. Classification of mouse Vk groups based on the partial amino acid sequence to the first invariant tryptophan: impact of 14 new sequences from IgG myeloma proteins. *Mol. Immunol.*, **19**, 1619–30 (1982).
80. Richards, F. F., and Konigsberg, W. H. Speculations: how specific are antibodies? *Immunochemistry*, **10**, 545–53 (1973).
81. Richter, A. W., and Hedin, H. I. Dextran hypersensitivity. *Immunol. Today*, **3**, 132–8 (1982).
82. Roitt, I. M., Male, D. K., Guarnotta, G., deCarralho, L. D., Cooke, A., Hay, F. C., Lydyard, P. M., Thanavala, Y., and Ivanyi, J. Idiotypic networks and their exploitation for manipulation of the immune response. *Lancet*, **I**, 1041–5 (1981).
83. Roitt, I. M., Thanavala, D. K., and Hay, F. C. Anti-idiotypes as surrogate antigens: structural considerations. *Immunol. Today*, **6**, 265–7 (1985).

84. Rubinstein, L. J., Goldberg, B., Hiernaux, J., Stein, K. E., and Bona, C. A. Idiotype-antiidiotype regulation. V. The requirement for immunization with antigen or monoclonal antiidiotypic antibodies for the activation of β2 → 6 and β2 → 1 polyfructosan-reactive clones in BALB/c mice treated at birth with minute amounts of anti-A48 idiotype antibodies. *J. Exp. Med.*, **158**, 1129–44 (1983).
85. Ruckel, E. R., and Schuerch, C. Chemical synthesis of a stereoregular linear polysaccharide. *J. Am. Chem. Soc.*, **88**, 2605–6 (1966).
86. Sacks, D. L., Kirchhoff, L. V., Hievy, S., and Sher, A. Molecular mimicry of a carbohydrate epitope on a major surface glycoprotein of *Trypanosoma cruzi* by using anti-idiotypic antibodies. *J. Immunology*, **135**, 4155–9 (1985).
87. Sarff, L. D., McCracken, G. H., Jr., Schiffer, M. S., Glode, M. P., Robbins, J. B., Ørskov, I., and Ørskov, F. Epidemiology of *Escherichia coli* K1 in healthy and diseased newborns. *Lancet* I, 1099–104 (1975).
88. Saxon, A., and Barnett, E. Human autoantiidiotypes regulate T cell mediated reactivity to tetanus toxoid. *J. Clin. Invest.*, **73**, 342–8 (1984).
89. Schiemann, O., and Casper, W. Sind die spezifisch pracipitabelen Substanzen der 3 Pneumokokkentypen Haptene? *Z. Hyg. Infekt. Krank.*, **108**, 220–57 (1927).
90. Sege, K., and Peterson, P. A. Use of anti-idiotypic antibodies as cell-surface receptor probes. *Proc. Natl. Acad. Sci. USA*, **75**, 2443–7 (1978).
91. Sharon, J., Kabat, E. A., and Morrison, S. L. Studies on mouse hybridomas secreting IgM or IgA antibodies to α(1 → 6)-linked dextran. *Molec. Immunol.*, **18**, 831–46 (1981).
92. Sharon, J., Kabat, E. A., and Morrison, S. L. Immunochemical characterization of binding sites of hybridoma antibodies specific for α(1 → 6)-linked dextran. *Molec. Immunol.*, **19**, 375–88 (1982).
93. Sharon, J., Kabat, E. A., and Morrison, S. L. Association constants of hybridoma antibodies specific for α(1 → 6)-linked dextran determined by affinity electrophoresis. *Molec. Immunol.*, **19**, 389–97 (1982).
94. Sidebotham, R. L. Dextrans. *Adv. in Carb. Chem. Biochem.* **30**, 371–444 (1953).
95. Sikder, S. K., Akolkar, P. N., Kaladas, P. M., Morrison, S. L., and Kabat, E. A. Sequences of variable regions of hybridoma antibodies to α(1 → 6)dextran in BALB/c and C57BL/6 mice. *J. Immunol.*, **135**, 4215–21 (1985).
96. Stein, K. E. Network regulation of the immune response to bacterial polysaccharide antigens. *Current Topics in Microbiol. Immunol.*, **119**, 57–74 (1985).
97. Stein, K. E., and Soderstrom, T. Neonatal administration of idiotype or antiidiotype primes for protection against *Escherichia coli* K13 infection in mice. *J. Exp. Med.*, **160**, 1001–11 (1984).
98. Stein, K. E., Zopf, D. A., Johnson, B. M., Miller, C. B., and Paul, W. E. The immune response to an isomaltohexosyl-protein conjugate, a thymus-dependent analogue of α(1 → 6)dextran. *J. Immunol.*, **128**, 1350–4 (1982).
99. Sugg, J. Y., and Hehre, E. J. Reactions of dextrans of *Leuconostoc mesenteroides* with the antiserums of leuconostoc and of types 220 and 72 pneumococcus. *J. Immunol.*, **43**, 119–28 (1942).
100. Suh, S.-W., Bhat, T. N., Navia, M. A., Cohen, G. H., Rao, D. N., Rudikoff, S., and Davies, D. R. The galactan binding immunoglobulin Fab 539: an x-ray diffraction study at 26A resolution. *Proteins: Structure Function and Genetics*, **1**, 74–80 (1986).
101. Thanavala, Y. M., Brown, S. E., Howard, C. R., Roitt, I. M., and Steward, M. W. A surrogate hepatitis B virus antigenic epitope represented by a synthetic

peptide and an internal image antiidiotype antibody. *J. Exp. Med.*, **164**, 227–36 (1986).
102. Turvey, J. R., and Whelan, W. J. Preparation and characterization of isomalto-dextrans. *Biochem. J.*, **67**, 49–52 (1957).
103. Urbain, J., Francotte, M., Franssen, J. D., Hiernaux, J., Leo, O., Moser, M., Slaoui, M., Urbain-Vansanten, G., Acker, A. V., and Wikler, M. From clonal selection to immune networks: induction of silent idiotypes. *Annal N.Y. Acad. Sci.*, **418**, 1–8 (1983).
104. Uytdehaag, F. G. C. M., Bunschoten, H., Weijer, K., and Osterhaus, A. D. M. E. From Jenner to Jerne: towards idiotype vaccines. *Immunological Rev.*, **90**, 93–113 (1986).
105. Wood, C., and Kabat, E. A. Immunochemical studies on conjugates of isomaltosyl oligosaccharides to lipid: specificities and reactivities of the antibodies formed in rabbits to stearylisomaltosyl oligosaccharides. *Arch. Biochem. Biophys.*, **212**, 262–76 (1981).
106. Wood, C., and Kabat, E. A. Immunochemical studies on conjugates of isomaltosyl oligosaccharides to lipid: fractionation of rabbit antibodies to stearylisomaltosyl oligosaccharides and a study of their combining sites by a competitive binding assay. *Arch. Biochem. Biophys.*, **212**, 277–89 (1981).
107. Wu, T. T., and Kabat, E. A. An analysis of the sequences of the variable regions of Bence Jones proteins and myeloma light chains and their implications for antibody complementarity. *J. Exp. Med.*, **132**, 211–50 (1970).
108. Wyle, F. A., Artenstein, M. S., Brandt, B. L., Traumont, E. C., Kasper, D. L., Alteri, P. L., Berman, S. L., and Lowenthal, J. P. Immunologic response of man to group B meningococcal polysaccharide vaccine. *J. Infect. Dis.*, **126**, 514–22 (1972).

DISCUSSION – Chaired by Dr J. Howard

HOWARD: Thank you very much Professor Kabat for such a comprehensive retrospective and update of this work. Do you know why it is that the specificities of your hybridomas have almost always turned out to be either hexa- or hepta-saccharide, even though other antibody molecules with a tri-, or a tetra-specificity are also produced following immunization. Is it anything to do with the dose of antigen that you have immunized with?

KABAT: This is always a problem, there are so many parameters in immunization and there are so many species differences. The rabbit behaves quite differently, and I would like just to say that one of my graduate students, Paula Borden, has just sequenced W3129, which is the only monoclonal anti-dextran with a cavity-type site specific for the non-reducing end of the dextran. W3129 is different from all the other anti-dextrans sequenced to date. Thus we have a real difference between what we call cavity-type and groove-type sites. The rabbit makes largely cavity-type sites, but there is not an easy way of getting hybridomas in rabbits.

From our studies in the human, we have shown that you can have antibody-combining sites which are complementary to somewhere between one and two glucoses as a lower limit, and those complementary to six and seven as the upper limit. We have a myeloma protein, which is complementary to five. One of these hybridomas is complementary to four. I think what we are dealing with is the statistics of getting a random sample in one species or another. That is why we intend to go to these other methods of immunization for trying to get a better approximation of the total repertoire.

HOWARD: Do you recall the immunization experiments of G. I. Vicari? As I recall, when he immunized mice with dextran B512 the antibody-secreting cells he produced were predominantly isomaltohexaose specific. If he increased his immunizing dose a hundredfold he had a predominance of thc isomaltotetraose specificity.

KABAT: Well this is certainly another parameter to investigate. I suppose I could spend the rest of my life investigating it, and I may damn' well do it!

HANDMAN: I wonder if more important than the immunization protocol may be the selection protocol for the hybridomas. How did you select those hybridomas?

KABAT: We selected them in two ways. One, we plate the clones in soft agar, cover them with a cellulose filter impregnated either with dextran-BSa or with a mouse IgA. The anti-dextran is taken up by the filter at the site of each producing clone. Then we take dextran, couple it with red cells then we cover the closed filter with dextran-coated red cells, allow them to attach, and wash the filter gently. We identify red spots with the colonies which produce anti-dextran. The other way is merely screening by agglutination with dextran-coated red cells. There are other ways of screening, but I think one will always have this same type of problem.

MÄKELÄ: You emphasized the heterogeneity of the heavy chains and I agree that it was impressive. I also think there was an impressive lack of heterogeneity in the light chains. Wasn't it true that several antibodies had almost the same sequence?

KABAT: I should have mentioned that these all are kappa antibodies. One major group is identical with Cesar Milstein's anti-oxazolones. They use the same germ-line gene in BALB/c, the J is different from Milstein's J of his anti-oxaxolones, but our C57 black uses the same J as Cesar Milstein's and that is absolutely identical nucleotide for nucleotide for nucleotide over the entire V-region. I think V kappa chains give a limited view, because in most of our animals we are getting out this germ-line kappa sequence exactly. I do not know why are they are using the same germ-line almost all the time under these particular conditions. The second group is just as different from the first family as it could possibly be. Moreover, it has seven extra amino acids in CDR 1. I think if we had other methods of immunization we could get different chains. This second group which got glycolipid, gives you a very different germ-line gene. I think that what one has seen so far is essentially

a Maxwell Demon selection in which we see one major germ-line gene family and perhaps one germ-line gene subfamily, or a somatic mutation pattern.
SÖDERSTRÖM: Do you have any information on the subclasses of the hybridomas?
KABAT: I am sorry I forgot to mention it. We have some 40-odd hybridomas, half are IgM and half are IgA. We have had one, and now we have another, IgG_3 resulting from an incredibly large amount of screening which was unsuccessful, except in these two cases. Everybody says that the major hybridoma response that one gets to the carbohydrate antigens is IgG_3 and, of course, we have been at this now for 6 years, and Dr Chen in our laboratory got an IgG_3 just a few months ago. I don't know why we are not getting it – it can be the method of selection.
MOSIER: Dr Kabat, you had several antibody sequences that had a minor number of mutations, do you know if those mutations increased the binding affinity for the hexasaccharide?
KABAT: In many cases they don't. I think when we get more, if we have the luck of the draw, we will be able to tell you which amino acid substitutions do nothing and which amino acid substitutions are functional. One of the great questions, which again I did not mention when I showed you this carbohydrate-binding site, is: is there carbohydrate there? And that is the one where the binding constant goes up almost a hundredfold compared to some of the others. You could think of this particular substitution giving you the increased binding constant, but you could equally well think that carbohydrates might open the site by pulling it away so that things got in better, and we are trying to determine the carbohydrate. Unfortunately, since we don't have IgGs where there is no carbohydrate in CH 1 but IgA and IgM also have carbohydrates in CH 1, it is a terribly difficult problem to be sure that you get rid of the pieces of the chain which come from CH 1, to be sure that you have carbohydrate in V, but we are getting there, I think.
MOSIER: Perhaps I could just comment that we screened a very large number of antiphosphorylcholine hybridomas generated following T-independent immunization for somatic mutation and increases in affinity, and it is exceedingly rare to find such an antibody. We have one that we have now sequenced, but it's certainly an exception to the rule.
KABAT: The antibody differs how, I didn't quite get that?
MOSIER: The antibody differs by having an increased affinity for phosphorylcholine from the germ-line sequence. It is sequenced.
GEYSEN: Dr Kabat, could you please comment on something, since you used choline structure as part of your talk. On reading the paper I was very interested to see some of their own assessments of that structure. I mean, I think if I remember the figures right, there are 17 amino acids on the lysozyme that are considered in contact with the antibody. That is a glutamine, in actual fact, that fits down into the cavity, it is the one residue that

is pulled out. If you look at the specificity they claim for the monoclonal from which the Fab was taken, it does not react with two other avian lysozymes which have a single amino acid change which correlates with that glutamine. The change is a glutamine to a histidine. However, when they looked at the structure of the cavity, and they did some modelling work, they assessed themselves that the histidine would fit in where the glutamine went and it would make the same hydrogen bond in the floor of the cavity that the glutamine makes. So all the other 17 residues are conserved and yet that monoclonal does not bind to avian lysozyme in which there has been a single change from glutamine to histidine, and the histidine can't be assessed as precluding binding. This would suggest that the binding is based on a single residue and that the other residues don't contribute any net binding energy. Could you comment on that?

KABAT: They didn't draw this interpretation, certainly.

GEYSEN: I think it is in their paper. All that information is spelled out very carefully in that Science paper.

KABAT: Well it is quite interesting and surprising. The fact that histidine fits into the site of the glutamine may not mean that it is actually inside in the way the contour of this particular complementarity determining stretch.

GEYSEN: Obviously, there has to be a reason for why it doesn't react. One of the other observations is that I think, these days, we would have to consider that the antigen-combining sites of antibodies are soft. They are not rigid, they are soft. The assessment was that there are three phenyl rings which close about, particularly, the methylene groups of the glutamine and the glutamine penetrates through the sort of collar of phenyl rings and makes a hydrogen bond on the floor of the cavity. As they stated themselves in the paper, they couldn't see a good reason why the histidine wouldn't do the same thing and make the same hydrogen bond, yet it will not bind to that lysozyme. So one residue changes overriding the seventeen conserved chains . . .

KABAT: But one residue could change the conformation of the CDR, substantially perhaps, so that it wouldn't be in exactly the same position for interacting with the lysozyme. These are all questions to which we will have to learn the answers from more cases. There were two other lysozyme structures which David Davies has in which the complementarity-determining residues are quite different and directed toward a different part of the molecule. In one case, I believe it is sufficiently close, so it forms a site involving some of the same residues.

ROBBINS: Dr Kabat, one of the startling things about some of these monoclonals is the narrow pH range at which they show activity. Have you ever thought that that pH range might be an expression of the charged quality of the side chain of the amino acid that might be doing the direct binding? Is there any way, by looking at the old titration data with enzymes to figure out what might be the active site just by that?

KABAT: Well that question almost sends me into anaphylactic shock because we had two antibodies to *Klebsiella*. After several years of work, we found that one was completely insensitive to a pH range of 4–8, whereas the other one only reacted at pH 4 and, of course, we were mostly working in neutral solution. It took us a long time to figure out what was going on. It turned out actually that almost all of our polysaccharides to *Klebsiella*, which people were working with and sent us, were the sodium salt but one person had sent us the free acid and, since we were working in this case with a purified antibody and not in whole serum, there was no buffering power so it was at pH 4 and we couldn't figure out what was going on until we found that this antibody had a different pH. You can see why it sent me into anaphylactic shock.

Towards Better Carbohydrate Vaccines
Edited by R. Bell and G. Torrigiani

Published by John Wiley & Sons Ltd

8

Subsite mapping of monoclonal antipolysaccharide antibodies

C. P. J. GLAUDEMANS
National Institutes of Health, Bethesda, Md., USA

Our laboratory has been studying the interaction of a series of monoclonal antibodies with specificity for a β(1,6)-D-galactopyranan [1, 4]. One of these antibodies in particular – IgA J539 – has been studied. Findings can be summed up as follows (the reader is referred to one of the latest papers [2] for previous references).

The specificity of the antibody is high, β-1,4 or β-1,3 galactoses do not appear to bind. The combining site of the antibody can accommodate four sequentially linked β-1,6-D-galactopyranosyl residues. The conformation of the saccharide antigen is such that the ring oxygen of the sugar is one side of the polysaccharide chain for one residue and on the other side of the chain for the next residue, and so on. The antibody-combining site binds to only *one* side of the saccharide chain, indicative of binding on the antibody *surface*. This was confirmed by measuring the binding of IgA J539 with the saccharide now carrying large bulky substituents on the solvent side of the antigen (substituents not capable themselves of binding to the antibody)and finding these substituents to have no influence of the binding strength.

Secondly, it was shown that a linear polysaccharide, a β-1,6-D-galactopyranan from P. Zopfii (whose structure was shown by Manners *et al.* [6]) bound antibody *along* its polysaccharide chain and not only at its terminal end. In an attempt to probe possible hydrogen bonding between saccharide and antibody a series of simple methyl β-galactopyranosides were prepared bearing a deoxyfluoro group at C-2, C-3, C-4 and C-6, and it was found [3] that the 2- and 3-deoxyfluoro methyl β-D-galactopyranosides did not show binding to the antibody. A deoxyfluoro group in the antigen, in lieu of a hydroxy group, could facilitate binding if hydrogen bonding took place from the antibody → saccharide, but would eliminate hydrogen bonding from the saccharide → antibody. Thus the protein bound galactose in its highest binding subsite mediated by hydrogen bonding. Synthesizing a large number of galactosyl oligosaccharides linked 1,6 and bearing a 3-deoxyfluoro galactoside at various parts of the molecule was undertaken [5]. The binding of each oligosaccharide with antibody was measured and interpreted as follows:

The antibody is incapable of binding the deoxyfluoro galactose of the oligosaccharide in its highest binding subsite. Thus it will shift the oligosaccharide along the four subsites in order to maximize the binding energy, while at the same time avoiding contact of the highest binding subsite with the fluoro-galactose residue within the oligosaccharide ligand. By measuring the affinity of a series of oligosaccharides – each having fluoro-galactose residue(s) at different locations in the sequence – it was possible to assign an affinity to each subsite with which it binds its galactosyl residue. If these subsites are labelled CABD (in sequence) in going from the heavy (H) to the light (L) chain across the face of the antibody combining area, the relative affinity of each subsite for 'its' galactosyl residue decreases in the order A > B > C > D. The subsite A, which is therefore internal in the sequence of subsites, accounts for *circa* 50% of the total binding free energy of the maximally binding tetrasaccharide determinant. The Ka's for a galactosyl residue for each subsite are: A(10^3), B(47), C(10) and D(1.3). The binding of this antibody then can be pictured as taking place mostly through hydrogen bonding in one subsite. The other three residues of the galactan bind to the antibody, possibly through van der Waals' or hydrophobic forces.

REFERENCES

1. Glaudemans, C. P. J. Immunodominance of terminal sugars revisited. *Molec. Immun.*, **23**, 917–18 (1986).
2. Glaudemans, C. P. J., Bhattacharjee, A. K., and Manjula, B. N. Monoclonal anti-galactan IgA J539 binds intercatenarily to its polysaccharide antigen. Observations on the binding of antibody to a macromolecular antigen. *Molec. Immun.*, **23**, 655–60 (1986).
3. Ittah, Y., and Glaudemans, C. P. J. Preparation of two methyl deoxyfluoro-beta-D-galactan-specific immunoglobulin A J539 (Fab'). *Carbohydr. Res.*, **95**, 189–94 (1981).
4. Jolley, M. E., Rudikoff, S., Potter, M., and Glaudemans, C. P. J. Spectral changes on binding of oligosaccharides to murine immunoglobulin A myeloma proteins. *Biochem.*, **12**, 3039–44 (1973).
5. Kovac, P., and Glaudemans, C. P. J. Confirmation of the location of subsite D in monoclonal IgA J539. *J. Carbohydr. Chem.*, **4**, 613–26 (1986).

6. Manners, D. J., Pennie, I. R., and Ryley, J. F. The molecular structures of a glucan and a galactan synthesized by *Prototheca zopfli*. *Carbohydr. Res.*, **29**, 63–77 (1974).

DISCUSSION – Chaired by Dr J. B. Robbins

ROBBINS: Have you tried to prepare your haptenic substances with atoms that more resemble oxygen than fluorine, for instance is it possible to substitute some of these hydroxyls with sulphhydryls?

GLAUDEMANS: Fluorine actually has the same size as a hydroxyl and it is highly electro-negative. It may accept hydrogen bonding and bind more strongly; it will of course not donate hydrogen bonding because it doesn't have hydrogen. It has been shown by R. Murray that, in crystals, when you substitute hydroxyls for fluorine, there is no change in the crystal structure of saccharides so that they do not influence shape-wise and size-wise any binding phenomenon. We have not done any sulphhydryls.

ROBBINS: The reason I asked that is that the traditional approach has been to choose substitutes which would eliminate binding, therefore, to understand better the contribution of the original antigen, I wonder whether it would be possible to substitute materials that might bind better to the antibody in order to understand their interaction?

GLAUDEMANS: As Dr Kabat knows, we are now studying together his dextran system and, in that case, you can make glycosides of glucose, and in certain positions where we have put fluorine we already get an increased binding, showing that at least one of the hydrogen bonds of the antibody may be from the protein donation to the ligand. So there is a case where we get it the other way around.

ROBBINS: I don't think you have to apologize for the relevance of what you said about the need for understanding the vaccine action; if we could define the effects of our vaccines on antibody synthesis with that degree of precision, I am sure we would make better vaccines.

Towards Better Carbohydrate Vaccines
Edited by R. Bell and G. Torrigiani

Published by John Wiley & Sons Ltd

9

Peptides which mimic carbohydrate antigens

H. Mario Geysen, Rod Macfarlan, Stuart J. Rodda, Gordon Tribbick, Thomas J. Mason, and Peter Schoofs
Department of Molecular Immunology, Commonwealth Serum Laboratories, 45 Poplar Road, Parkville, Victoria 3052, Australia

In recent years it has been clearly demonstrated that the immune response to carrier-coupled peptides includes antibodies which react with the complete or native protein antigen [1, 6]. This observation was surprising only in the context of an older proposal that immunoglobulins require an absolute structure or conformation for the residues comprising the epitope. The finding that the binding interaction between the antigen and immunoglobulin results in conformational changes in the antigen and probably in the antigen-combining site also, relaxes the constraints placed on the use of peptides as immunogens [3–5, 8–9]. There are two necessary conditions for a binding interaction to occur: (1) that a sufficient degree of complementarity between the contact surfaces is maintained; and (2) that the overall change in the free energy of the system is negative. This suggested a possible strategy for directly identifying small peptides able to bind with specificity to antibodies, namely the screening of a large repertoire of peptides to satisfy the above criteria [7]. A modified approach was subsequently demonstrated in which antibody-binding peptides were delineated in a stepwise procedure from an optimum binding dipeptide [5].

In order to apply this 'mimotope' strategy, the only starting requirement is an antibody (preferably a monoclonal) to the antigen of interest. As there is no reason to believe that antibodies to polysaccharides differ in any fundamental way from antibodies to protein antigens, antibody-binding peptides can also be identified for antibodies raised to polysaccharide antigens. An obvious benefit from this approach to small synthetic antigens is that the requisite synthetic procedures have been 'translated' from complex carbohydrate chemistry to the well-developed chemistry of peptides.

The present article describes the delineation of a small family of peptides showing the specificity attributes of the polysaccharide epitope or determinant associated with the human blood group, type A. In addition to binding to the defining monoclonal antibody, these peptides also bound a second monoclonal antibody of comparable specificity. In contrast a monoclonal antibody of blood group type B specificity failed to react. This example provides some optimism for the concept that peptide mimics of polysaccharide epitopes may eventually form the basis of a new generation of vaccines.

GENERAL STRATEGY FOR 'MAPPING' THE ANTIGEN-COMBINING SITE

The ideal strategy begins with the selection of an antibody having an optimal set of properties as defined by suitable tests; for example, neutralization of an essential biological activity, or an appropriate specificity for distinguishing between antigens in a diagnostic test. The antigen-combining site of the chosen antibody defines the epitope of interest and is used to select suitable ligands from a sufficient number of peptides to comprise an effective screen. Given that this strategy is not compromised by an unknown factor, it obviates the need to isolate or even to identify the appropriate antigen. It also sidesteps the issue of the spatial geometry of the inducing epitope, i.e. whether or not the epitope was continuous (linear) or discontinuous (assembled). Furthermore, it would appear to be independent of the composition of the inducing epitope, i.e. as to whether or not it was composed of amino acids or carbohydrate moieties or a combination of both.

The antigen-combining site as a template

We adopted the view that an antibody represents a selected product of the immune system, and as such its antigen-combining site is complementary to one of the potential epitopes on the inducing antigen. This complementarity has two definable components:

1. A complementarity for the shape (e.g. the envelope defined by rolling a sphere the size of a water molecule over the contact surface of the antigen [2]), which may or may not bear a recognizable relationship to the original

antigen shape, depending on whether or not a conformational change was induced in the antigen on binding by antibody [5].
2. A complementarity for full and partial charge centres, for hydrogen-bonding centres and for regions of hydrophobicity.

Determination of the optimum antibody-binding peptide element

It is almost axiomatic that longer peptides provide more definitive information in the primary screen. For example, each residue (spacer-residues excepted) in a peptide would be expected to contribute to the overall specificity, as well as the total binding energy of the interaction of the antibody. At the same time, the more extensive the repertoire of residues, the greater is the probability of achieving a close to optimum 'fit' of peptide into the antigen-combining site of an antibody. This is achieved by the use of a more extensive set of amino acids than is represented by the 20 genetically coded L-amino acids. The variety of shapes and chemical characteristics of individual side-chains is extended by the inclusion of unusual amino acids and by D-optical isomers.

Whilst the previous paragraph describes the ideal, clearly the size of an initial screen using dipeptides increases with the square of the number of included residues. This affects both the number of peptides required to be synthesized and the quantity of antibody necessary for testing in the primary screen. From the finding that antibodies bind in a reproducible manner to dipeptides, an effective compromise is to use an initial screen of 1600 dipeptides. This screen comprises all possible dipeptide combinations of the D and L-optical isomers of the 20 genetically coded amino acids (for ease of organization the optically inactive glycine is used as if it were active).

Extending an antibody-binding peptide element by one residue

Subsequent to the determination of the preferred dipeptide element from the primary screen, a new screen is synthesized to provide a number of possible modes of extension of this element. Again a compromise is reached between the number of peptides synthesized and sufficient variability to achieve an effective 'fit' to the antigen-combining site. Figure 1 illustrates the relationships between the set of extended tetrapeptides and the preferred tripeptide element. It is seen that both a direct extension and an indirect extension (the addition of a beta-alanine spacer between the added residue and the dipeptide to either the amino-terminal or the carboxy-terminal side) are provided for. The repetitive application of the procedure then 'adds' residues one at a time and is continued until there is no further improvement

	Direction of extension	
	Amino-terminal	Carboxy-terminal
Direct	A_N–$R_1\star R_2\star R_3$	$R_1\star R_2\star R_3$–A_C
Indirect	$R_1\star R_2\star R_3$	$R_1\star R_2\star R_3$
	A_N	A_C

Figure 1. The set of systematically extended peptides one residue longer (spacer residue beta-amino alanine excluded) than the parent peptide, $R_1\star R_2\star R_3$. Each of the longer peptides is systematically derived from the parent by the addition of a residue at either the amino (A_N) or carboxy-terminal (A_C) side, directly adjacent or spaced by a beta-alanine for greater conformational freedom. The beta-alanine is represented as a flexible bend which allows the added residue to lie alongside R_1 or R_3 respectively. A_N and A_C are taken from the set which includes, in addition to both the L- and D-optical isomers of the 20 genetically coded amino acids, some non-natural amino acids

in the affinity (as inferred from the relative extinctions obtained in the ELISA) or specificity for the defining antibody.

Selection of the optimum peptide element for extension

In the majority of examples to date, there was a multiplicity of choices of peptides for extension. This suggests that small peptides sharing a fixed binding element accommodate to the antigen-combining site with some tolerance for the added residue. It also suggests, as was found by Edmundson *et al.* [3, 4, 9] in studying the binding of ligands by the Mcg light-chain dimer, that immunoglobulin binding cavities are 'soft' and able to adjust to the inserted peptide with some latitude for the residues present.

The choice of dipeptide for extension is generally aided by the finding of a clear bias for one amino acid, often with an absolute optical isomeric preference, as was the case with the example cited in Table I.

The interpretation of the results obtained from the testing of a set of extended peptides is again aided by trends in the data. A 'successful extension' is defined as a longer peptide with higher affinity than the previous optimum peptide (parent peptide). In the first instance the frequency of successful amino-terminal *versus* carboxy-terminal extensions, without regard to their being direct or indirect (spaced), is assessed for all peptides giving extinctions higher than the parent peptide. This frequency defines the

Table I. Identification of antibody-binding peptides for two monoclonal antibodies

Peptides tested[a]	Monoclonal antibody	
	No. 1	No. 2
Dipeptides	wV	wl
	wA	
	wH	
	wl	
	wI	
	wv	
Extensions of wl	**wlD** (2.6)	wlP (4.6)[b]
	wl–F (2.5)	wlG
	wl–E (2.5)	**wl–E** (4.4)
	wlG	**wl–q**
	wl–V	**wl–D**
	wl–I	**wl–Q**
	wlE (2.3)	**wl–N**
	wlP	**wlQ**
	wl–e (2.3)	E–**wl**
		wlE (3.7)
Extensions of wl–E	**wl–Em** (1.3)	**wl–E–I** (1.3)
	wl–EM	**wl–El**
	wl–Eq	wl–E–p
	wl–EK	
	wl–E–p	
	wl–Ea	
Extensions of wlE	**wlE–a** (1.3)	**wlE–a** (1.4)
	wlE–v	**wlE–I**
	wlE–q	**wlEA**
		wlE–n
		wlES
Extensions of wlE–a	**wlE–am** (1.5)	**wlE–al** (1.3)
	wlE–al	wlE–aD
	wlE–a–s	wlE–aT
	wlE–a–I	**wlE–a–L**
	wlE–a–V	**wlE–a–l**

[a] Identification of progressively longer peptides binding to either of the two monoclonal antibodies of human blood group type A specificity. Amino acids are identified by the single-letter code. Upper-case letters are used to identify the L-optical isomer and lower-case letters the D-optical isomer. Those peptides reacting most strongly with either antibody, and giving a higher optical density in an ELISA test than the parent, are shown in descending order of optical density. A '–' indicates the incorporation of the spacer residue, beta-amino alanine. The peptides within each group of extensions containing physicochemically related added residues are shown in bold face, for example, the related set D, E, Q and N.

[b] Numbers in parentheses are the ratio of the optical density obtained in the ELISA test to the optical density for the parent for that group. At each step the dilution of hybridoma culture supernatant tested was chosen to ensure ELISA values that were on scale (<2.0). The dilution ranged from 1/20 for the initial testing, to 1/2000 for testing against the longer peptides.

Related interactions		Non-related interactions	
MAb No. 1	MAb No. 2	MAb No. 1	MAb No. 2
Dipeptide interactions			
wV	**wl**		tY
wA	WE		kG
wH	wA		aV
wl			
wI			
wv			
Extensions of wl			
wlD	**wl–E** (4.5)	wl–F (2.5)	wlP (4.6)
wl–E (4.4)	wl–e	wlG	wlG
wlE (2.4)	wl–q	wl–V	
wl–e	wl–D	wl–I	
wl–D	wl–Q	wlP	
	wl–N	wlA	
	wlQ		
	E–wl		
	wlE (3.7)		
Extensions of wl–E			
wl–Em (1.3)	wl–E–I (1.3)	wl–Eq (1.1)	w1–E–p (1.3)
wl–EM	wl–El	wl–EK	wl–ES
wl–El		wl–E–p	wl–ET
wl–Ea		wl–EQ	Gwl–E
			P wl–E
Extensions of wlE			
wlE–a (1.3)	**wlE–a** (1.4)	wlE–q (1.2)	wlEt (1.2)
wlE–v	wlE–I	wlE–t	wlET
wlEA	wlEA	wlEq	wlES
	wlEm	wlE–n	
	wlE–L	wlES	
Extensions of wlE–a			
wlE–am (1.5)	wlE–al (1.3)	wlE–a–s (1.4)	wlE–aD (1.3)
wlE–al	wlE–a–L	wlE–aq	wlE–aT
wlE–a–I	wlE–a–l		wlE–a–d
wlE–a–V	wlE–am		QwlE–a
wlE–a–m			wlE–aE
w1E–aA			
w1E–a–l			

'preferred' side for extension. The data obtained for successful extensions on the preferred side are then assessed for frequency of direct *versus* indirect (spaced) extensions. Finally, the frequency of occurrence in successful extensions of each added amino acid, without regard to optical isomerism, is determined. At this stage of the analysis, frequent occurrence of residues which are conservative analogues of the most frequently occurring residue are taken as additional evidence supporting its choice.

Choice of antibody

Polysaccharide antigens are widespread, both as components of infectious micro-organisms and as markers on mammalian cells. In order to test out the 'mimotope' strategy on antibodies known to be against polysaccharide antigens, two monoclonal antibodies (MAbs) with specificity for the human blood group, type A, were selected.

Determination of the optimum antibody-binding dipeptide

Both MAbs (No. 1 and No. 2) were reacted with the set of dipeptides as described above. Table I illustrates the choices made in progressing from the primary screen through multiple extensions to reach the longer antibody-binding peptide. The results from the initial screen clearly identified the D-optical isomer of tryptophan as the prime requirement for interaction at the dipeptide level. Taking the results obtained for both MAbs into account, wl (see Table I for nomenclature) was selected as the optimum antibody-binding dipeptide for further extension.

Elucidation of longer antibody-binding peptides

Tripeptides giving a significantly greater extinction than the dipeptide wl are listed in Table I and show the following trends: (1) a clear preference for the 'added' amino acid to be carboxy-terminal with respect to the parent dipeptide (wl); (2) a significant bias for the 'added' amino acid to be spaced from the parent dipeptide, i.e. an indirect extension; and (3) that the 'added' amino acid giving the most useful degree of cross-reactivity when comparing the two MAbs is L-glutamic acid.

The choice of glutamic acid (E) is well supported by both the frequency of occurrence of glutamic acid (as either the D- or L-optical isomer) and the occurrence of related residues such as aspartic acid, glutamine and asparagine. However, despite the seemingly clear choice for extension of wl, namely wl–E, we elected to try for further extensions with wlE also.

Extensions of either wl–E or wlE failed to identify a peptide with greatly improved binding (Table I). Furthermore, there was only a weak bias for residue 'type' added, i.e. extensions grouped on the basis of adding (to the parent peptide) a large hydrophobic residue, such as methionine, leucine, isoleucine or valine, are not clearly better than an alternative grouping comprising more polar residues such as glutamine, lysine or serine. By choosing for further extension the peptide wlE–a, in which the small residue, D-alanine, occurs adjacent to the beta-alanine as an indirect extension of wlE, we expected a much clearer pattern for a preferred residue to emerge from the next series of extensions than was actually observed. Again, peptides giving an improved signal over the parent include both hydrophobic and polar residues as the 'added' amino acid, see Table I.

Further work

The failure to identify a clear preference for a single or closely related set of amino acids suggests that: (1) inherent in the 'mapping' of antibodies to carbohydrate epitopes are the difficulties of adequately mimicking the polysaccharide surface with a molecule restricted to the amino acid set used in this study; and (2) some optimization of the peptide element **wl–E** is necessary before proceeding with the extension strategy. In order to achieve this optimization, we normally synthesize the complete set of analogues differing from the parent sequence by a single residue change [7]. Analysis of the dependence of antibody binding on the identity of the residue(s) at each position, in the context of the remaining residues, may yield a better understanding of the results presented above and suggest a preferred peptide with which to continue the extension strategy.

DISCUSSION

The observation that peptides will bind with specificity to an antibody which is nominally specific for a carbohydrate epitope is consistent with the observations of others. Edmundson *et al.* [4] convincingly demonstrated that a Bence-Jones light-chain dimer bound a range of molecules which included, in addition to numerous peptides (endorphines, chemotactic), diverse organic molecules such as single- to multi-ring aromatic (e.g. 6-carboxy-tetramethylrhodamine) and the commonly used haptenic molecule, bis-DNP-lysine. Further examples of antibodies of one generic specificity, binding to molecules of another completely different specificity, are found in the more recent descriptions of anti-idiotypic antibodies generated to anti-polysaccharide antibodies [10]. This latter anti-idiotypic approach to alternative vaccines shares many aspects with the 'mimotope' strategy, in that both bypass the necessity of identifying the actual epitope for a given antibody. However, whereas the anti-idiotypic approach selects an antibody-binding molecule from the antibody repertoire itself, the 'mimotope' strategy selects a binding molecule from a suitably large repertoire of chemically synthesized peptides.

It would now appear that the 'mimotope' strategy, as outlined above, will be applicable to the large majority of antibody molecules. We are at present evaluating the potential of these mimotopes to mimic the actual epitope in inducing the equivalent antibody in animals. It is also clear that with the use of an extended set of 'molecular building blocks', i.e. D-amino acids and non-natural amino acids, it is feasible to construct mimotopes with possibly advantageous properties such as an increased biological stability. This may lead not only to a new generation of vaccines but to vaccines that can be administered by alternative routes, for example, orally or intranasally.

ACKNOWLEDGEMENTS

The authors are particularly indebted to the Director of CSL, Dr N. McCarthy, for his support, advice and encouragement, and to Steve Laurie, Heather Forsyth, Kim Lund and Mary Bullas for their enthusiastic and skilled assistance. We also thank Allen Edmundson for critical evaluation of the manuscript.

REFERENCES

1. Alexander, H., Johnson, D. A., Rosen, J., Jerabek, L., Green, N., Weissman, I. L., and Lerner, R. A. Mimicking the alloantigenicity of proteins with chemically synthesized peptides differing in single amino acids. *Nature (Lond.)*, **306**, 697–9 (1983).
2. Connolly, M. L. Solvent-accessible surfaces of proteins and nucleic acids. *Science*, **221**, 709–13 (1983).
3. Edmundson, A. B., and Ely, K. R. Binding of N-formylated chemotactic peptides in crystals of the Mcg light chain dimer: similarities with neutrophil receptors. *Molec. Immun.*, **22**, 463–75 (1985).
4. Edmundson, A. B., Ely, K. R., and Herron, J. N. A search for site-filling ligands in the Mcg Bence-Jones dimer: crystal binding studies of fluorescent compounds. *Molec. Immun.*, **21**, 561–76 (1984).
5. Geysen, H. M. Antigen–antibody interactions at the molecular level: adventures in peptide synthesis. *Immun. Today*, **6**, 364–9 (1985).
6. Geysen, H. M., Meloen, R. H., and Barteling, S. J. Use of peptide synthesis to probe viral antigens for epitopes to a resolution of a single amino acid. *Proc. Natl. Acad. Sci. USA*, **81**, 3998–4002 (1984).
7. Geysen, H. M., Rodda, S. J., and Mason, T. J. A priori delineation of a peptide which mimics a discontinuous antigenic determinant. *Molec. Immun.*, **23**, 709–15 (1986).
8. Geysen, H. M., Tainer, J. A., Rodda, S. J., Mason, T. J., Alexander, H., Getzoff, E. D., and Lerner, R. A. Chemistry of antibody binding to a protein. *Science*, **235**, 1184–90 (1987).

9. Herron, J. N., Ely, K. R., and Edmundson, A. B. Pressure-induced conformational changes in a human Bence-Jones protein (Mcg). *Biochemistry*, **24**, 3453–9 (1985).
10. Kennedy, R. C., Dreesman, G. R., and Kohler, H. Vaccines utilizing internal image anti-idiotypic antibodies that mimic antigens of infectious organisms. *BioTechniques*, **3**, 404–8 (1985).

DISCUSSION – Chaired by Dr J. Howard

ROBBINS: A terrific presentation. Have you had a chance to immunize with any of these peptides that have the D-amino acids? It is said that D-amino acid polymers are poor immunogens, in some case tolerogens. I wonder if the introduction of the amino acids might serve as an inhibitor against active immunization?

GEYSEN: I am aware of that statement. At this stage, I would say that we appear to get the same level of responses to peptides that contain D-amino acids as *L*-amino acids. To us, that is not particularly surprising in that the peptides that were used with the D-amino acids are confirmed to bind antibodies. I think that, from the results to date, we could certainly suggest peptides that would be non-immunogenic, based on the composition of those peptides. For argument's sake, we have not yet ever found a peptide or an epitope for which arginine is a content substitute. I think that some of the previous results using D-amino acids may have just used the wrong balance of residues. We are not guessing here. We are first determining something which binds to an antibody and it is not surprising to us that, if we use that as an immunogen, we generate very acceptable antibody responses at least, back to those peptides, irrespective of whether they have got D-amino acids or non-natural amino acids. We use quite a repertoire of non-natural amino acids.

ROBBINS: When these experiments were done with the D-amino acid peptides, it was said that the processing mechanism, considered to be an essential part of immunogenicity, would not work because there were no host enzymes that could degrade D-amino acid peptide bonds.

GEYSEN: I think that the evidence for processing, at least for protein antigens, has to be called into question a little bit. We ourselves thought that the observation that a lot of our contact residues were large hydrophobic residues, which was not consistent with what we knew about protein folding, was a function of prior antigen processing before the immune response or the fragments, i.e. that what was buried in the total structure was obviously not buried after antigen processing. But, in all cases that we have looked at, we can show competition in solution phase in the native antigen. So, clearly, it is not necessary for interaction with an antibody to get any kind of processing whatsoever, either by denaturation of the antigen or by, let's say, proteolytic cleavage. Again, all I can say is that, on that basis it would not surprise us that you could more or less make any kind of molecule. This has been observed in the hapten, you can make antibodies to all sorts of haptens. One does not believe that a lot of those haptens are capable of enzymatic degradation. I think it is in fact consistent with more evidence, than it is inconsistent.

MOSIER: Let me clarify this issue of non-immunogenicity of D-glutamic acid – D-lysine, which is the prototype for a D-amino acid conjugate that is tolerogenic. First of all, to be tolerogenic it has to exist as a very long random copolymer of approximate molecular weight 60 000. Lower molecular weight conjugates are not tolerogenic and, in fact, can be immunogenic. The second thing is that, while that molecule cannot be processed naturally, one can make small molecular weight fragments of DNP-D-GL, treat macrophages with these fragments and generate an antibody response to the hapten, coupled to D-GL. So, in certain circumstances it can be immunogenic, so that the tolerogenic capability of these molecules depends upon their being of large molecular weight. Certainly the processing of the D-GL conjugate is much, much slower than the processing of the L-amino acid copolymer.

GEYSEN: I suggest there is another possible explanation. If you look through the literature, the bulk of the polymers that have been used, at least as the base polymer, for testing the immunogenicity of, particularly, the hapten group, have been lysine-type polymers, at least with a reasonable frequency of inclusion of lysine, largely because it provides a very convenient coupling group, the epsilon amino group of lysine. In a study we have just completed, we found that which tends to support a hypothesis I put forward a couple of years ago, that for something to be immunogenic, it was very important that it had the correct overall charge. I hesitate to generalize from a single study, particularly the study of this protein, also the protein itself has an overall negative charge, but when we identified what we considered to be the immunodominant epitopes on that protein, as distinct from the immunosilent ones, there was an excellent correlation with the field strength and the direction of the field in that all immunodominant epitopes had associated with a negative electrostatic field, and all the silent ones had associated with a positive electrostatic field. My suggestion is that it may be that, if you use a lysine-type polymer, that you may in actual fact end up with something that is not particularly immunogenic because, overall, you have given it the wrong charge.

FEIZI: I wanted to ask you whether this peptide reactivity applies to one anti-A, or whether you have looked at other anti-A antibodies?

GEYSEN: The delineation was done simultaneously, assessing it against two completely distinct monoclonals that had the same overall specificity to type A. In actual fact, when you screen them against the peptides, you can see that there are differences. They share at least a certain reactivity with common peptides. The peptide itself because, of course, we do all the screening with the peptides remaining, or at very small quantities coupled to the tips of these pins. When we have finished our screening procedure, we then synthesize the peptides in larger quantities by conventional methodology. Then we are able to do a lot of other types of test with it and it is being synthesized at the moment, at least at the pentapeptide level. That will be provided to our typing group within the laboratory where I work, to see whether, in actual fact, against a lot of the polyclonal reagents it still shows exactly the same specificity pattern, but that has not been completed yet with the bulk peptide.

SÖDERSTRÖM: These two monoclonals, were they specific for any of the blood group A families, 1, 2, 3 or 4, or were they shared determinants?

GEYSEN: I cannot really answer that, in that I am not quite sure of the fine data of how you define specificity for blood group determinants. They were provided to us by the group that does all the blood typing at the Commonwealth Serum Laboratories as being very characteristic for the human blood group A. They are both IgMs, in that particular instance, and they are used normally to do typing. On that basis, we chose them to try the methodology because we at least believed that the blood group A is a polysaccharide, but the fine specificity I really cannot tell you.

KABAT: Were these monoclonals that you used?

GEYSEN: They were both monoclonal antibodies.

KABAT: Of what class?

GEYSEN: IgM.

KABAT: All workers seem to have got only IgM hybridoma antibodies to blood group A and B.

GEYSEN: One can use the strategy for polyclonal sera, but it becomes a little bit more complicated because, clearly, you end up with signals at the beginning and you have to guess a little bit about which are the useful ones. It works with polyclonals, but it is easier to work with monoclonals.

ROBBINS: Since you have been crazy enough to look at peptides as a method of making antibodies to carbohydrates, have you restricted this kind of approach to amino acids? Polymer chemists use carbon chains of four to seven, that have different structures to synthesize polymers like nylon and other plastics. Have you considered using other small molecules, that may not be natural substances, to see if they might be better inducers? Have you had a chance to look at that?

GEYSEN: We use quite a repertoire of non-natural amino acids and we also used a number of amino acids which have real constraints on the geometry. We have a number which are based on cyclohexane or cyclopentol rings, in which the amino group in the carboxylic acid group are adjacent but, so far, we have to use amino acids because the chemistry does not allow you to vary the type of link and it is just a very convenient way. It is very much like stringing beads on a necklace. The repertoire is only dictated by the different beads that you use, but you must stick with the same linking. In fact, we cannot show much involvement of the main chain for the binding. Therefore, I think it is perfectly feasible, if you have the chemistry, to string things together without relying on peptide bonds. Of course you can see very clear advantages in that, you could theoretically make very stable molecules that still show the correct attributes.

KABAT: When you put your spacer on, this represented just one amino acid?

GEYSEN: Yes. We used that as the general strategy. Now, the earliest mimotope that we made, in actual fact, where we found the need to incorporate a spacer, we have a series which go from a single glycine spacer to four beta alanine spacers which, linearly, is very long and it makes very little difference. In fact, the optimum was the two-beta alanine and close to that was three-beta alanines. I think all that is telling us is that it is folding back on itself, and that the link, or the spacer, is hanging outside the antigen-combining site and plays no major role. Now that has been confirmed for a number of them by using a peptide, containing a cyclohexile spacer instead of a beta alanine, and they interact almost indistinguishably from the ones with the beta alanine. So that, in most cases where we find the beta alanine occurring, we believe that it is just allowing the peptide to fold back so that we see the epitope as being across two chains which lie parallel to one another. What we usually find is that the two sides of a spacer have an opposite requirement for the stereo chemistry. In other words, one side will usually be D-amino acids and the other side L, or they will both be LS. One can interpret that as to whether the main chain was parallel in the original epitope or anti-parallel because, clearly, the peptides that fold are always anti-parallel and one can correct for the fact that they were parallel in the folded protein by just changing the optical summaries of all the residues that occur on one side of the folded peptide. They are indistinguishable, in a geometrical sense, from the case where it is made up of all Ls and the two main chains run parallel to one another.

FEIZI: Dr Geysen's approach is reminiscent of the approach that Frank Richards used some years ago when he tested the binding of a number of organic compounds (DNP and many other compounds) to mouse myeloma proteins. He could classify the myeloma proteins on the basis of their ability to bind these. My question is whether the peptide binding you describe is just a property of one particular monoclonal antibody, or whether other antibodies with the same specificity show binding?

GEYSEN: We are approaching ten fairly well characterized mimotopes. When we compare the series, going from the smallest to the longest, in terms of a titre with defining antibody *versus* titres of any randomly selected antibody, we find invariably that with a non-relevant antibody there is no detectable titre. With the defining antibody, we routinely get titres well over one in a million of a fairly typical ascites fluid for the correct identity. Allen Edmundson is currently in our laboratory for a small sabbatical and we have access to some of the Mcg light-chain dimer, which is one of the Bence-Jones proteins and, of course, Allen has spent a number of years now perfusing ligands into the crystal of the light-chain dimer, locating exactly the orientation in which it binds and drawing conclusions about how soft the cavity is and so on, and so on. We have actually applied the strategy to the light-chain dimer and we now have a family of peptides, starting from scratch, which also bind with absolute specificity to the light-chain dimer, and they do not have any real relationship. There are two families that we have identified, one has some relationship to some of the known peptides that bind the light-chain dimer and another set does not. Allen will take these peptides back with him to fuse them into the crystal and really tell us exactly what orientation the series adopts as you go from the dipeptide element up to the longer ones. The question that is of prime interest is: do the two residues at the dipeptide level take up the same orientation as the same two residues as part of the tetrapeptide, or do the additional residues actually start to distort the orientation of the original two that you started delineating the site from? That, of course, is very important from our point of view. However, we suspect that when we try to put into the cavity, the tetrapeptide, that it will not work; that it will actually destroy the crystal, because he knows from his own work that if the ligand he tries to go in is too big, and it still has binding affinity for it, i.e. as detected in the solution phase it will, in fact, distort the cavity to such an extent that the crystal literally blows apart. So, based on the size limitations that he has determined, we suspect that the tetrapeptide – and we have actually got up to the hexapeptide with the light-chain dimer because it is quite a large cavity – will in, actual fact, destroy the crystal, so we may only get information at the dimer tripeptide level. But it does seem to work. Let me just add that I have shown you data for antibodies which have a fairly well-defined binding function but, in actual fact, the same strategy is applicable with receptor molecules and things like viruses directly. For the haemagglutinin, we are well on the way to identifying a peptide which binds to the haemagglutinin molecule of either isolated haemagglutinin or to the virus itself and we think, because it is independent of the strain of haemagglutinin, that it binds into the top of the trimer and, possibly, this constitutes a peptide antibiotic, because if we can make a binding strong enough, we ought to be able to preclude the influenza virus from binding to the cell-surface protein that is the first part of the infectious procedure. So the strategy seems to work with any molecule that has a binding capability, and just start from scratch.

ROBBINS: Amino acid, the bacterial diamopimelic acid confers a lot of structure to the cell wall of bacteria. Have you had a chance to look at this amino acid?

GEYSEN: No. That is the simple answer! I think there must be very many good examples that one could look at with this strategy but, despite the fact that we are now a group of about 20 people, there is still only a certain number of things that we can do. We try actually to demonstrate that the technology is applicable over a broad range, for obvious reasons, but I welcome any useful suggestion because I think our experience also dictates a little bit the narrowness of our view in what we think is applicable and what we think is not applicable.

KABAT: I do not quite have a visual picture of how you put the different amino acids on the tips each time. It seems to me that you could very easily get mixed up.

GEYSEN: Actually, it is self-correcting. The synthesis schedule, if you like, has never been done by hand. I actually wrote some programmes and it is all handled by computer, and all the data are fed straight back into the computer. We only see the final output and it is all closely correlated. Strictly speaking, when you go to do the additions and we do use computer assistance in making the additions, i.e. the reaction trays have eight matrices of holes, they sit into a plotting bed and, instead of having a pen in there, it just has a pointer, so somebody just goes with a multiple-delivery system and adds an activated alanine, for instance, into all the wells that the pointer points to. Then you go through all your amino acids like that. It is self-correcting because, if you have made a mistake, you are going to try and add into a well that is already full and, at the end of it, you are going to have an empty well. It is always very obvious if there is a mistake. But you are right, there is no identity in the end. You have got to do it correctly, otherwise you have lost the sense, but the blocks themselves have three legs on one end and two legs on the other, it is impossible to put them in upside down. They are all etched, or at least we use a scribe to identify them very carefully, and they match and it is double checked.

KABAT: Are some of these sets going to be manufactured so that you can produce a set of reproducible dipeptides or tripeptides etc., so that almost anyone could do this without actually going through the whole works?

GEYSEN: The hardware, plus the software package and the method is going to be commercially available from Cambridge Research Biochemicals Ltd. We supply the components for that, but they actually market it. One cannot make available the tripeptide sets, for the obvious reason that you have got to do the original assessment as to which is the best dipeptide. You can use the same set of dipeptides for the universal screen if you like. From that point onwards, one has to follow each test with a synthesis and it is frustrating in that it might take you 6–8 days, for instance, to do the synthesis of the longer set. You do one test before you can designate the next synthesis, so it takes about 6–8 weeks to run through the full set of extensions to delineate a mimotope. But we can do upwards of ten simultaneously, though not all our efforts are put into mimotopes, we have other fields for which we require synthesis, but it is a reasonably efficient process.

KABAT: You are never going to market 20^8.

GEYSEN: I think, actually, the synthesis of large numbers is not the problem, so much as the testing, and the quantity of material that you need for the testing. To get a signal from a dipeptide you need to start with the dilution of ascites of about one in a thousand, so you would need quite large volumes of ascites if you were going to test, for argument's sake, 100 000. We actually considered synthesizing a total repertoire of tripeptides and our major repertoire has 48 components to it, that is the DS and the LS plus nine non-natural amino acids, which makes 125 000 tripeptides. We could synthesize that in about 3 months, but we do not consider that we could test it effectively, so we are still trying to work from a dipeptide screen, but there are some disadvantages to doing that, it is not quite as efficient as going from a tripeptide.

Towards Better Carbohydrate Vaccines
Edited by R. Bell and G. Torrigiani

Published by John Wiley & Sons Ltd

10

Anti-idiotypes as surrogate polysaccharide vaccines

TOMMY SÖDERSTRÖM
Department of Clinical Immunology, Sahlgrenska Hospital and the University of Göteborg, Göteborg, Sweden

INTRODUCTION

The receptor – ligand recognition is, by nature, a three-dimensional process. Clearly, the interaction between epitopes and paratopes represents a process in which specificity requires a functional spatial complementarity. Several experimental models have demonstrated that it is possible to substitute biologically active molecules with anti-idiotype antibodies, for example in the anti-anti-insulin model, where antibodies could mimic the effect of insulin on the blood glucose levels [38]. Such findings have contributed to a less antigen-centred view of the immune system. Since carbohydrates may serve as antigens triggering synthesis of protein antibodies, it is not difficult to envisage the possibility of protein images of specific carbohydrate structures. Similarly, complementary protein images of protein structures are easily conceived. In fact, Jerne's formulation of the network concept suggests the presence of an internal image of the universe of external antigens [17]. Since it is clear that the network comprises not only B cells and B-cell products, but also T cells, endogenously stimulated idiotype-related regulatory circuits, may be an important part of long-term immunological memory.

Clearly it would be of importance to substitute antigens with, for example, anti-idiotype antibodies in situations where antigen is sparse or dangerous to handle, or where more efficient regulatory pathways for the immune response could be activated. Polysaccharides are poor immunogens among children under 2 years of age, the period with the highest incidence of infections from encapsulated bacteria. Since anti-carbohydrate antibodies are highly protective, capsular polysaccharides clearly represent antigens for which alternative ways to induce protective immunity, also in infants, should be explored.

In this chapter some of the characteristics of anticarbohydrate responses will be discussed, especially in regard to the possibility of increasing the immune response via network manipulation.

ANTI-POLYSACCHARIDE RESPONSIVENESS DURING ONTOGENY AND IN PATIENTS WITH IgG SUBCLASS DEFICIENCIES

The immunoglobulin synthesizing capacity of peripheral blood lymphocytes from infants varies for different classes and subclasses [1]. B lymphocytes from new-borns can be stimulated to synthesize IgM at adult rates, whereas total IgG production reaches adult levels around the age of 24 months, when IgA production is still reduced. The capacity to synthesize IgG subclasses also shows variation with age, inasmuch as IgG_1 and IgG_3 secretion comes within 12 months after birth, and IgG_2 and IgG_4 production is still low at 24 months. Furthermore, T cell-dependent activation of plaque-forming cells with pokeweed mitogen fails to induce immunoglobulin synthesis in lymphocytes from newborns and infants up to the age of 6 months.

Adult levels of immunoglobulin secretion are thus not reached until about the age of 2 years. This parallels the age of aquisition of capacity to respond against most carbohydrate antigens. Since IgG anti-carbohydrate antibodies in normal adults often appear in the IgG_2 subclass, the late aquisition of IgG_2 synthesizing cells probably contributes to the late appearance of antibody responses to polysaccharides. Children preferentially express anticarbohydrate antibodies of the IgG_1 subclass [14], a pattern we also observe among IgG_2 subclass-deficient individuals. Recently, Hammarström *et al.* proposed a model for the maturation and subclass restriction of the antibody repertoire in man [14]. They predicted that IgG anti-carbohydrate antibodies in infants utilize a heavy chain variable region (V_H subgroup) 3′ of those expressed in the IgG_2 subclass, with a low affinity for carbohydrate antigens. Such antibodies would be less efficient for protection than the ‘adult-type’ IgG_2 antibodies, albeit the same antigen specificity. Recent findings among subclass-deficient patients may be fitted into their model (Söderström *et al.*, manuscript in preparation).

Different V_H genes may thus be expressed in the respective IgG subclasses, and lack of responsiveness in a certain subclass may indicate a restriction in the available V-gene repertoire. Further knowledge about the regulatory defects in patients with subclass-associated immunodeficiencies may help understand how V_H genes coding for high affinity anti-polysaccharide paratopes can be activated.

CHARACTERISTICS OF IMMUNE RESPONSES TO POLYSACCHARIDES

Besides the idiotype restriction and the late development during ontogeny discussed above a number of characteristics distinguish polysaccharide-driven immune responses from anti-protein responses. This has recently been reviewed by K. E. Stein [41] (Table I). Of great importance for a possible use of polysaccharide vaccines to induce protective immunity are factors like thymus independence and lack of memory which, in comparison with protein-based vaccines, make polysaccharide vaccines less efficient.

Table I. Characterization of immune responses against polysaccharide antigens (modified from Stein [41])

Thymus independence [25]
Failure to stimulate a memory response [4, 19]
Failure to undergo affinity maturation [4, 19]
Late development in ontogeny [2, 13, 25, 30]
Requirement for a specific B lymphocyte subset [26]
Isotype restriction [3, 31, 48]
Idiotype restriction [6, 15, 21, 31, 42, 47]

Inherent characteristics of polysaccharides may strongly influence the antibody responses. Examples of such factors could be resistance to degradation by mammalian enzymes, the structure of the repeat units, and 'loose' structure of polysaccharides in solution [33]. Furthermore, the 'molecular size' of the capsular polysaccharides seems to be directly related to their immunogenicity [33]. Not only antigen size, however, but also availability of functioning non-suppressed antibody V-regions for specific epitopes may influence the outcome of immunization. This was demonstrated for the bacterial levan system, where two antibody families are produced in mice [22]. The $\beta 2 \rightarrow 6$ fructosan binding clones can be expanded at birth, whereas an ontogenic delay has been reported for the clones specific for $\beta 2 \rightarrow 1$ [16].

Interestingly, different regulatory mechanisms seem to control systemic *versus* mucosal anti-polysaccharide responses. Thus, antibodies against the $\alpha 2 \rightarrow 8$ *N*-acetyl neuraminic acid polymer constituting the *Escherichia coli* K1 and the *Neisseria meningitidis* Group B capsular antigens can be demonstrated in human breast milk, also in women with no or very little serum antibodies [12].

The K1 antigen illustrates another important characteristic of environmental polysaccharide antigens. Developing human and rat brains contain unique $\alpha 2 \rightarrow 8$ linked polysialic acid chains cross-reacting with the polyclonal antiserum to meningococcal type B polysaccharide [10]. Using monoclonal anti-type B antibodies, we showed reactivity with the human gangliosides GD3 or GM3. Monoclonal antibodies against the B capsule reacting with terminal $\alpha 2 \rightarrow 8$ sialic acid epitopes, as well as antibodies requiring a repeated sialic acid sequence, were found. The difference in paratope specificity between such clones, all reacting with a K1 antigen, could thus be expected to differ in reactivity against autoantigens. It would be very important to establish methods to selectively induce non-autoreactive clones, for example through network manipulation.

ANTI-IDIOTYPE ANTIBODIES AND ANTIGEN–ANTIBODY INTERACTIONS

The antibodies synthesized upon antigen administration (Ab1) have the capacity to bind to the specific antigen determinants. These immunoglobulin molecules possess V-region associated determinants (idiotypes). These idiotypes may function as antigens eliciting anti-idiotype antibodies (Ab2). Monoclonal Ab2 react with single epitopes and are frequently referred to as anti-idiotopes. The Ab2 antibodies react with the corresponding Ab1 and may be involved in the regulation of Ab1 synthesis during an immune response [23]. As stated in the network hypothesis, Ab2 antibodies may also function as immunogens, inducing synthesis of Ab3 [5, 17, 45]. A portion of Ab3 antibodies may mimic Ab1 antibodies. Anti-idiotype antibodies constitute a heterogeneous population of molecules classified into three major types (Table II). Ab 2α are anti-framework antibodies which may suppress or enhance the response of cells with the corresponding idiotype. Ab2α may thus be used to prime for a specific response, following binding to the immunoregulatory idiotypes of specific cell clones.

Table II. Classification of anti-idiotype antibodies (modified from Rubinstein *et al.* (1984) [35])

Anti-idiotype designation	Characteristics
Ab2α	Recognizes 'conventional' idiotypes on the immune receptor of T and B lymphocytes
Ab2β	True internal images Stimulate antigen-specific clones via epitope receptors
Ab2ϵ	Epibodies, binding to epitopes as well as idiotopes

To mimic the three-dimensional structure of the antigen (internal image) it is likely that the anti-idiotype must be paratope-associated. Such Ab2β antibodies have several advantages as vaccine candidates [29] since they can mimic microbial antigens in addition to hormones and drugs in the binding to specific cell-bound receptors. Compared to anti-idiotypes of the Ab2α type, Ab2β should not only be able to prime normal animals but also to induce an antigen specific response. Furthermore, Ab2β should have the capacity to stimulate cell clones with the corresponding idiotype as well as antigen-specific clones with other idiotypes (unrestricted response). The frequency of Ab2β in the anti-idiotype response has, however, been predicted to be very low [37].

NEONATAL PRIMING WITH IDIOTYPE OR ANTI-IDIOTYPE FOR PROTECTION AGAINST *E. COLI* K13 INFECTION

Chemical composition of the *E. coli* K13 polysaccharide

Escherichia coli K13 are frequently isolated from urinary tract infections in humans [18], and the bacteria have little invasive capacity compared to, for instance *E. coli* K1. The K13 capsule consists of a homopolymer of 3)-β-ribofuranosyl-(1 → 7)-β-KDO-(2 → and is acetylated (Table III). We have previously published the structures of the *E. coli* K20 and K23 antigens which have a similar basic structure as K13 [46].

Table III. Composition of the *E. coli* K13, K20 and K23 polysaccharides (from Vann *et al.* (1983) [46])

K13	3)-β-Ribofuranosyl-(1 → 7)-β-KDO-(2 → 4 (of KDO) ↑ Acetyl
K20	3)-β-Ribofuranosyl-(1 → 7)-β-KDO-(2 → 5 (of Ribofuranosyl) ↑ Acetyl
K23	3)-β-Ribofuranosyl-(1 → 7)-β-KDO-(2 →

Characteristics of anti-K13 antibodies

The characteristics of the K13 epitopes were investigated in detail using monoclonal antibodies prepared in BALB/c mice [39, 40]. Antibodies differentiating between the K13, K20 and K23 antigens were found. We chose to study further an IgM antibody, 150C8, which was shown to be bactericidal and to confer passive protection against infection with *E. coli* 06 : K13 : H1 [40].

Characteristics of the anti-150C8 (anti-idiotype) antibodies

Monoclonal antibodies against the 150C8 antibody were prepared in A/He mice following fusion with the SP2/0 cell line [43]. An IgG_1 antibody, 5868C, was chosen for further studies since it fulfilled the criteria of probable relevance for induction of protective immunity (Table IV). The 150C8 idiotype was found in pre-immune sera of several mouse strains, showing an early increase following immunization with K13 polysaccharide or a whole-cell vaccine, and the idiotype was also present in rat hyperimmune sera (43). These findings suggested that 5868C had the characteristics of an anti-idiotype containing a 'related epitope' [29].

Table IV. Characteristics of anti-idiotypes to be used for induction of protective immunity (modified from Stein and Söderström (1984) [43])

1. Antibodies expressing the corresponding idiotype should confer passive protection
2. The interaction between the idiotype and the anti-idiotype should be inhibited by antigen
3. Immunization with antigen or natural infection should give rise to an increase in idiotype-expressing antibodies

The interaction between the 150C8 idiotype and 5868C anti-idiotype was studied. Double diffusion analysis showed that the two antibodies formed a precipitate in agarose. The idiotype–anti-idiotype interaction was further studied using 5868C-coated erythrocytes. The agglutination by 150C8 was specifically inhibited by the K13 polysaccharide, although a weak cross-reactivity was detected for the K13-related polysaccharides K20 and K23 (Table V). The unrelated *E. coli* K1 and *Haemophilus influenzae* type b/Hib polysaccharides, on the other hand, did not inhibit.

Neonatal priming with idiotype or anti-idiotype for protection against infection with *E. coli* K13

BALB/c mice were injected within 24 hours after birth with anti-idiotype antibodies (5868C) or idiotype (150C8) in sterile saline. The mice were

Table V. Inhibition of idiotype–anti-idiotype by antigen (from Stein and Söderström (1984) [43])

Polysaccharide[a]		HAI titre[b]
K13	3)-β-Ribofuranosyl-(1 → 7)-β-KDO-(2 → 4 (on KDO) ↑ Acetyl	44
K20	3)-β-Ribofuranosyl-(1 → 7)-β-KDO-(2 → 5 (on Ribofuranosyl) ↑ Acetyl	5
K23	3-β-Ribofuranosyl-(1 → 7)-β-KDO-(2 →	6
K1	8)-α-NeuNAc-(2 → 8)-α-NeuNAc-(2 →	1
Hib	3(-β-Ribofuranosyl-(1 → 1)-Ribitol-5-(PO_4 →	1

[a] The starting concentration of polysaccharide was 10 mg/ml and serial twofold dilutions were used for inhibition.
[b] Log 2.

Table VI. Effect of neonatal priming with idiotype and anti-idiotype when BALB/c mice were challenged at 5 weeks of age (from Stein and Söderström (1984) [43])

Treatment at birth	Immunization at 4 weeks of age	No. of mice	% survival
Experiment 1			
—[a]	—	6	0[b]
—	K13 vaccine	9	44
K13 Ps, 2.5 μg	K13 vaccine	6	33
150C8, 1 μg	K13 vaccine	15	87
5868C, 50 ng	K13 vaccine	15	93
5868C, 10 μg given to mothers after delivery[c]	K13 vaccine	6	83
Experiment 2			
Saline	K13 Ps, 2.5 μg	6	0[d]
K13 Ps, 2.5 μg	K13 Ps, 2.5 μg	6	33
150C8, 1 μg	K13 Ps, 2.5 μg	8	75
150C8, 50 ng	K13 Ps, 2.5 μg	10	40
5868C, 1 μg	K13 Ps, 2.5 μg	5	80
5868C, 50 ng	K13 Ps, 2.5 μg	9	78

[a] — = no injection
[b] Mice were challenged with 20 × LD_{50} live *E. coli* 06 : K13.
[c] Anti-idiotype was injected intraperitoneally into the mother within 24 hours after delivery of her pups.
[d] Mice were challenged with 30 × LD_{50} live *E. coli* 06 : K13.

immunized at 4 weeks with killed *E. coli* K13 (experiment 1) or purified K13 polysaccharide (experiment 2). One week after the immunization the mice were challenged intraperitoneally with 20 or 30 × LD_{50} *E. coli* 06 : K13 : H1. The percentage of mice surviving 24 hours after challenge is shown in Table VI. Mice primed with idiotype as well as mice given anti-idiotype were protected. One group was included where the mother was given a high dose of anti-idiotype within 24 hours after delivery. The protection observed in her pups suggests priming via the milk (Table VI).

Delaying the vaccinations until the mice were 12 weeks old, mice neonatally given anti-idiotype survived a 50 × LD_{50} *E. coli* K13 challenge dose (Table VII). At this age we saw no effect of priming with idiotype. The anti-idiotype priming effect was not directly reflected as increased anti-K13 antibody titres in the primed animals. The relative proportion of the anti-K13 antibodies carrying the 150C8 idiotype used for priming, however, was strongly enhanced by priming with anti-idiotype.

Table VII. Effect of idiotype and anti-idiotype priming when BALB/c mice were challenged at 13 weeks of age

Treatment at birth	Immunization at 12 weeks of age	No. of mice	% survival[a]
—[b]	—	9	0
—	K13 Ps, 2.5 μg	20	25
150C8, 1 μg	—	5	0
150C8, 1 μg	K13 Ps, 2.5 μg	27	22
5868C, 1 μg	K13 Ps, 2.5 μg	19	16
5868C, 50 ng	K13 Ps, 2.5 μg	30	78

[a] Mice were challenged with 50 × LD_{50} live *E. coli* 06 : K13.
[b] — = no injection.

OTHER EXPERIMENTAL SYSTEMS WITH IMMUNITY AGAINST MICROBES INDUCED BY ANTI-IDIOTYPE

There have been several reports of enhanced immunity against parasitic, viral and bacterial antigens following anti-idiotype administration [20, 24, 27, 32, 36]. The antibacterial systems include priming with anti-idiotype for anti-polysaccharide responses against the Group A streptococcus [9], and *Streptococcus pneumoniae* [24, 44]. In the *S. pneumoniae* system, a monoclonal anti-idiotype coupled to keyhole limpet haemocyanin induced antibodies to the immunodominant part of the cell-wall C polysaccharide and, in addition, protection against infection with *S. pneumoniae* was induced without antigen administration [24].

The work by D. L. Sacks *et al.* in a parasite model, *Trypanosoma cruzi* concerns anti-idiotype-induced immunity to a carbohydrate epitope [36]. Xenogenic Ab2 were raised in rabbits against a mouse monoclonal antibody with specificity for an epitope of a 72K glycoprotein specific for *T. cruzi*. In a number of assays, including interspecies immunization, the purified Ab2 was shown to contain antibodies demonstrating molecular mimicry of the carbohydrate epitope (Ab2β).

DISCUSSION

Little is known about the regulatory role of anti-idiotype antibodies in human anti-microbial immune responses. In fact, only a few well-documented systems with human auto-anti-idiotypic antibodies have been described, for example the casein system of Cunningham-Rundles [7], the tetanus toxoid system by Geha [11] and the myasthenia gravis system studied by Dwyer *et al.* [8].

Clearly there is a need for improved procedures to increase the immunogenicity in humans of a number of critical carbohydrate epitopes, especially in infants and, as suggested above, also in patients with various immunodeficiencies. Recent data suggest that specific unresponsiveness against polysaccharides may be common also among infection prone individuals without known immunodeficiency (R. Geha, personal communication). As mentioned above, different V-regions may be used for production of different classes and subclasses of antibodies against a given antigen, as exemplified by the failure of infants and IgG_2-deficient adults to produce the ‘adult type’ of high-affinity IgG_2 anti-carbohydrate antibodies. Little is known about the regulatory defects behind the unresponsiveness. Animal data, however, suggest the possibility of successfully manipulating the V-region repertoire available upon antigen stimulation. The correlation of high-affinity variable region activation to specific isotypes may perhaps be utilized in the search for useful anti-idiotype probes.

One example may be the studies of Nishinarita *et al.* [28], demonstrating an idiotype determinant consisting of the cross-reactive T15-idiotype and a portion of the constant region of IgA. Only IgA T15-positive anti-phosphorycholine antibodies inhibited the monoclonal anti-idiotype. Possibly human anti idiotype antibodies used as alternative polysaccharide vaccines should include an epitope formed by an Ab2β against a ‘protective idiotype’ in combination with a portion of the constant region of an ‘adult high-affinity subclass type’ constant immunoglobulin region.

Although great progress has been achieved in the manufacturing of effective and safe vaccines, there are numerous biological functions to be considered in the immune response, for example complement fixation, opsonization, binding to acute phase proteins and avoidance of induction of antibodies binding to autoantigens. It seems likely that in the future such events can be reproduced by, for instance, recombinant DNA products.

The molecular mimicry or internal images of anti-idiotypes of the respective antigens obviously does not require resemblance in the overall structure, but merely in the contact sites with the idiotype. Appropriately placed amino-acid residues constitute an idiotype, but other residues in the same antigenic area may be involved in binding to other antibodies. This may, as suggested by Roitt *et al.* [34], mean that a cocktail of anti-idiotypes would be required to compete successfully with antigen in recognition of B-cell receptors. Since anti-idiotypes may substitute for carbohydrate antigens (Ab2β), the internal image concept must be restricted to physico-chemical similarities between the contact residues in their bonds, be they of the ionic, hydrogen, hydrophobic or van der Waals' forces as discussed by Roitt *et al.* [34].

As demonstrated in the *E. coli* K13 systems as well as in other experimental systems (Stein 1985 [41], for review), presentation of maternal idiotypes to the foetus or new-born may favour the expansion of clones positive for the respective idiotypes upon antigen stimulation. Thus passively administered antibodies may not only protect the new-born directly against infection, but also prime the immune system to an efficient response upon later encounter with the antigen. Possibly synthetic idiotypes may soon be available also for use in humans. Much remains to be understood, however, about the mechanisms by which anti-idiotypes may influence anti-polysaccharide responsiveness before such reagents can be used as alternative vaccines in humans. Increased knowledge about microbial epitopes optimal for protection, hybridoma technology and amino-acid sequencing, may soon make synthetic oligopeptides, possibly linked to immunopotentiating carrier structures, available for experimental use. Such reagents should have a great potential as tailor-made tools for specific immune intervention.

ACKNOWLEDGEMENTS

The valuable collaboration of a number of colleagues involved in these studies is gratefully acknowledged. Parts of this study have been supported by grants from the Swedish Board for Technical Development (STU), the Swedish Medical Research Council (No. 315) and the Ellen, Walter and Lennert Hesselman Foundation.

REFERENCES

1. Anderson, U., Bird, G., and Britton, S. A sequentional study of human B lymphocyte function from birth to two years of age. *Acta Paediatr Scand.*, **70**, 837–42 (1981).
2. Baker, P. J., Morse, H. C. III., Cross, S. S., Stashak, P. W., and Prescott, B. Maturation to regulatory factors influencing magnitude of antibody response to capsular polysaccharide type III *Streptococcus pneumoniae*. *J. Infect. Dis.*, **136**, 20–4 (1977).
3. Der Balian, G. P., Slack, J., Clevinger, B. L., Bazin, H., and Davie, J. M. Subclass restriction of murine antibodies. III. Antigens that stimulate IgG3 in mice stimulate IgG2c in rats. *J. Exp. Med.*, **152**, 209–18 (1980).
4. Briles, D. E., and Davie, J. M. Clonal dominance. I. Restricted nature of the IgM antibody response to group A streptococcal carbohydrate in mice. *J. Exp. Med.*, **141**, 1291–307 (1975).
5. Cazenave, P. A. Idiotypic-antiidiotypic regulations of antibody synthesis in rabbits. *Proc. Natl. Acad. Sci. USA*, **74**, 5122–6 (1977).
6. Cramer, M., and Braun, D. G. Genetics of restricted antibodies to streptococcal group polysaccharides in mice. II. The Ir-A-CHO gene determines antibody levels, and regulatory genes influence the restriction of the response. *Eur. J. Immunol.*, **5**, 823–30 (1975).
7. Cunningham-Rundles, C. Naturally occurring autologous anti-idiotypic antibodies. Participation in immune complex formation in selective IgA deficiency. *J. Exp. Med.*, **155**, 711–19 (1982).
8. Dwyer, D. S., Bradley, R. J., Urquhart, C. K., and Kearney, J. F. An enzyme-linked immunosorbent assay for measuring naturally occurring anti-idiotypic antibodies in myasthenia gravis patients. *Nature (London)*, **301**, 601–14 (1983).
9. Eichman, K. Idiotype suppression. I. Influence of the dose and of the effector functions of anti-idiotypic antibody on the production of an idiotype. *Eur. J. Immunol.*, **4**, 296–302 (1974).
10. Finne, J., Leinonen, M., and Mäkelä, P. H. Antigenic similarities between brain components and bacteria causing meningitis. *Lancet*, **ii**, 235–7 (1983).
11. Geha, R. S. Presence of circulating anti-idiotype bearing cells after booster immunization with tetanus toxoid (TT) and inhibition of anti-TT antibody synthesis by auto-anti-idiotypic antibody. *J. Immunol.*, **130**, 1634–9 (1983).
12. Glode, M. P., Sutton, A., Robbins, J. B., McCracken, G. H., Gotschlich, E. C., Kaijser, B., and Hanson, L. A. Neonatal meningitis due to *Escherichia coli* Kl. *J. Infect. Dis.*, **136**, 93–7 (1977).
13. Gold, R., Lepow, M. L., Goldschneider, J., and Gotschlich, E. C. Immune response of human infants to polysaccharide vaccines of groups A and C *Neisseria meningitidis*. *J. Infect. Dis.*, **136**, 531–5, Suppl. (1977).
14. Hammarström, L., Lefranc, G., Lefranc, M. P., Persson, M. A. A., and Smith, C. I. E. Aberrant pattern of anti-carbohydrate antibodies in immunoglobulin class or subclass-deficient donors. In *Immunoglobulin Subclass Deficiencies* (ed. L. A. Hanson, T. Söderström and V.-A. Oxelius), Vol. 20, Karger, Basle, 1986, pp. 50–6.
15. Hansburg, D., Clevinger, B., Perlmutter, R. M., Griffith, R., Briles, D. E., Davie, J. M. Analysis of the diversity of marine antibodies to $\alpha(1 \rightarrow 3)$ dextran. In *Cells of Immunoglobulin Synthesis*, (ed. B. Pernis and H. J. Vogel) Academic Press, New York, 1979, pp. 295–308.
16. Hiernaux, J., Bona, C., and Baker, P. J. Neonatal treatment with low doses of

anti-idiotypic antibody leads to the expression of a silent clone. *J. Exp. Med.*, **153**, 1004–8 (1981).
17. Jerne, N. K. Towards a network theory of the immune systems. *Ann. Immunol. (Paris)*, **125C**, 373–9 (1974).
18. Kaijser, B., Hanson, L. A., Jodal, V., Lidin-Jansson, G., and Robbins, J. B. Frequency of *E. coli* K antigens in urinary tract infections in children. *Lancet*, **i**, 664–6 (1977).
19. Käyhty, H., Karanko, V., Peltola, H., and Mäkelä, P. H. Serum antibodies after vaccinations with *Haemophilus influenzae* type b capsular polysaccharide and responses to reimmunization: no evidence of immunologic tolerance or memory. *Pediatrics*, **74**, 857–65 (1984).
20. Kennedy, R. C., Tonesco-Malia, J., Sanchez, J., and Dreesman, G. R. Detection of interspecies idiotypic cross-sections associated with antibodies to hepatitis B surface antigen. *Eur. J. Immunol.*, **13**, 232–5 (1983).
21. Kunkel, H. G., Mannik, M., and Williams, R. C. Individual antigenic specificity of isolated antibodies. *Science*, **140**, 1218–19 (1963).
22. Lieberman, R., Potter, M., Humphrey, W. Jr, Mushinsky, E. B., and Vrana, M. Multiple individual and cross-specific idiotypes on 13 levan-binding myeloma proteins of BALB/c mice. *J. Exp. Med.*, **142**, 106–19 (1975).
23. McKearn, T. J. Antireceptor antiserum causes specific inhibition of reactivity to rat histocompatibility antigens. *Science*, **183**, 94–6 (1974).
24. McNamara, M. K., Ward, R. E., and Kohler, H. Monoclonal idiotype vaccine against *Streptococcus pneumoniae* infections. *Science*, **226**, 1325–6 (1984).
25. Mosier, D. E., Zaldivar, N. M., Goldings, E., Mond, J., Scher, J., and Paul, W. E. Formation of antibody in the newborn mouse: study of T-cell-independent antibody response. *J. Infect. Dis.*, **136**, 14–19 (1977).
26. Mosier, D. E., Zitron, J. M., Mond, J. J., Ahmed, A., Scher, J., and Paul, W. E. Surface immunoglobulin D as a functional receptor for a subclass of B lymphocytes. *Immunological Rev.*, **27**, 89–104 (1977).
27. Nepom, J. T., Werner, H. L., Dichter, M. A., Tarchien, M., Spriggs, D. R., Graunn, C. F., Powers, M. L., Fields, B. N., and Greene, M. J. Identification of a hemagglutinin-specific idiotype associated with reovirus recognition shared by lymphoid and neural cells. *J. Exp. Med.*, **115**, 155–67 (1982).
28. Nishinarita, S., Claflin, J. L., and Lieberman, R. IgA isotype restricted idiotypes associated with T15 Id^+ PC antibodies. *J. Immunol.*, **134**, 2544–9 (1985).
29. Nisonoff, A., and Lamoyi, E. Hypothesis. Implications of the presence of an internal image of the antigen in anti-idiotypic antibodies: possible applications to vaccine production. *Clin. Immunol. Immunopathol.*, **21**, 397–406 (1981).
30. Peltola, H., Käythy, H., Sivonen, A., and Mäkelä, P. H. *Haemophilus influenzae* in children: a double-blind field study of 100 000 vaccinees 3 months to 5 years of age in Finland. *Pediatrics*, **60**, 730–7 (1977).
31. Perlmutter, R. M., Hansburg, D., Briles, D. E., Nicolotti, R. A., and Davie, J. M. Subclass restriction of murine anti-carbohydrate antibodies. *J. Immunol.*, **121**, 566–72 (1978).
32. Reagan, K. J., Wurmer, W. H., Wiktor, T. J., and Koprowski, H. Anti-idiotypic antibodies induce neutralizing antibodies to rabies virus glycoproteins. *J. Virol.*, **48**, 660–6 (1983).
33. Robbins, J. B. Vaccines for the prevention of encapsulated bacterial diseases: current status, problems and prospects for the future. *Immunochemistry*, **15**, 839–54 (1978).
34. Roitt, I. M., Thanavala, Y. M., Male, D. K., and Hay, F. C. Anti-idiotypes

as surrogate antigens: structural considerations. *Immunology Today*, **6**, 265–7 (1985).
35. Rubinstein, L. J., Bonilla, F. A., Manheimer, A. J., and Bona, C. A. Characterization of immunochemical and molecular properties of monoclonal anti-idiotypic antibody carrying the internal image of bacterial levan. In *High Technology Route to Virus Vaccines*, Houston, American Society for Microbiology, Washington DC, pp. 167–77, 1985.
36. Sacks, D. L., Esser, K. M., and Scher, A. Immunization of mice against African trypanosomiasis using anti-idiotypic antibodies. *J. Exp. Med.*, **155**, 1108–19 (1982).
37. Schuler, W., Weiler, E., and Kolb, H. Characterization of syngeneic anti-idiotypic antibody against the idiotypic antibody against the idiotype of BALB/c myeloma protein J558. *Eur. J. Immunol.*, **7**, 649–59 (1977).
38. Sege, K., and Peterson, P. Use of anti-idiotypic antibodies as cell-surface receptor probes. *Proc. Natl. Acad. Sci. USA*, **75**, 2443–7 (1978).
39. Söderström, T., Brinton, C. C. Jr, Fusco, P., Karpas, A., Ahlstedt, S., Stein, K., Sutton, A., Hosea, S., Schneerson, R., and Hanson, L. Å. Analysis of pilus-mediated pathogenic mechanisms with monoclonal antibodies. In *Microbiology – 1982* (ed. D. Schlessinger), American Society for Microbiology, Washington DC, 1982, pp. 305–7.
40. Söderström, T., Stein, K., Brinton, C. C. Jr, Hosea, S., Burch, C., Hansson, H. A., Karpas, A., Schneerson, R., Sutton, A., Vann, W. J., and Hanson, L. Å. Serological and functional properties of monoclonal antibodies to *Escherichia coli* type 1 pilus and capsular antigens. *Progr. Allergy*, **33**, 259–74 (1983).
41. Stein, K. E. Network regulation of the immune response to bacterial polysaccharide antigens. In *Images of Biologically Active Structures in the Immune System* (ed. H. Koprowski and F. Melchers), Current Topics in Microbiology and Immunology, Vol. 119, Springer Verlag, Berlin 1985, pp. 57–74.
42. Stein, K. E., Bona, C., Lieberman, R., Chien, C. C., and Paul, W. E. Regulation of the anti-inulin antibody response by a nonallotype-linked gene. *J. Exp. Med.*, **151**, 1088–102 (1980).
43. Stein, K. E., and Söderström, T. Neonatal administration of idiotype or anti-idiotype primes for protection against *Escherichia coli* K13 infection in mice. *J. Exp. Med.*, **160**, 1001–11 (1984).
44. Trenkner, E., and Riblet, R. Induction of antiphosphorylcholine antibody formation by anti-idiotypic antibodies. *J. Exp. Med.*, **142**, 1121–32 (1975).
45. Urbain, J., Wikler, M., Franssen, J. D., and Collignon, C. Idiotypic regulation of the immune system by the induction of antibodies against antiidiotypic antibodies. *Proc. Natl. Acad. Sci., USA*, **74**, 5126–31 (1977).
46. Vann, W. F., Söderström, T., Egan, W., Tsui, F.-P., Schneerson, R., Orskov, J., and Orskov, F. Serological chemical and structural analyses of the *Escherichia coli* cross-reactive capsular polysaccharides K13, K20 and K23. *Infect. Immun.*, **39**, 623–9 (1983).
47. Wikler, M., and Urbain, J. Idiotypic manipulation of the rabbit immune response against *Micrococcus luteus*. In *Idiotypi in Biology and Medicine* (ed. H. Kohler, J. Urbain and P. A. Cazenave), Academic Press, New York, 1984, pp. 219–41.
48. Yount, W. J., Dorner, M. M., Kunkel, H. G., and Kabat, E. A. Studies on human antibodies. VI. Selective variations in subgroup composition and genetic markers. *J. Exp. Med.*, **127**, 633–46 (1968).

DISCUSSION – Chaired by Dr J. Howard

MOSIER: I would like to clarify two points and ask a question. One has to do with the ordering of expression of V-region changes in the mouse. You implied that there was a discrete order with 3′ V regions being expressed first. To my knowledge, that is only true for the Ly-1 B-cell subset and it is certainly not true for conventional B cells, even in the neonatal mouse. Also the order of V_H gene expression, while it begins with the 81X gene, the most 3′ member, is non-random but certainly not in the gene order thereafter. The second most frequently expressed family is the J558 family, which is many hundreds of kilobases 5′ of the 81X gene. The second point I wanted to make was to emphasize that the use of anti-idiotypes in place of antigens has some possible drawbacks. Certainly in the mouse, injection of the anti-T15 idiotype, the idiotype that recognizes phosphorocholine (PC), during the neotnatal period leads to a lifelong suppression of the ability to make anti-PC antibodies and, in our experience, there is simply no time at which that anti-idiotype will prime for an anti-PC response. The final question I had was that you suggested that the anti-idiotype that you administered might be working *via* an anti-idiotypic T-helper cell or an idiotypic T-helper cell. Do you have any evidence for that hypothesis?

SÖDERSTRÖM: As to the last point, I must have been unclear since anti-idiotypic priming in some models has been suggested to prime idiotype-specific B cells.

ROBBINS: If anti-idiotypes were considered as vaccines for humans, would you envisage that they would have to be homologous or heterologous anti-antibodies? The second question is, can you induce a booster or, if you will, a secondary response with anti-idiotypes?

SÖDERSTRÖM: We have analysed the appearance of antibodies and see only small differences in the total levels of anti-Kl3 between the groups. There is, however, a significant difference in the levels of the protective 150 C8 idiotype. We are currently looking at booster effects and also at the effects on secretory immunity using these anti-idiotypic antibodies.

CAPRON: I wonder if you would like, both Dr Geysen and yourself, to comment on what seems difficult to reconcile in the present state of our knowledge concerning anti-idiotypes and what we heard yesterday about mimotopes? In other words, it's currently admitted that anti-idiotype antibody would represent conformational structure which would mimic the antigen, and we were told yesterday that it was possible to produce linear cathidic structures which would also mimic this antigen. Would you like to comment on that, Dr Geysen?

GEYSEN: I think the major issue is: what's the necessity for the fidelity of the conformation of the antigen? I would argue that, if all the evidence that we look at says that the antigen that is normally responded to is responded to effectively with a different conformation, then you see it normally, let's say its low energy state however it circulates. If that is really true, then, clearly, conformation isn't important. It doesn't matter what the conformation is, the conformation will be effectively generated during the interaction at the time of the immune response to that particular antigen and I would argue that that means that it doesn't matter whether your antigen has a defined structure to start with, or whether it has no structure to start with. As long as one part of the equation has some structure, then thermodynamics tell you that, if the two interact, the half of the equation that has a structure will act as sink for the correct conformation. So that, effectively, a conformation-free peptide will fold into the cavity, without worrying about the conformation and, at the same time, something that already has a conformation will have its conformation altered as it also binds with the cavity. Now, all I can add to support that is that we've demonstrated that we get exactly the same response as analysed by the set of analogues, searching for contact residues, when we start from an epitope that is part of, say, a structured virus and from a small heptapeptide. They give indistinguishable responses as far as the immune response to those two very different structured antigens are concerned. So I don't really see it as a conflict, I think that it doesn't matter whether you start with a structured antigen or whether you start with an unstructured antigen. You will get what the immune response is prepared to give you and nothing else.

SÖDERSTRÖM: The idiotypic (anti-K13) antibodies had a profound effect in our model. Synthetic idiotypes would be an alternative vaccine approach. Such structures may be easier to handle than anti-idiotypic antibodies because of less risk of inducing suppression. Maybe part of the high efficacy of the protein–protein interaction, in comparison to the protein–carbohydrate interaction, may relate to the lower hydrophilicity of proteins.

CAPRON: Did you have any evidence of a particular antibody isotype which was produced in your Ab2 immunized animals? Preferential isotypic production?

SÖDERSTRÖM: This work is in progress, as is determination of the affinity of the antibodies.

CAPRON: Any adjuvant being used for immunization?

SÖDERSTRÖM: No.

HANDMAN: Is there any cross-reaction between the carbohydrates present on the original antibodies that you inject and the *E. coli* polysaccharides?

SÖDERSTRÖM: Well, you saw the structure of the K13 antigen. Does anyone know whether similar carbohydrates can be found on antibodies?

HANDMAN: But I am saying, are you in actual fact inducing an antibody to a carbohydrate determinant shared between the original antibody that you inject and the *E. coli* carbohydrate, and that is why it works?

ROBBINS: Well, if the antibody in this study, or the anti-idiotype is reacting with the polysaccharide that induced the anti-antibody . . .
SÖDERSTRÖM: We have no evidence that the anti-idiotype is interacting with the carbohydrate part of the idiotype.
HANDMAN: Right, that is what I am asking, basically.
GRIFFISS: The best evidence that that wouldn't be the case is, at least for IgG in man and rabbits, that the oligosaccharides are invariate among different antibody molecules and do not contain KDO. They are primarily high-mannose bi-antennary structures that end NeuNAc-(2 → 6)GalGlcNAc. That is the terminal trisaccharide on each branch. IgG and IgM have some galactose residues on binding site areas, but they are usually either mono or disaccharides, and it seems unlikely that they could function as antigens.
SÖDERSTRÖM: It was mentioned yesterday that one rarely sees precipitating monoclonal antibodies. The anti-idiotype and idiotype in the K13 system form precipitin lines in agarose.
ADA: John Robbins asked a question which wasn't answered. Let's talk just for one minute about the possibility of using anti-idiotypes as vaccines, which was behind John Robbins's question. The first question you asked was, would you use the homologous population? Would it be necessary to use human instead of the murine immunoglobulins? That is a very important question which needs to be answered. Secondly, even if you could do that, how practical is it to use anti-idiotypes as vaccines? Would somebody care to comment on those two points?
SÖDERSTRÖM: Polysaccharide responses are, probably not without reason, strictly regulated which could also make you pessimistic about the practical use of anti-idiotypes as alternative vaccines. On the other hand, they offer unique tools for immune intervention. At this stage of knowledge, the question about heterologous or homologous antibodies may not be so important.
ROBBINS: In consideration of a heterologous source of anti-idiotype antibodies as vaccines, it would be difficult for me to see how you would avoid inducing an immune response to the inducer which would make use of any other anti-idiotype, from that species at least or related species, no longer useful. The recipient would have an antibody to the inducing substance. If the anti-idiotype is from the human source acceptable for human experimentation (control of malignant or carcinogens being transformed along with them), what advantage would it have over using the antigen itself? I can't see the advantage of using an anti-idiotype over using the antigen presented in a more effective way. It seems to me that it is reacting the same way as an antigen, it is an antigen, only it is in the form of an antibody, made by a clever and ingenious way. Its action is that of an antigen, it combines with the receptor molecule which is an antibody on the surface of the cell. Presumably this anti-idiotype stimulation caps the membrane antibody which alters the structure of the membrane so that the intracellular metabolism of the

antibody-producing cell is activated. So I think anti-idiotypes are another form of an antigen, an ingenious one, but I don't see that this type of antigen has any advantage over the antigen itself.
SÖDERSTRÖM: If it is true that different antibodies with the same specificity but of different isotypes or different subclasses utilize different V_H genes and that the products differ qualitatively, it could be important to try to influence which type of antibodies are being produced. Also, there is evidence in other experimental models indicating that anti-idiotypic structures can prime in situations where antigens cannot; you know about the results in the Lyb5-positive and -negative cells indicating that anti-idiotypic structures can activate before the environmental antigens have tolerized this cell population. If this is true, there could be important differences between the response induced by an internal image as compared to the actual antigen.

MOSIER: I would just like to amplify on one or two points that you made, Dr Söderström. The primary advantage of an anti-idiotype vaccine, if you wish, is that it can engage a B cell that would not normally respond to carbohydrate. To my knowledge, all such idiotype or anti-idiotype primed responses are T-dependent and you in essence convert what would naturally be a T-independent antigen into a T-dependent form. A consequence of this is that heterologous anti-idiotypes are very much more potent at inducing B-cell priming than are homologous anti-idiotypes because they engender T-helper cells which recognize the heterologous immunoglobulin. Of course, there are many complications one can envisage of using heterologous anti-idiotypes in humans. On the other hand, one can genetically engineer a mouse variable region to a human constant region and get around most of the anti-heterologous protein response in the human but, by doing so, one again loses the advantage of some of the T-cell priming. So, while there are very many attractive aspects to this kind of approach to vaccine production, there are still some very thorny problems to be solved about how to actually use this in man.
SÖDERSTRÖM: We are collaborating with molecular biologists who are trying to produce clones utilizing the Fab part of mouse antibodies and the Fc part of human antibodies.
ROBBINS: I see no advantage provided by the use of anti-idiotypes over that by using the specific polysaccharide antigen presented in T-dependent form.
ADA: There is one other advantage in using an anti-idiotype as an alternative approach and that is when you can't produce enough of an antigen to make a vaccine.
SÖDERSTRÖM: I think that there may be additional reasons why one would consider utilizing this type of structure. The experiments should be done, comparing the responses following the administration of polysaccharides, conjugates, anti-idiotypes and idiotypes, looking in detail into isotype distri-

bution of the responses, the possibility to boost and the protective capacity of the antibodies.

Part III: Disease Agents and Current Prophylaxis

Towards Better Carbohydrate Vaccines
Edited by R. Bell and G. Torrigiani

Published by John Wiley & Sons Ltd

11

The pathogenetic basis of the distribution and epidemiology of diseases caused by encapsulated bacteria

J. McLeod Griffiss
The Centre for Immunochemistry and the Departments of Laboratory Medicine and Medicine University of California, San Francisco, CA 94143, USA

INTRODUCTION

Any discussion of the epidemiology of diseases caused by encapsulated bacteria must be based on the pathogenic potential conferred upon these bacteria by their capsules. In the simplest terms, capsular polysaccharides interfere with complement-mediated clearance of bacteria from the bloodstream [2, 6, 15, 19, 22, 29], but the molecular mechanism(s) by which, and the degree to which, they interfere varies greatly among different polysaccharides [19, 29].

Because capsules are highly polar and hydrophilic, they interfere with cell-to-cell interactions and are antiphagocytic [28]. When functionally deposited on to the cell surface, C3b components of complement form ligands that bind bacteria to the phagocytic cell surface through specific receptors and despite encapsulation [2, 21]. Antibodies binding to capsules negate charge and hydrophilicity, and may activate complement [22, 28]. The Fc regions of certain antibodies may also act as bacterial-cell-to-phagocytic-cell ligands [28]. *Neisseria meningitidis* of certain capsular serogroups and *Haemophilus influenzae* type b are not efficiently cleared through opsonophagocytic mechanisms. Their clearance requires insertion into their outer membranes of the membrane attack complex of activated C5–C9 and consequent immune lysis.

Most capsular polysaccharides confer no pathogenic potential; others do so only for infants [5, 14, 21, 25, 31]. A very few are potentially pathogenetic for individuals of any age who lack antibodies specific for them or for alternative surface antigens of the bacteria they encapsulate [11, 14]. Immunologically, some resemble common molecular species of the human and are not immunogenic: notably the 2 → 8 sialic acid capsule of Group B *N. meningitidis* and Kl *Escherichia coli*, the hyaluronic acid capsule of Group A *Streptococcus pyogenes* and the heparin-like capsule of K5 *E. coli* [14]. For these bacteria immunity depends upon antibody to alternative antigens [11, 14].

ANTI-COMPLEMENTARITY

Some polysaccharides are able to bind the first component of complement (Clq) directly, thereby generating surface-bound C3b through the classical pathway (CP) [21]; others require that antibody bind to them before the CP is activated [22]. Molecules of C3b that are spontaneously generated by the slow decay of circulating C3 (tick-over effect) randomly adhere to cell surfaces (alternative pathway (ACP)). Regardless of the pathway through which they are generated, deposited C3b attract and bind additional components. If either additional C3b or Bb molecules are bound, the CP or ACP C3 convertases are respectively formed and more C3b molecules generated ('up-regulation' of activation). Binding of H disassembles the ACP convertase, whereas that of I further cleaves bound C3b to inactive fragments ('down-regulation') [21–2].

Polysaccharides influence the affinity with which H binds to C3b and thus regulate whether Bb (up-regulation) or H (down-regulation) binds to deposited C3b [8]. Anti-complementarity, or down-regulation, has been demonstrated for both fluid-phase and cell-bound polysaccharides, and for both pathways of complement activation [7, 8, 15, 19]. Different polysaccharides vary in their ability to down-regulate complement activation, and this variation has chemical specificity that is separate from antigenic specificity [15, 19].

Both antibody and complement molecules recognize fine chemical structures, but they do not recognize the same structures. As the various polysaccharides are denominated by antigenic structure, the relationship of chemical structure to anti-complementarity is often obscured. For example, the capsules of Groups A and C *N. meningitidis* and of type III, Group B streptococcus, are equally able, on a weight basis, to interfere with complement, but the polysaccharide of Group B *N. meningitidis* is twice as effective as the other three [19]. A similar hierarchy of anti-complementarity explains differences in pathogenic potential among serotypes of *H. influenzae* [29].

The chemical specificity of down-regulation of the ACP appears to reside in carbonyl groups (acetyl substituents) [8, 19, 30]. Circulating polysaccharides decomplement the ACP of neonates during the pathogenesis of *E. coli* K1/ Group B *N. meningitidis*, and type III, Group B streptococcal disease [7, 14, 23].

EFFECT OF ANTIBODY

When antibody binds to a polysaccharide it may up-regulate complement activation and facilitate complement-mediated clearance [2, 22]. Whether or not an antibody facilitates clearance is a function in part of its molecular structure, as indicated by isotype, and in part of the site to which it binds. IgA molecules not only do not initiate complement-mediated immune effector mechanisms, but block their initiation by antibodies of other isotypes or by the cell surface directly [10, 12, 13, 17, 18]. Certain IgG isotypes active complement poorly and may not facilitate complement-mediated clearance. The most effective antibodies are those that bind to, or adjacent to, the chemical structures of the polysaccharides that down-regulate complement. Such antibodies mask the effector moiety, and substitute complement-binding sites within their molecular structures. Antibody molecules binding to structures removed from the sites of complement regulation probably have little if any effect on clearance.

The surface of a bacterium contains structures other than capsules that together constitute 'sub-capsular' or somatic antigens [11, 14]. For gram-negative bacteria, these molecules are the principal outer membrane glycolipids (lipopolysaccharides and lipo-oligosaccharides) and certain proteins, primarily the porin proteins [27, 32]. The lipo-oligosaccharides of *H. influenzae* and *N. meningitidis* provide an alternative set of carbohydrate antigens, the immunochemistry and pathogenic potential of which is only beginning to be explored [26, 27]. It is clear that these molecules are involved in pathogenesis [26] and that they largely determine the epidemiology and distribution of encapsulated bacteria that cause disease [11, 14, 23]. Antibodies binding sub-capsular determinants probably serve the same function and contribute to macro-epidemiology in the same way as those binding to capsular polysaccharides.

The pathogenesis of diseases caused by encapsulated bacteria, then, is a complex interaction between the variable expression of complement-regulating carbohydrate moieties on the cell surface; quantitative and qualitative variations in circulating complement components; and the presence or absence of antibodies that bind to the various carbohydrate moieties and variously effect their regulation of complement activation.

EFFECT OF AGE

The pathogenetic potential of capsular polysaccharides varies with the age of the host [3, 5, 14, 20, 25, 31]. Certain polysaccharides confer pathogenic potential to bacteria only when they colonize during the first month of life. Others are pathogenetic only for infants, for older children or for individuals at either extreme of life. In general, those capsules that provide pathogenic potential to bacteria colonizing neonates are non-immunogenic in adults or in the subset of women who give birth to susceptible infants. Group B streptococci, *E. coli* K1/Group B *N. meningitidis*, and type 5 *Streptococcus pneumoniae*, fall into this category [5, 14, 25, 31]. Other polysaccharides are immunogenic in older children and adults of childbearing age, but poorly in infancy. Bacteria bearing these polysaccharides cause disease during a 'window' of susceptibility between the decay of maternal antibody and the development of autonomous immunity. *H. influenzae* type b, Group C *N. meningitidis* and several of the pneumococcal serotypes fall into this category [14, 15, 21, 29]. Still other capsules induce poorly effective antibody during colonization, and the organisms they encapsulate remain pathogenic for life. Group A *N. meningitidis* and several pneumococcal serotypes are in this category.

As a result of age-specific differences in their immunochemistry, the distribution of disease-associated capsular polysaccharides within each pathogenic genus varies with the age of the population surveyed [14].

ENVIRONMENTAL EFFECTS

Environmental factors subtly affect the pathogenetic influence of capsules. Ecological conditioning of a population can permit outbreaks to occur, shift the age at which bacteria bearing certain polysaccharides cause disease [14] and even make possible causation of disease by poorly pathogenic capsular types [4, 5, 11, 20].

Epidemics of disease caused by encapsulated bacteria are time and space delimited [4, 11]. That is, they occur within a certain ecological focus, the epidemic environment, in which the necessary immunological conditioning takes place. Within this environment a single strain (clonotype), denoted by both capsular and often sub-capsular antigens, and called the epidemic strain, expresses the ability to cause disease among individuals who prior to, and after, the epidemic evidenced no susceptibility to it [1, 4, 11, 14, 16].

Ecological conditioning is most apparent in the epidemiology of Group A meningococcal disease in the African Sahel. In any area outbreaks occur at roughly 10 year intervals, but the distribution of disease in an area is not uniform. During the most recent outbreak in The Gambia, rates of disease in villages situated within 2 km of one another varied from 0 to 10% of the total population. Disease occurred in older children and young adults and spared infants <2 years of age. As is typical in the Sahel, disease occurrence abruptly stopped at the onset of the rains, only to reoccur during the following dry season. Carriage and transmission of the epidemic strain did not vary among villages or with the seasons. Thus, susceptibility to the pathogenetic influence of the Group A capsule varied with age, climate and immediate environment, despite constant exposure.

Epidemics can be recognized by an upward shift in the age-specific incidence of disease within a demographically delimited population, and by the emergence of the epidemic strain [14]. An upward shift in age-specific incidence occurs during epidemics caused by all capsular types, but as endemic age-specific incidences vary among types, the shift can be missed until the capsular type of the epidemic strain is appreciated [4].

Environmental conditioning way also shift downward the age-specific distribution of bacterial serotypes causing disease in a population. The incidence of disease caused by *H. influenzae* peaks in the United States of America and Europe in infants between 12 and 24 months of age, but in those 7 and 8 months of age in Africa [3, 5, 20]. As a similar, but slightly less pronounced, downward shift in the age-specific incidence of *Haemophilus* disease occurs among native Americans and Eskimos in the USA, it is unlikely to be genetically determined.

As we would expect, economic development alters the distribution of disease-associated capsules. In many less-developed areas, the lower serotypes, particularly 1, are the predominant causes of pneumococcal disease and Group A that of meningococcal disease [3, 5, 20]. In developed countries it is the higher serotypes of the pneumococcus that routinely cause disease, particularly in children [21], and Group A meningococci cause only occasional focal outbreaks [4].

As a result of environmental differences, capsular polysaccharide vaccines developed for use in economically advanced countries are less useful in less-developed areas. The polysaccharide vaccine that successfully controlled outbreaks of Group A meningococcal disease in Finland and the USA, has provided little enduring benefit in the Sahel [4, 24].

EFFECT OF POLYMICROBIAL PRESENTATION OF CARBOHYDRATE ANTIGENS

The same, or immunologically indistinguishable antigens can be expressed by several different bacteria that normally colonize different anatomic sites

[9, 11]. In fact, most antibody to capsular polysaccharides is not acquired during encounters with potentially pathogenic bacteria, but during those with non-pathogenic bacteria that bear the same antigens. In the epidemic environment, enteric colonization by 'cross-reactive' bacteria is the rule [9, 11], and it is thought that faecal–oral spread of these bacteria conditions the population to express epidemic susceptibility by inducing circulating IgA [9–13, 17, 18]. In this setting, the epidemic strain will express the cross-reacting antigen [9, 11, 33]. This phenomenon was clearly shown during an outbreak of Group A, type L10 meningococcal disease among Skid Row *habitués* in the USA Pacific North-west [9, 11, 33]. A strain of *Streptococcus faecalis* that bears both the Group A capsular polysaccharide and the L10 lipooligosaccharide antigens enterally colonized the population at the same prevalence (4%) as the epidemic meningococcal strain [4, 9].

EFFECT OF VARIATIONS IN PREVALENCE OF ANTIBODY

Regardless of how it is required, the age-specific prevalence of antibody varies in any population [14]. As a result, the prevalence of disease caused by bacteria bearing the corresponding antigens varies counter-cyclically [33]. For example, the prevalence of type 2 pneumococcal disease in Dakar, Senegal, varied from 0 to 11.6% of all cases of pneumococcal disease between 1977 and 198s, whereas that of type 5 pneumococcal disease varied from 1.1 to 16%. Data such as these make clear that the distribution or prevalence of capsules associated with disease in an area cannot be predicted from data pooled from various parts of the world and from different times.

SUMMARY

The distribution of disease-associated bacterial capsular polysaccharides is a function of the immunoepidemiology of these antigens and of the pathogenic potential that they confer on a bacterium. In the absence of maternally derived antibody, an infant must rely on complement alone to clear invading bacteria and the relative ability of capsular polysaccharides to down-regulate complement determines their prevalence. Some polysaccharides are not immunogenic, and levels of maternal antibody specific for immunogenic ones vary over time in a cyclical fashion. Disease distribution reflects this. Bacteria bearing non-immunogenic capsules cause disease during infancy; the capsule-specific incidences of diseases in older children vary counter-cyclically with levels of antibody in the population. Populations with adequate levels of immunity against one bacterium can be rendered susceptible by enteric co-colonization with a different bacterium that bears similar antigens and induces circulating IgA. In that setting, the antigens of the cross-reacting bacteria determine the distribution of capsular and sub-capsular disease-associated antigens. Finally, the ecology of developed countries tends to shift upward the age-specific incidences of diseases, delays the acquisition of specific antibody and renders unlikely disease caused by bacteria bearing certain capsules. Vaccine-development programmes must take into account these time and place differences and the immunoepidemiology that determines them.

REFERENCES

1. Broud, D. D., Griffiss, J. McL., and Baker, C. J. Heterogeneity of serotypes of *Neisseria meningitidis* causing endemic disease. *J. Infect. Dis.*, **140**, 465–70 (1979).
2. Brown, E. J., Hosea, S. W., and Frank, M. M. The role of antibody and complement in the reticuloendothelial clearance of pneumococci from the bloodstream. *Rev. Infect. Dis.*, **5**, 5797–805 (1983).
3. Cadoz, M., Denis, F., and Mar, I. D. Etude épidémiologique des cas de méningites purulentes hospitalisés à Dakar pendant la décennie 1970–1979. *Bull. Org. Mond. Santé*, **59**, 575–84 (1981).
4. Counts, G. W., Gregory, D. F., Spearman, J. G., Lee, B. A., Filice, G. A., Holmes, K. K., and Griffiss, J.McL. Group A meningococcal disease in the U.S. Pacific Northwest: epidemiology, clinical features, and effect of a vaccination control program. *Ref. Infect. Dis.*, **6**, 640–8 (1984).
5. Denis, F. A., Greenwood, B. D., Rey, J. L., Prince-David, M., M Boup, S., Lloyd-Evans, N., Williams, K., Benbachir, I., El Ndaghri, N., Hansman, D., Omanga, V., Krubwa, K., Duchassin, M., and Perrin, J. Etude multicentrique des serotypes de pneumocoques en Afrique. *Bull. Org. Mond. Santé*, **61**, 661–9 (1983).
6. Di Ninno, V. L., and Chenier, V. K. Activation of complement by *Neisseria meningitidis. FEMS Microbiol. Lett.*, **12**, 55–60 (1981).
7. Edwards, M. S., Nicholson-Weller, A., Baker, C. J., and Kasper, D. L. The role of the alternative complement pathway in opsonophagocytosis of type III, group B streptococcus. *J. Exp. Med.*, **151**, 1275–87 (1980).
8. Fearon, D. T. Regulation by membrane sialic acid of β1H-dependent decay-dissociation of amplification C3 convertase of the alternative complement pathway. *Proc. Natl. Acad. Sci. USA*, **75**, 1971–5 (1978).
9. Filice, G. A., Hayes, P. S., Counts, G. A., Griffiss, J. McL., and Fraser, D. W. Risk of group A meningococcal diseases: bacterial interference and cross-reactive bacteria among mucosal flora. *J. Clin. Microbiol.*, **22**, 152–6 (1985).
10. Griffiss, J. McL. Bactericidal activity of meningococcal antisera: blocking by IgA of lytic antibody in human convalescent sera. *J. Immunol.*, **114**, 1779–84 (1975).
11. Griffiss, J. McL. Epidemic meningococcal disease: synthesis of a hypothetical immunoepidemiologic model. *Rev. Infect. Dis.*, **4**, 159–71 (1982).
12. Griffiss, J. McL. Biologic function of the serum IgA system: modulation of complement-mediated effector mechanisms and conservation of antigenic mass. *Ann. NY. Acad. Sci.*, **409**, 697–707 (1983).
13. Griffiss, J. McL., and Bertram, M. A. Immunoepidemiology of meningococcal disease in military recruits. II. Blocking of serum bactericidal activity by circu-

lating IgA early in the course of invasive disease. *J. Infect. Dis.*, **136**, 733–9 (1977).
14. Griffiss, J. McL., and Brandt, B. L. Nonepidemic (endemic) meningococcal disease: pathogenetic factors and clinical features. In *Current Clinical Topics in Infectious Diseases* (ed. J. S. Remington and M. N. Swartz), McGraw-Hill, New York, 1986, pp. 27–50.
15. Griffiss, J. McL., Brandt, B. L., Broud, D. D., Goroff, D. K., and Baker, C. J. Immune response of infants and children to disseminated *Neisseria meningitidis* infection. *J. Infect. Dis.*, **150**, 71–9 (1984).
16. Griffiss, J. McL., Broud, D. D., Silver, C. A., and Artenstein, M. S. Immunoepidemiology of meningococcal disease in military recruits. I. A model for serogroup independency of epidemic potential as determined by serotyping. *J. Infect. Dis.*, **136**, 176–86 (1977).
17. Griffiss, J. McL., and Goroff, D. K. IgA blocks IgM and IgG-initiated immune lysis by separate molecular mechanisms. *J. Immunol.*, **130**, 2882–5 (1983).
18. Griffiss, J. McL., and Jarvis, G. A. Interaction of serum IgA with complement components: the molecular basis of IgA blockade. In *Proceedings of the International Congress of Mucosal Immunology*, 29 June–3 July 1986, Niagara Falls, New York, 1986, in press.
19. Griffiss, J. McL., Schecter, S., Eads, M. M., Yamasaki, R., and Jarvis, G. A. Regulation of complement activation on bacterial surfaces. In *Proceedings of the 10th International Convocation on Immunology*, 14–17 July 1986, Buffalo, New York, 1986, in press.
20. Guirguis, N., Hafez, K., El Kholy, M. A. Robbins, J. B., and Gotschlich, E. C. Bacterial meningitis in Egypt: analysis of CSF isolates from hospital patients in Cairo, 1977–78. *Bull. WHO.* **61**, 517–24 (1983).
21. Hostetter, M. K. Serotypic variations among virulent pneumococci in deposition and degradation of covalently bound C3b: implications for phagocytosis and antibody production. *J. Infect. Dis.*, **153**, 682–93 (1986).
22. Jarvis, G. A., and Vedros, N. A. Sialic acid of group B *Neisseria meningitidis* regulates alternative complement pathway activation. *Infect. Immun.*, 55, 174–80 (1987).
23. Levy, N. J., Nicholson-Weller, A., Baker, C. J., and Kasper, D. L. Potentiation of virulence by group B streptococcal polysaccharides. *J. Infect. Dis.*, **149**, 851–60 (1984).
24. Reingold, A. L., Broome, C. V. Hightower, A. W., Ajello, G. W., Bolan, G. A., Adamsbaum, C., Jones, E. E., Phillips, C., Tiendrebeogo, H., and Yada, A. Age-specific differences in duration of clinical protection after vaccination with meningococcal polysaccharide A vaccine. *Lancet*, **2**, 114–18 (1985).
25. Robbins, J. B., McCracken, G. H., Gotschlich, E. C. Ørskov, F., Ørskov, I., and Hanson, L. A. *Escherichia coli* K1 capsular polysaccharide associated with neonatal meningitidis. *N. Engl. J. Med.*, **290**, 1216–20 (1974).
26. Schneider, H., Griffiss, J. McL., Mandrell, R. E., and Jarvis, G. A. Elaboration of a 3.6-kilodalton lipooligosaccharide, antibody against which is absent from human sera, is associated with serum resistance of *Neisseria gonorrhoeae. Infect. Immun.*, **50**, 672–7 (1985).
27. Schneider, H., Hale, T. L., Zollinger, W. D., Seid, R. C. Jr, Hammack, C. A., and Griffiss, J. McL. Heterogeneity of molecular size and antigenic expression within the lipooligosaccharides of individual strains of *Neisseria gonorrhoeae* and *N. meningitidis. Infect. Immun.*, **45**, 544–9 (1984).
28. Stendahl, O., Tagesson, C., and Edebo, L. Influence of hyperimmune immuno-

globulin G on the physico-chemical properties of the surface of *Salmonella typhimurium* 395 MS in relation to interaction with phagocytic cells. *Infect. Immun.*, **10**, 316–1 (1974).
29. Sutton, A., Schneerson, R., Kendall-Morris, S., and Robbins, J. B. Differential complement resistance mediates virulence of *Haemophilus influenzae* type b. *Infect. Immun.*, **35**, 95–104 (1982).
30. Varki, A., and Kornfeld, S. An autosomal dominant gene regulates the extent of 9-0-acetylation of murine erythrocyte sialic acids. A probable explanation for the variation in capacity to activate the human alternate complement pathway. *J. Exp. Med.*, **152**, 532–44 (1980).
31. Wilkinson, H. W., Facklam, R. R., and Wortham, E. C. Distribution by serologic type of group B streptococci isolated from a variety of clinical material over a five-year period (with special reference to neonatal sepsis and meningitis). *Infect. Immun.*, **8**, 228–35 (1973).
32. Wilson, M. E., and Morrison, D. C. Evidence for different requirements in physical state for the interaction of lipopolysaccharides with the classical and alternative pathways of complement. *Eur. J. Biochem.*, **128**, 137–41 (1982).
33. Yamasaki, R., O'Brien, J. P. Mandrell, R. E., Schneider, H., Ruis, N., Sugasawara, R. J., Sippel, J. E., and Griffiss, J. McL. Lipooligosaccharides (LOS) of individual strains of *Neisseria meningitidis* consist of multiple discrete oligosaccharides that account for LOS M_r heterogeneity, antigenic and serotypic diversity and epidemiologic relatedness. In *The Pathogenic Neisseriae: Proceedings of the Fourth International Symposium* (ed. G. K. Schoolnik, G. F. Brooks, S. Falkow, C. E. Frasch, J. S. Knapp, J. A. McCutchan and S. A. Morse), American Society for Microbiology, Washington, DC, 1985, pp. 550–5.

DISCUSSION – Chaired by Professor A. Capron

JENNINGS: The actual structural basis of the inhibition of complement activation in all the polysaccharides you have shown on your slide could be that each one of them contains terminal sialic acid. It is from previous work with bacterial erythrocytes that terminal sialic acid is able to function as an inhibitor of complement activation. Of interest would be that, if you acetylated the terminal sialic acid, this might also modify the complement activation. One of the things I would like to suggest is you could actually test this hypothesis in an experiment involving the partial peroxidation of the B polysaccharide where, by specifically destroying the polysaccharide's terminal sialic acid residues, the inhibition should disappear completely.
GRIFFISS: The problem is of course that the sialic acid is also *N*-acetylated, and there is evidence that for the erythrocytes it is the *N*-acetyl group, and not the carboxyl group, that controls complement activation. What one has to be acreful of is that one reduces the carboxyl group of sialic acid preferentially over the carbonyl group of *N*-acetyl. The alternative appraoch that we use, since we are not terribly good chemists, is to use different polysaccharides, and if one recalculates those inhibitions using moles of *N*-acetyl rather than moles of carbohydrate, the polysaccharides are the same, whereas if

you use moles of sialic acid they are not. What I don't know is whether GLc–NAc and Gal–NAc invariably have the same function as Man–NAc (Group A polysaccharide), or whether it has everything to do with its chemical environment. For instance, it could well be, as you have shown, that the hydrogen bonding that may exist between the carbonyl and carboxyl carbons may, in fact, be as important as the presence of *N*-acetyl group. That is, there may be some conformational constraints on whether or not the down-regulation occurs. It is approachable though, that's the important thing.

JENNINGS: Dennis Kasper has shown that if you reduce the carboxylate on the type III Group B streptococcal polysaccharide, which also contains an *N*-acetyl, then complement activation occurs immediately. So I don't think the carbonyl of the *N*-acetyl group is an important factor.

GRIFFISS: But how could you do that without reducing the carbonyl carbon?

JENNINGS: Well, under the conditions that we use, you don't reduce the carbonyl. This is known. In model compound studies when you reduce the carboxyl, you don't reduce the carbonyl group.

GRIFFISS: In Kasper's studies, as I recall, and my lab was right next to Dennis's when he did them, he never checked to see whether, in fact, the carbonyl carbon had not been reduced under the conditions of the carbodiormide reduction he used.

JENNINGS: That may be true. It is very very difficult to verify this on the cell surface, but we've done it using the polysaccharide itself. Also, another point to remember is that the structural basis of the inhibition of complement activation is probably even more complex than that, because, if you take the example of *Haemophilus influenzae* type b, it contains neither carboxylate nor *N*-acetyl groups and yet also has the ability to inactivate complement activation.

MORENO: You believe that when you examine and compare C polysaccharide with B polysaccharide for sectional mobility in the absence of *O*-acetyl groups you are going to find results that would account for the quantitative difference in the capacity of both polysaccharides to fix complement. Is that correct?

GRIFFISS: It's theoretically correct, and the calculations that your laboratory has done suggest that it is correct. If one looks at a Driden model, there is considerable motion at those points. But if you try to measure motion by NMR, the problem is that you see an average signal from across a large molecule, and the effector moment within that molecule may be far too small to be seen in NMR spectra. So, rather than dogmatically state one way or the other, I think it is up to us to determine how $2 \rightarrow 8$ and $2 \rightarrow 9$ sialic acid homopolymers can have a shared epitope, and how they can function to down-regulate complement.

MORENO: Just a remark to follow that. It would be necessary to make the measurements with similar or very similar chain lengths because the terminal residues would have a tremendous influence. I would suggest including K92 in that analysis, if you intend to follow it up, because in *E. coli* K92 polysaccharide there are alternating $\alpha 2 \rightarrow 8$ and $\alpha 2 \rightarrow 9$ linkages and you could have both B- and C-like residues along the same molecule. As we have demonstrated, with John Lindon and R. Lifely, the mobility of the residues along that chain changes. The C-like residues are more mobile and flexible than the B-like residues.

GRIFFISS: Which is what you would predict. But it seems to me to be less than you would predict.

KABAT: There is no cross-reaction with our human anti-Group B with either of those two polysaccharides, the Group C or the alternating $\alpha 2 \rightarrow 8$, $\alpha 2 \rightarrow 9$ structure.

MORENO: That's quite correct, although in some instances you find that some anti-C polysaccharides do cross-react with K92 and we have monoclonal antibodies that do show that.

ROBBINS: We made about 12 rabbit and 1 burro hyperimmune antisera by injection of formalin-treated K92 *E. coli.* In all instances, we could only demonstrate reactivity with the Group C, the $\alpha 2 \rightarrow 9$, and none with B (α-$2 \rightarrow 8$). We thought we had an answer to the Group B problem when we identified the alternating B and C type linkages on the K93 capsular polysaccharide of *E. coli.* But it is curious that something that should have such an alternating linkage with specifically only induced antibodies that would react with the $2 \rightarrow 9$ and not with the $2 \rightarrow 9$ linkages, in addition to itself. Just to the other point, we have never seen a cross-reaction with C and B. It must be that the monoclonals may have a very specific reaction we have not observed with ordinary immunization techniques.

GRIFFISS: Actually, that is not completely true, John. From the beginning when Mal Artenstein first started this, we always found a low level of cross-reacting antibodies in the people immunized with the C polysaccharide. Mal got around this by titering the sera, before the radioactive antigen-binding assay was developed. When the RABA test was developed, it was just ignored. But if one looks carefully at those data, you find a very low level of cross-reacting antibody. The point I want to make is that we have several monoclonal antibodies that only see what you and I would call B and that do not see K1 or K92. They are very specific. We also have monoclonals that see both B and C, and we have four monoclonals that see different epitopes on C. So the point is that these polysaccharides are a basket of epitopes. It is up to us to sort that basket out and find those that are responsible for the effects we are interested in. When one starts talking about mimotope and idiotope vaccines, then this sorting process becomes a critical issue.

EASMON: To go back to the question of the age distribution of the appearance of disease, particularly in *H. influenzae*, you seem to be ascribing this entirely to possible exposure of the population from different parts of the world. I just wondered if you had taken into account the very great differences in nutritional and environmental factors. You were comparing the United States of America with Africa, and I would imagine that the African populations, as young children, are going to be in a far less satisfactory nutritional state, which might allow the disease to appear earlier, once the decrease in maternal antibody made them susceptible.

GRIFFISS: We always trot that out as an explanation for these things, but it is certainly true that conditions on Indian reservations in the USA are considerably worse than in Dakar. And it does seem to me that nutrition during the first year of life in the major cities of Africa, where they are not undergoing starvation conditions at all, is likely to be fairly good, inasmuch as it is going to be derived primarily from the mother. This would not be the case in a refugee camp somewhere in the Sahel, but in Dakar it seems unlikely that nutrition alone would do it. It also seems unlikely that it would do it in Alaska; in Eskimos who live in a far less sterile environment than in the rest of the USA, but whose nutrition is not bad.

SÖDERSTRÖM: I have two comments. In the series of monoclonal antibodies which we have raised against the meningococcal B, or the *E. coli* K1, there are a couple that also bind to the human gangliosides GD3 and GM3. We have data suggesting that some antibodies require only the terminal sialic acid for binding, whereas others require a repeated sequence. Our approach is to see if any of these monoclonal antibodies will interfere with the complement effects we heard about. Furthermore, we have raised anti-idiotypic antibodies against the ones that require the repeated sequence as well as against the one binding to terminal sialic acid. It will be interesting to see whether we have the tools to preferentially induce antibodies against terminal sialic, or against the repeated sequence using these anti-idiotypic antibodies. It may be possible to include in the idiotypic structures not only antigen but also heavy chain epitopes. This could lead to development of anti-idiotypic antibodies inducing a specific class or subclass of antigen-specific antibodies.

MÄKELÄ: You want to raise antibodies to the precise structures on the polysaccharide that are important for, for instance, down-regulation of the complement. It could be argued, on the other hand, that the repeating unit is so small that, no matter which part of it bound the antibody, as long as the antibody was tightly bound, the steric hindrance would be sufficient to prevent the function of the polysaccharide.

ROBBINS: It just occurred to me, with what Dr Söderström said, that it might be an argument for the use of an idiotypic vaccine. If there are cross-reactive structures on this very unusual and important polysaccharide that induce antibodies reactive with tissue factors, the avoiding antibodies directed to that specificity might be best accomplished with an idiotype vaccine.

SÖDERSTRÖM: That is the background for the studies I mentioned.

MORENO: But most of the antibodies produced under normal conditions against this polysaccharide do not cross-react with the glycolipids. The cross-reactivity that you are mentioning is quite unusual. We have one monoclonal antibody that was produced against meningococcal Group B polysaccharide and shows a very modest reaction with C. Most of the B specificities are probably conformational and require a three-dimensional structure. The one that you mention, it is not even a specific for the 2 → 8 linkage because, if I remember correctly, it reacted with GM1 ganglioside.
SÖDERSTRÖM: The monoclonal antibodies that we are using to induce the anti-idiotypic antibodies are protective in the infant rat model.
ROBBINS: Carlos, what is a 'modest reaction'?
MORENO: You are referring to the cross-reactivity of C? Well, simply that the agglutination, or antigen-binding capacity of the monoclonals at the same concentration of antigen was one order of magnitude lower, that is all.
SÖDERSTRÖM: Can I briefly mention that we have tried additional approaches related to the Kl antigen. As you know, there are bacteriophages specific for the K1 structure, thus in a way 'mimicking' the idiotype in specific binding to K1. We have raised antibodies against the bacteriophages as a short cut to obtain anti-idiotypic antibodies.
ROTTA: I just wish to refer to another part of your exposé, and the study of Group B streptococci. We are getting a number of strains in my laboratory for typing, and we see that a large number do carry the protein antigens, starting R, X and C, originally called 1BC. Now we call it C, because of protein antigen. I wonder whether some of the effects of the surface activation that you are talking about could not be some sort of interference by the presence of this protein antigen? I was also very interested to see the data on the frequency of pneumococcus types in different parts of the world, such as in Dakar. It is hard for me to believe that there could be such a big difference from one year to the other in the occurrence or the frequency of type 5. Could you comment on this?
GRIFFISS: Type 5 is a relatively uncommon cause of disease in many parts of the world and this may represent an especial West African circumstance. My purpose in showing that was twofold. First, to point out that if one looks at the neonatal period, one can make inferences about the immunogenicity of a capsule. Second, a point that I want to make over and over again: that if one wishes to know the serotypes causing disease in a certain part of the world, one must go there and sample. One cannot infer from large collections, collected in ways which are usually not clear, and pooled from different parts of the world. The distribution of capsules reflects, in part, ecological circumstances. When a streptococcus bearing the same antigen(s) as the Group A meningococcus is being faecally/orally spread in the Pacific Northwest of the USA, one gets Group A meningococcal disease – a type that had not been seen in the USA for 30 years before, and has not been seen

since. When one is talking about delivering vaccines specific for antigens occurring in different parts of the world, there is no substitute for knowing what is going on in that area. That there are time-to-time differences in pneumococcal serotypes and in meningococcal serogroups is quite clear. It can be shown in *any* country – if one does longitudinal studies. However, there are few longitudinal studies, and the pools of strains that have been studied are often pools from different times.

As for the Group B streptococcus, I will defer to John Robbins, who knows more about it than I.

ROBBINS: There are only certain types of pneumococcus that cause disease; among the 86 now discovered about 95% are caused by about 25 or 26 types. This has not changed in any part of the world, although the distribution within that 25 may change.

I think that there are two types of pneumococcal disease. One type that we saw in the USA in the 1930s, and continues to be seen in underdeveloped countries, is due to migration of the pneumococci from the nasopharynx into the lungs. This occurs in children, especially children who have to sleep every night in houses where there is smoke, due to inadequate ventilation and burning of organic matter that generates irritants. That is aspiration pneumonia, with a pneumococcus that is capable of causing disease. Those types that we had in our country, and that are still prevalent in underdeveloped countries, types 1, 2, 5, seem to occur under those conditions more often. I suggest there is another type of pneumococcal disease which occurs in all infants and children that do not have pre-existing antibody and carry around these pneumococci all the time. There is a pneumococcal carrier state; an additional factor, such as a respiratory infection by a virus that disturbs the equilibrium with the pneumococcus in the nasopharynx can cause disease by causing bacteriaemia. The types causing this second form of pneumococcal disease are the ones that we see in our country more often; 6, 14, 19, 23, which comprise 80% of the disease isolates in infants. Pneumococcus types in healthy individuals throughout the world may be different, but these types 6, 14, 19, 23, are universal. It is when you look at the types from children who are ill, or from patients, from spinal fluid or from blood, that you see the differences and I think that it is due to two types of disease: one, aspiration pneumonia, and the other bacteraemic pneumonia. That is conjecture.

GRIFFISS: So long as we are conjecturing, we might also say that because every IgG molecule that a mother passes transplacentally to her foetus is an anti-idiotype, that mothers can transfer to the infant a ‘cultural’ memory of those antigens that she, herself has encountered, and that some of the variations over time may represent ‘forgetfulness’. For instance, one could make the following hallucinatory argument about Group B streptococcal diseases. Since that organism is primarily a cause of mastitis in cows, we routinely immunized everyone enterally in the developed world until penicillin, and proscriptions against milking cows with mastitis, came along. We are now creating an increasingly large pool of women of childbearing age who were born of mothers who had never seen this antigen at the gut level, and who therefore passed no idiotype memory of it to their daughters who are now unable to recognize it, and unable to respond to it. It would be simply an alteration in the idiotype repertoire of the population caused by alterations in our environment. I would submit that that is an equally attractive hypothesis to explain these variations.

SÖDERSTRÖM: Can I bring up one additional point? Using the neonatal rat model for *E. coli* K1 infections, we studied the effect of BCG administration to new-born rats, anticipating non-specific protection. Instead we found that BCG significantly increased the number of pups developing *E. coli* K1 sepsis. We do not know why BCG administration, in doses per kg body weight comparable to what is used in humans, would make the rat pups susceptible to disease.

Towards Better Carbohydrate Vaccines
Edited by R. Bell and G. Torrigiani

Published by John Wiley & Sons Ltd

12

Profiles of diseases caused by encapsulated bacteria

C. S. F. Easmon
Department of Medical Microbiology, Wright–Fleming Institute, St Mary's Hospital Medical School, London W2 1PG, UK

INTRODUCTION

A number of the bacterial pathogens causing acute invasive disease carry carbohydrate capsules. These serve as virulence factors inhibiting antibody and complement-mediated phagocytosis.

Capsules can work in several ways. At the physico-chemical level their presence renders the bacterial surface relatively non-hydrophobic, thus reducing the likelihood of hydrophobic interactions with phagocytic cells, resulting in ingestion and intracellular killing. They may limit the activation of complement and deposition of C3b on the bacterial surface. Capsules may also prevent the binding of antibody to underlying cell-wall structures. Finally, large capsules may allow binding of antibody and complement to the cell wall, but then interfere mechanically with the recognition of these bound opsonins by Fc and C3b receptors on phagocytic cells.

My aim in this chapter is twofold: first, to give a brief profile of the types of diseases caused by encapsulated bacteria; second, to consider pathogenic and pathophysiological factors that may be relevant to epidemiology and immunity in these diseases.

STREPTOCOCCUS PNEUMONIAE

Streptococcus pneumoniae is a commensal of the upper respiratory tract. Most of the diseases associated with it are directly related to colonization of this site.

The polysaccharide capsule is a major determinant of virulence, enabling the organism to resist opsonization, ingestion and clearance from the bloodstream.

Virulence is associated with both capsule composition and size. As with other encapsulated organisms, the precise reason why some capsular types are more virulent than others is unclear. Complement is necessary for optimal opsonization of pneumococci. Patients with deficiencies of C3 and C3b inactivator in particular are subject to recurrent pneumococcal infections [1] as are those with hypogammglobulinaemia.

Differences in the rate of C3b to the pneumococcal surface and mechanical interference with the recognition of cell-bound C3b by C3b receptors on phagocytic cells may well account for differences in serotype virulence [26].

Initially, antibiotic resistance was not a problem with *S. pneumoniae*. However, since 1965, there have been reports of strains showing *in vitro* intermediate resistance, not only to penicillin, but also to a range of other antibiotics [24]. In some cases, *in vitro* resistance has been associated with failure of therapy. More recently, highly resistant pneumococci have been seen with penicillin minimum inhibitory concentrations of 2–10 mg/l. Resistant strains can cause bacteraemia, meningitis and pneumonia. However, it is difficult to assess whether antibiotic-resistant *S. pneumoniae* are any more or less virulent than fully sensitive strains of the same capsular type. Resistance to penicillin results from alterations to the penicillin binding proteins of the same serotype [28].

Pneumonia

Streptococcus pneumoniae is the most common cause of bacterial pneumonia, whether community or hospital acquired, lobar or bronchopneumonia. Finland has estimated that pneumonia accounts for one-third of all pneumococcal infection.

Attack rates of pneumonia are greatest at the extremes of life. Untreated, the mortality rates for pneumococcal pneumonia range from 15 to 35%, the higher rates being seen in cases associated with bacteraemia (about one-third of all cases of pneumococcal pneumonia). Even in the absence of antibiotic-resistant strains, the mortality of untreated pneumococcal pneumonia is still 4–8% while in bacteraemic cases it can exceed 15%. Even more significantly, chemotherapy appears to have little effect in reducing deaths in the early phase of infection [3]. Underlying conditions, such as diabetes mellitus, unrelated pulmonary disease and malignancy, increase the severity of pneumococcal pneumonia.

From this it can be seen that pneumococcal pulmonary infection is an aggressive process. The limited success of chemotherapy suggests that pulmonary defences against newly encountered capsular types are not very effective once infection is established. In experimental infections Coonrod and Yoneda [4] have shown that complement levels in broncho-alveolar secretions are low and opsonization far less effective in this milieu than in serum. In the absence of anticapsular antibody, virulent pneumococci find little in the lungs to impede their multiplication.

Local host defences may also contribute to the pathology of pneumococcal pulmonary disease. Both oxidative and non-oxidative phagocytic killing systems can produce considerable tissue damage. Phagocyte contents will act on the complement and kinin systems, increasing the inflammatory response and attracting even more cells [12].

Otitis media

The majority of children have at least one attack of otitis media before they reach school age. In at least 50% of cases *S. pneumoniae* is the principal pathogen [8]. As well as the pain and inflammation of the acute disease, otitis media can, if untreated, become chronic, with deafness, mastoiditis and, more rarely, cerebral complications. There is a link between otitis media and upper respiratory tract viral infection. A limited range of pneumococal types [6, 14, 19, 23] are usually involved [9].

Using an experimental model of infection in chinchillas, Giebink has analysed factors involved in pneumococal otitis media. Compromised middle-ear ventilation, impaired local and systemic humoral immunity and the presence of *S. pneumoniae* in the nasopharynx [7]. His work supports clinical observations by Howie *et al.* [11] that otitis media can be controlled by immunization.

Bacteriaemia and meningitis

As described above, bacteraemia is a common complication of pneumococcal pneumonia, its presence making the prognosis for the patient worse. Bacteraemia may, however, occur without preceding pneumonia or any obvious focus. These cases may run a more benign course. High-grade pneumococcal bacteraemia is seen in splenectomized patients and in sickle-cell disease, but this is discussed more fully below.

Streptococcus pneumoniae is one of the main causes of acute bacterial meningitis, together with *Haemophilus influenzae* type b and *Neisseria menin-*

gitidis. The mortality of pneumococcal meningitis remains high, despite modern chemotherapy.

Pneumococcal meningitis may result from preceding bacteraemia/pneumonia with seeding of bacteria across the blood–brain barrier. How exactly this occurs is not known. More rarely, direct spread can occur from mastoiditis. The third way in which meningeal infection can be initiated is through a traumatic or congenital communication between sinuses, cribriform plate, orbit or middle ear. Those patients with a CSF leak are particularly at risk. Skull fractures are often very minor and difficult to localize on X-ray.

As in other sites, local CSF defences against *S. pneumoniae* depend on complement, antibody and phagocytic cells. Normal CSF contains no phagocytic cells, very low levels of IgG and negligible levels of complement. During the inflammation that follows acute meningitis, IgG and phagocytic cells accumulate in the CSF, although complement opsonic activity remains far below that in serum. However, there does appear to be a lag phase and pneumococci, once in the CSF, probably have a crucial period during which host defences are minimal [21].

Pneumococcal infection in splenectomized patients and in sickle-cell disease

Following splenectomy, patients, particularly young children, are susceptible to overwhelming pneumococcal bacteraemia. Levels of 10^5 organisms/ml of blood can be found. Patients present with fever, abdominal pain, hypotension and, occasionally, even a haemorrhagic skin rash. The syndrome may be indistinguishable from classical gram-negative shock seen with organisms like *N. meningitidis*. A similar pattern of disease can be seen in patients with sickle-cell disease who have a non-functional spleen and deficient serum opsonic activity for *S. pneumoniae* [20, 27].

The spleen is important, both as a means for phagocytosis and clearance of bacteria from the circulation and as a site of antibody production [23]. The clearance function of the spleen is thought to be important in coping with poorly opsonized particles. Loss of these protective functions would render the individual suscpetible to encapsulated virulent bacteria. Although *S. pneumoniae* is responsible for the majority of infections in these patients, the other main pathogens are also encapsulated, i.e. *H. influenzae* type b and *N. meningitidis*.

HAEMOPHILUS INFLUENZAE

Haemophilus influenzae exists in both capsulated and uncapsulated forms. The latter do not usually cause invasive disease, being normally associated with acute exacerbations of chronic bronchitis.

There are six capsular types, a–f. All six capsules consist of negatively charged polysaccharides. One of the six, type b, is the cause of nearly all serious *H. influenzae* infections. Why virulence should be seen exclusively with just this one type is not known. However, unlike the other types, type b organisms are resistant to complement-mediated lysis, requiring anti-capsular antibody in addition. *Haemophilus influenzae* type b causes two types of invasive disease, both associated with bacteraemia – meningitis and epiglottitis [22].

Meningitis

Haemophilus influenzae type b meningitis primarily affects infants and children between the ages of 3 months and 2–3 years. The organism invades from the upper respiratory tract mucosa, causes a bacteraemia and spreads to meninges. It is not known how invasion occurs, but experimental work in infant rats suggests a role for concomitant upper respiratory tract viral infection.

Although *in vitro* antibodies against *H. influenzae* type b are bactericidal in the presence of complement, the spleen plays an important part in controlling bacteraemia in both animals and man. This may indicate an important role for opsonization rather than bacterial lysis [2]. *Haemophilus influenzae* meningitis is not associated with defects in the terminal complement components necessary for lysis, as is meningococcal meningitis.

In rats meningitis only occurs when bacteraemia reaches 10^3 organisms/ml for at least 6 hours [17].

The age pattern of *H. influenzae* type b meningitis is related to levels of protective anti-capsular antibody. Infants less than 3 months old still have circulating maternal antibody. However, in common with other polysaccharide antigens, children below the age of 18–24 months respond poorly to the type b antigen. As their immunity develops thereafter, the incidence of *H. influenzae* type b diseases drops sharply.

As a gram-negative organism, *H. influenzae* contains lipopolysaccharide in its outer envelope. Occasionally this can precipitate bacteriogenic shock with hypotension, focal haemorrhages in skin and viscera, thrombocytopaenia and clotting abnormalities. The prognosis in these cases is poor. Otherwise the mortality from meningitis has stayed at similar levels since the introduction of effective chemotherapy. However, there is a significant morbidity with both physical and mental sequelae.

Antibiotic resistance is variable. Beta-lactamase producing strains of *H. influenzae* appeared about 13 years ago. In some areas 15% of isolates may produce this enzyme, but resistance is patchy. Chloramphenicol resistance has been described, but is still rare. However, this problem is likely to grow.

Epiglottitis

Epiglottitis is the other serious consequence of *H. influenzae* type b bacteraemia. Children progress rapidly from minimal upper respiratory tract symptoms to severe airway obstruction within a few hours. Inflammation is restricted to the epiglottis and immediate surrounding area. *Haemophilus influenzae* type b is almost invariably isolated from the blood.

Whisnant *et al.* [25] analysed and compared the demographic features, pre-existing and subsequent type b anti-capsular antibody levels and host genetic factors in children presenting with haemophilus meningitis and epiglottitis. Those with epiglottitis were older, had higher pre-existing antibody levels and a better post-infection antibody response. There were also differences in host-cell markers. From this they concluded that host factors might play a role in determining the pattern of invasive *H. influenzae* disease.

NEISSERIA MENINGITIDIS

Neisseria meningitidis is the third major cause of meningitis. As with *S. pneumoniae* and *H. influenzae* type b, meningitis results from invasion from respiratory tract mucosa and bloodstream dissemination. Meningococcaemia can exist without concomitant meningitis, and is just as serious.

It appears that *N. meningitidis* adheres to mucosal epithelium by means of fimbriae. Organisms are ingested by epithelial cells and transported in an orderly fashion. The capsule does not seem to play any role in this process.

All serogroups can cause invasive disease. The disease occurs in infants, children and young adults, particularly in army camps and schools. Meningococcal meningitis is an epidemic disease and, where there are cases, there will be asymptomatic carriers. There is no non-human reservoir of infection.

Bacterial lysis does appear to be important as a defence in meningococcal infection. Individuals with defects of C7 and C8 whose serum is incapable of lysing *N. meningitidis* are unduly susceptible to meningococcal infection. The importance of bacteriolysis and opsonization *in vivo* is unclear, but in both processes anti-capsular antibodies are important.

Meningococcal meningitis and bacteraemia are particularly associated with haemorrhagic skin rashes, focal haemorrhages in many organs, including the adrenals, and with other features of bacteriogenic shock. As in all cases of this syndrome, mortality is high and in meningococcal disease shock can occur when the patient appears to be making a good recovery.

The Group B meningococcus is the major current problem. The Group B polysaccharide is a polymer of *N*-acetylneuraminic acid (it is chemically identical to the K1 antigen of *Escherichia coli*). It is poorly immunogenic, stimulating at best short-lived IgM responses, usually of poor affinity. *N*-

acetyl neuraminic acid on the bacterial surface prevents activation of the alternative pathway, thus blocking the protective effects of the complement system in non-immune individuals.

GROUP B STREPTOCOCCUS

The Group B streptococcus (GBS) is a normal inhabitant of the gastrointestinal tract and is commonly isolated from the lower female genital tract. It has a range of type-specific capsular polysaccharide antigens which appear to act as virulence factors in that antibodies directed against them are protective. These polysaccharides have a terminal *N*-acetyl neuraminic acid moiety [14]. This may be related to virulence, as it prevents activation of the alternative complement pathway and recruitment of complement-mediated phagocytosis in those babies with no protective antibody [5].

Although the organism can cause invasive disease in adults, particularly in women in labour and diabetics, neonatal septicaemia and meningitis are the most serious GBS diseases. Two forms are recognized: so-called 'early-onset' and 'late-onset' disease. Both occur in babies who have received no protective anti-capsular opsonic antibody from their mothers across the placenta.

Early-onset infection

As its name suggests, early-onset disease is usually seen within the first 72 hours of life. Organisms invade from the respiratory tract mucosa, a prime site of neonatal GBS colonization. Bacteraemia is accompanied by respiratory distress and hypotension and the picture may be confused with non-infective causes of respiratory distress. Infection rates vary from 0.25 to 5 or more cases/1000 live births. Even with prompt diagnosis and treatment, mortality can exceed 50%.

Meningitis can occur in early-onset infection, but is of less importance than in late-onset disease. The neonate, even at full term, is not immunocompetent and the high mortality of early-onset disease reflects this.

Late-onset infection

Meningitis following bacteraemia is the main feature of late-onset disease. This usually affects older infants, up to 6 weeks of age. Mortality is far lower than with early-onset infection, although still appreciable. The meningitis has no special features and the portal of entry of infection is unclear. There is a strong association between GBS meningitis and strains of type III, but the reason for this is unknown.

ESCHERICHIA COLI

Escherichia coli causes a very wide range of infections. The capsular K antigens are only related to a few of these, and I will only deal with those where K antigens are relevant.

Bacteraemia and meningitis

The K antigens are acid polysaccharides. K1 is identical to the Group B meningococcal capsular antigen. We have recently surveyed a range of adult sera for the presence of opsonic or bactericidal antibodies to K1-containing *E. coli* strains and invariably found little or no activity. In infant rats, K1-containing strains can invade the gut wall causing bacteraemia and meningitis.

Escherichia coli K1 is, with GBS, the most common cause of neonatal meningitis.

Urinary tract infections

There is an association between certain K antigens and cystitis and pyelonephritis [10]. However, many other factors are involved and the exact role of the capsule in these infections is not clear. Antibodies directed against K antigens can protect rats against ascending pyelonephritis [13].

BACTEROIDES FRAGILIS

Non-sporing anaerobes are involved in a wide range of infections such as bacteraemia, brain abscesses, dental infections, intra-abdominal sepsis and infections of the female genital tract. The mouth, gastrointestinal tract and female genital tract have an extensive microflora.

Of all anaerobes *B. fragilis* is the most common species causing bacteraemia. However, it is not the most common *Bacteroides* found as part of the normal flora in any of these sites. This disproportionate association with infection suggests that *B. fragilis* has specific virulence factors [16].

What seems to distinguish *B. fragilis* from the rest is the presence of a capsule that can be identified microscopically and immunologically [15], using the rat as an experimental model of intra-abdominal sepsis, the virulence of encapsulated as opposed to uncapsulated *B. fragilis* has been demonstrated [18, 19]. The capsule inhibits phagocytosis.

A serological response to *B. fragilis* capsular material has also been shown in women with pelvic inflammatory disease [16]. This study suggested that *B. fragilis* was in fact more important than *Neisseria gonorrhoeae* in this condition.

REFERENCES

1. Alper, C. A., Colten, H. R., Rosen, F. S., Rabson, A. R., MacNab, G. M., and Gear, J. S. S. Homozygous deficiency of C3 in a patient with repeated infections. *Lancet*, **ii**, 1179–81 (1972).
2. Anderson, P., Johnston, R. B. Jr, and Smith, D. H. Human serum activities against *Hemophilus influenzae* type b. *J. Clin. Invest.*, **51**, 31–8 (1972).
3. Austrian, R. Pneumococcal infections. In *Bacterial Vaccines* (ed. R. Germanier), Academic Press, London, 1984, pp. 257–88.
4. Coonrod, J. D., and Yoneda, K. Complement and opsonins in alveolar secretions and serum of rats with pneumonia due to *Streptococcus pneumoniae*. *Rev. Infect. Dis.*, **3**, 310–22 (1981).
5. Edwards, M. S., Kasper, D. L., Jennings, H. J., Baker, C. J., and Nicholson-Weller, A. Capsular sialic acid prevents activation of the alternative complement pathway by type III group B streptococcus. *J. Exp. Med.*, **121**, 1275–81 (1980).
6. Finland, M. Conference on the pneumococcus. Summary and contents. *Rev. Infect. Dis.*, **3**, 358–71 (1981).
7. Giebink, G. S. The pathogenesis of pneumococcal otitis media in chinchillas and the efficacy of vaccination in prophylaxis. *Rev. Infect. Dis.*, **3**, 342–52 (1981).
8. Giebink, G. S., and Quie, P. G. Otitis media: the spectrum of middle ear inflammation. *Ann. Rev.*, **29**, 285–306 (1978).
9. Grönroos, J. A., Vihma, L., Salmivalli, A., and Berglund, B. Co-existing viral (respiratory syncytial) and bacterial (pneumococcus) otitis media in children. *Acta Otolaryngol (Stockh.)*, **65**, 505–17 (1968).
10. Howard, C. J., and Glynn, A. A. The virulence for mice of strains of *Escherichia coli* related to the effects of K antigens on their resistance to phagocytosis and killing by complement. *Immunology*, **20**, 767–77 (1971).
11. Howie, G. M., Ploussard, J. H., and Sloyer, J. L. Immunisation against recurrent otitis media. *Ann. Otol. Rhinol. Laryngol.*, **85** (Suppl. 25), 254–8 (1976).
12. Johnston, R. B. Jr The host response to invasion by *Streptococcus pneumoniae*: protection and the pathogenesis of tissue damage. *Rev. Infect. Dis.*, **3**, 282–8 (1981).
13. Kaijser, B., Larsson, P., Nimmich, W., and Söderström, T. Antibodies to *Escherichia coli* K and O antigens in protection against acute pyelonephritis. *Prog. Allergy*, **33**, 275–88 (1983).
14. Kasper, D. L., Baker, C. J., and Jennings, H. J. Cell structure and antigenic composition of GBS. In *Neonatal Group B Streptococcal Infections* (ed. K. K. Christensen, P. Christensen and P. Ferrieri), Karger, Basle, 1985, pp. 90–100.
15. Kasper, D. L., Hayes, M. E., Reinap, B. G., Craft, F. O., Onderdonk, A. B., and Polk, B. F. Isolation and identification of encapsulated strains of *Bacteroides fragilis*. *J. Infect. Dis.*, **136**, 75–81 (1977).

16. Kasper, D. L., Onderdonk, A. B., Polk, B. F., and Bartlett, J. G. Surface antigens as virulence factors. In *Anaerobic Bacteria Selected Topics* (ed. D. W. Lambe, R. J. Genco and K. J. Mayberry-Carson), Plenum Press, New York, 1979, pp. 173–92.
17. Moxon, E. R., Zwahlen, A., and Rubin, L. G. Pathogenesis of *Haemophilus influenzae* meningitis: use of a rat model for studying microbial determinants of virulence. In *Bacterial Meningitis* (ed. M. A. Sande, A. L. Smith and R. K. Root), Churchill Livingstone, Edinburgh, 1985, pp. 23–36.
18. Onderdonk, A. B., Bartlett, J. G., Lovie, T. J., Sullivan-Siegler, N., and Gorbach, S. L. Micorbial synergy in experimental intraabdominal abscess. *Infect. Immun.*, **13**, 22–6 (1976).
19. Onderdonk, A. B., Kasper, D. L., Cisneros, R. L., and Bartlett, J. G. The capsular polysaccharide of *Bacteroides fragilis* as a virulence factor: comparison of the pathogenic potential of the encapsulated and unencapsulated strains. *J. Infect. Dis.*, **136**, 82–9 (1977).
20. Pearson, A. H., Spencer, R. P., and Cornelius, E. A. Functional asplenia in sickle cell anaemia. *N. Engl. J. Med.*, **281**, 923–6 (1969).
21. Scheld, W. M. Pathogenesis and pathophysiology of pneumococcal meningitis. In *Bacterial Meningitis (ed. M. A. Sande, A. L. Smith and R. K. Root), Churchill Livingstone, Edinburgh, 1985, pp. 37–69.*
22. *Turk, D. C., and May, J. R. Haemophilus influenzae: Its Clinical Importance.* English Universities Press, London, 1967, pp. 27 and 58.
23. Wara, D. W. Host defence against *Streptococcus pneumoniae*: the role of the spleen. *Rev. Infect. Dis.*, **3**, 299–309 (1981).
24. Ward, J. Antibiotic-resistant *Streptococcus pneumoniae*: clinical and epidemiologic aspects. *Rev. Infect. Dis.*, **3**, 254–66 (1981).
25. Whisnant, J. K., Rogentine, G. N., Gralnick, M. A., Schlesselman, J. J., and Robbins, J. B. Host factors and antibody response in *Haemophilus influenzae* type b meningitis and epiglottitis. *J. Infect. Dis.*, **133**, 448–55 (1976).
26. Winklestein, J. A. The role of complement in the host's defense against *Streptococcuspneumoniae. Rev. Infect. Dis.*, **3**, 289–98 (1981).
27. Winklestein, J. A., and Drachman, R. H. Deficiency of pneumococcal serum opzonizing activity in sickle cell disease. *N. Engl. J. Med.*, **279**, 459–66 (1968).
28. Zighelboim, S., and Tomasz, A. Multiple antibiotic resistance in South African strains of *Streptococcus pneumoniae*. Mechanism of resistance to β-lactam antibiotics. *Rev. Infect. Dis.*, **3**, 267–76 (1981).

DISCUSSION – Chaired by Professor A. Capron

ROTTA: I have three comments. Number one: the absence, if I understood it correctly, of type III antibodies in new-borns, to which you ascribe the frequent morbidity of new-borns due to type III, is due probably to the fact that, as has been shown, type III antibody is the least transferable *per* placenta, compared with types Ia, Ib and II. The second comment I wish to make concerns the occurrence of Ibc antigen, which is now called C. It is a protein like antigens X and R. We have shown in my laboratory that this C protein can be encountered in all types, Ia, Ib, II and III, and even the newly identified and accepted types IV and V. As far as the source of infection of the new-borns is concerned, of course, it is the mother, and the presence of Group B streptococci on the vaginal mucosa. We now actually consider Group B infection a sexually transmitted infection. An asymptomatic carriership in the urethra of the man may occur. You did not indicate the other sources of infection of the new-borns as they are in the hospital environment.

EASMON: Perhaps I could respond to that. I think difficulty of transfer of the type III antibody might partly account for the importance of type III organisms in the general causation of Group B streptococcal disease. However, if you look at the types of organisms responsible for early-onset disease, there is a very even distribution with no predominance of type III strains. It is when you look at the late-onset meningitic disease that you get this very remarkable predominance of type III. What you are suggesting may have some role, but I don't think it entirely explains the close association between type III strains and the meningitic form of late-onset disease.

On the second point, I agree entirely that the C antigen protein can be associated with any of the polysaccharides and certainly our streptococcal reference laboratory in the United Kingdom is now beginning to report the full range so you can have a IIR, a III3X, a III3C isolate. In our experience, C antigen does seem to be more stable in association with the polysaccharide antigens than either R or X. Could you remind me of your third point?

ROTTA: The source of the infection, the reservoir.

EASMON: Again, with the collaboration of the streptococcal reference laboratory, we have been able to study this quite extensively, using phage typing. One of the problems of the serotyping system for Group B streptococci is even distribution of the strains among serotypes and very poor discrimination. There is a phage-typing system now available that will effectively give 94 serophage groups and, using this, we have been able to document hospital-acquired transmission of the organism in up to 30% of babies that become colonized in hospital. It is very variable, it is controllable by simple hygiene, such as hand washing, but nosocomial transmission can be a major factor in acquisition of the organism.

SÖDERSTRÖM: You asked whether there are any possibilities of identifying the mothers who will fail to respond to the polysaccharides. It seems that patients with relative deficiency in isolated IgG subclasses are common. The most frequent diagnosis we find in paediatric patients with subclass deficiencies are otitis media and upper or lower respiratory tract infections. Often, encapsulated organisms are involved. We have also looked at complications to vascular surgery in Göteborg. In a controlled study, the patients who had the worst infectious complications were those who had the lowest individual IgG subclass levels prior to operation. Also in the normal population, without any subclass deficiencies, you will find individuals who respond poorly to polysaccharides. We find that IgG-deficient individuals respond extremely poorly, not only in serum but also on the mucosae. If, on the other hand, they have a combined IgG_2 and IgG_3 deficiency, they respond normally. Subclass determination could be a clue to looking into which patients will respond.

EASMON: I think there is a paper recently in the literature which actually looks at IgG subclasses. I am not sure if it is in relation to natural infection or in relation to actual immunization with the type III capsular polysaccharide. This suggested that there were not any marked differences between those women that were good and bad responders.

SÖDERSTRÖM: There definitely seems to be in our and other studies which are soon to be published.

Towards Better Carbohydrate Vaccines
Edited by R. Bell and G. Torrigiani

Published by John Wiley & Sons Ltd

13

Attenuated live bacteria: vaccine efficacy and shortcomings

ANNE MORRIS HOOKE
The Departments of Pediatrics and Microbiology, Georgetown University School of Medicine, Washington, DC 20007, USA

ABSTRACT

Live, attenuated vaccines were among the first preparations ever used to induce immunity to infectious diseases. The early vaccines of Pasteur were developed on the basis of pragmatic laboratory and field observations, without benefit of the knowledge we have today of the complexity of the immune system and the immunogenicity of different molecules.

With the exception of BCG, live vaccines fell into disfavour during the second quarter of this century, only to be revived in the 1960s, when their superiority over inactivated vaccines became clearer. Today, armed with the knowledge denied the early workers and the sophisticated techniques of molecular biology, we can address the shortcomings of some of the live vaccines and successfully exploit genetic attenuation based upon sound scientific reasoning.

INTRODUCTION

The basic requirements for any vaccine are that it should:

(i) contain the necessary antigenic determinants to induce formation of protective immunity in the vaccinee;
(ii) possess high immunogenic potential;
(iii) be safe for administration without any risk of clinical infection for the recipient or susceptible contacts of the recipient;

(iv) be devoid of any toxic side-effects from defined or ill-defined contaminants of otherwise pure preparations;
(v) be suitable for inoculation by the most appropriate route (oral, intranasal, topical or parenteral);
(vi) mimic closely, by its mode of administration, the circumstances of natural infection;
(vii) be stable under conditions of long-term storage; and,
(viii) be compatible with the usual inert vaccine carriers.

Live bacterial vaccines readily satisfy most of these requirements, at least in theory. The major stumbling-block for many has been the problem of reversion to virulence, resulting in the potential for causing disease in the vaccinee.

This chapter will describe briefly some of the problems associated with the use of killed cells or purified component vaccines, the various methods used in the past to attenuate live, bacterial pathogens, some of the new approaches being explored today and work from our laboratory on the development of temperature-sensitive (ts) vaccines for *Haemophilus influenzae*, *Pseudomonas aeruginosa* and *Salmonella typhi.*

CONVENTIONAL VACCINES

With the notable exception of BCG, most bacterial vaccines used worldwide have relied upon heat-killed or chemically inactivated whole cells or purified, detoxified preparations of cellular components or products. The use of killed cells is usually accompanied by a loss of immunogenic potential, because the killing process (physical or chemical treatment) often alters or destroys many of the surface antigenic determinants necessary for the induction of specific protective antibodies in the vaccinee. The antibodies produced in response to such altered antigens have reduced affinity for the molecular structures on the surface of the live organism and, therefore, may be less effective against the invading pathogen.

Vaccine use of antigenic components or products of bacteria is also often compromised by the effect of the purification and/or detoxification procedures on the three-dimensional arrangement of the antigenic determinants, and diminution of their inherent immunogenicity following removal from their natural positions in or on the cell. In spite of this, two obviously successful detoxified vaccines are, of course, diphtheria and tetanus toxoids, but it should be noted that these both require multiple administrations and derive enhanced immunogenicity from the pertussis component of the vaccine preparation. The pertussis component itself is responsible for considerable reactogenicity and is the target of concerted efforts for improvement.

Purified polysaccharides from *Neisseria meningitidis* and *H. influenzae*, when used as vaccines, almost always fail to elicit significant antibody responses in very young children – often the group most at risk for contracting disease. This defect appears to be related to the immaturity of the infant's immune system, and can be effectively overcome by the covalent coupling of the polysaccharide to T-dependent protein antigens or by its natural presentation as part of the cell [2, 3, 7, 23, 25, 28, 30, 33].

HISTORY OF LIVE VACCINES

Following, albeit by almost a century, the first observations and experiments of Jenner with cowpox virus, Louis Pasteur discovered accidentally that extended laboratory passage of chicken cholera cultures rendered the organisms avirulent. These attenuated cultures were, however, capable of inducing protection from the disease when injected into chickens. Within a few years Pasteur devised three different techniques for attenuating bacterial pathogens: laboratory passage (chicken cholera), incubation at high temperature (anthrax) and passage through rabbits (swine erysipelas). Not only did Pasteur's vaccines induce protection in experimental situations, they also were successful in highly publicized field trials, although he met considerable scepticism and criticism from his fellow scientists. Other live vaccines devised during the first years of microbiology include Haffkine's heat-passaged *Vibrio cholerae* and a live preparation of *V. cholerae* used by a Spanish physician who did not describe the details of his attenuating method [4].

The next milestone in live vaccine development occurred in 1922, with the production of the Bacille Calmette-Guérin (BCG), a strain of *Mycobacterium bovis* which had been attenuated by more than 200 passages in laboratory media. In spite of some setbacks due to contamination of vaccine lots with virulent *M. tuberculosis*, and some less-than-optimal preparations, widespread use of BCG is credited by many for the decrease in tuberculosis in Europe and Asia over the last 50 years [6].

Streptomycin-dependent mutants of *Shigella sonnei*, *S. flexneri* and *Salmonella typhi* were isolated following chemical mutagenesis, characterized and tested by oral administration to animals and humans in the 1960s and 1970s [8, 20, 21, 31]. For reasons ranging from the loss of immunogenicity upon lyophilization to unacceptable reversion frequencies (*circa* 10^{-10}), these strains did not gain wide acceptance.

CURRENT ATTENUATED VACCINES

The *galE* strain of *S. typhi* developed by Germanier and Fürer (Ty 21a) in the 1970s was derived following sequential steps of mutagenesis with nitrosoguanidine which caused mutations rendering the organism 'suicidal' in the presence of galactose [11]. In the complete absence of galactose the mutant is unable to synthesize complete LPS, an important antigen for protection, but in the presence of controlled amounts of the exogenous sugar the strain is smooth, until it lyses under the pressure of accumulated galactose-l-phosphate and UDP-galactose. Ty 21a is currently being evaluated as an oral vaccine in extensive field trials in Egypt and Chile [35]. There is considerable (90–99%) loss of viability following lyophilization, and it has so far only been tested in areas where typhoid is endemic and, therefore, its success has possibly depended upon anamnestic responses. Indeed, a recent report suggests that use of the *galE* vaccine in completely naïve (with respect to *S. typhi* exposure) individuals does not always provide protection [14]. Furthermore, the Ty 21a vaccine strain lacks the polysaccharide capsule (Vi antigen), thought by some to be important for inducing protection [32], although its absence could also contribute to the avirulence of any *galE* revertants, should they arise. The reversion rate of Ty 21a is estimated at 10^{-14}.

Nitrosoguanidine-mediated mutagenesis also led to the isolation of an attenuated strain of *V. cholerae* by Honda and Finkelstein in 1979, an A^-/B^+ mutant named Texas Star-SR whose avirulence is based upon its inability to make the A subunit of cholera toxin [16]. Although oral immunization of experimental animals with Texas Star-SR induced significant protection from virulent challenge, it also caused significant diarrhoea in volunteers and the protection seen in immunized humans did not equal that induced by natural disease [22].

An entirely different approach to attenuation was used by Hoiseth and Stocker [15] who constructed a deletion mutant by insertion of aro A554::tn10 into the genome of *S. typhimurium* causing requirements for *p*-aminobenzoic acid and 2,3-dihydroxybenzoate, compounds not available in vertebrate tissues. The *aroA* mutant is avirulent, induces protection in mice and is genetically stable because of the deletion. A similarly constructed *aroA* mutant of *S. typhi* is currently being tested in human volunteers (Stocker and Levine, personal communication).

Advances in molecular biology and recombinant DNA technology have resulted in many other sophisticated approaches to live vaccine development. The genes for *Shigella* surface antigens have been introduced into an avirulent *Escherichia coli* and the Ty 21a mutant of *S. typhi* [10, 19]. The hybrid *E. coli* vaccine strain, however, when administered orally to volunteers failed to induce protection, even when low challenge doses were used. The *Shigella*-

–*Salmonella* hybrid, on the other hand, has induced significant protection in mice, and is currently being tested in humans.

Kaper and Levine, Manning's group in Australia and Pearson and Mekalanos have used cloning techniques to manipulate *V. cholerae* genes in *E. coli* [18, 24, 29]. Expression and stabilization of some of the genes in these hybrid strains have proved troublesome, but ingenious solutions are already being found to overcome these problems.

TEMPERATURE-SENSITIVE ATTENUATED VACCINES

Temperature sensitivity as a form of genetic attenuation offers several specific advantages over other types. First, ts mutants with lesions in essential gene products cannot sustain growth at the restrictive temperature in any nutritional environment because the effect of the mutation cannot be corrected by exogenous supplies. Second, surface antigens remain intact and immunogenicity is uncompromised by incomplete expression of genes. Third, the method used for isolating ts mutants can be manipulated to yield strains ('coasters') which are capable of limited replication in the vaccinee, thus mimicking the initial stages of natural infection, allowing more prolonged stimulation of the immune system and, perhaps more importantly, permitting the expression of genes coding for antigens which are only synthesized *in vivo*.

The vaccine potential of ts strains was first explored by Fahey and Cooper in 1970 [9] with *S. enteritidis*. Later, Chanock and his colleagues investigated the immunogenicity of ts mutants of *Mycoplasma pneumoniae* and *Streptococcus pneumoniae* [12, 13]. In every case ts mutants proved immunogenic and capable of inducing protection from virulent challenge. The reversion rates (*circa* 10^{-7}) of the ts mutants, however, rendered them unsuitable for further development as human vaccines.

The problem of genetic instability can be overcome by the combination in one strain of two or more mutations of identical phenotype, thus reducing the reversion frequency to negligible levels (*circa* 10^{-21}). The difficulty of identifying recombinants whose phenotype is identical to that of the parental strains can be alleviated by exploiting linkage of the ts mutations to positively selectable chromosomal markers. The feasibility of this approach to vaccine development has been demonstrated in studies from our laboratory, using *H. influenzae* as a model [26], and the method is currently being applied to the development of ts vaccine strains of *P. aeruginosa* and *S. typhi*.

EXPERIMENTAL OUTLINE

The strains used throughout these studies are listed in Table I, together with their phenotypes and source.

Table I. *H. influenzae*, *P. aeruginosa* and *S. typhi* strains

Strain	Phenotype	Source
Rd-001	Unencapsulated mutant of type d *H. influenzae*	J. J. Scocca (from the collection of R. Herriott)
EKNSV	Transformant of Rd-001, chromosomally resistant to the antibiotics Em,[a] Km, Nb, Sm and Vm	J. J. Scocca
EKNSVNal	Spontaneous mutant of EKNSV, resistant to nalidixic acid	This study
Eagan	Encapsulated type b *H. influenzae*	J. B. Robbins
P. aeruginosa	Immunotype 1	C. Heifetz
S. typhi Ty 2	09, 12; Vi$^+$	ATCC

[a] Em: erythromycin; Km: kanamycin; Nb: novobiocin; Sm: streptomycin; Vm: viomycin

Isolation of temperature-sensitive mutants

Temperature-sensitive mutants of *H. influenzae*, *P. aeruginosa* and *S. typhi* were isolated after mutagenesis with nitrosoguanidine (NG) and two cycles of enrichment during temperature shift with penicillin, cefazolin or D-cycloserine [26, 27]. Because it may be necessary to colonize the nasopharynx or gastrointestinal tract *temporarily* with the vaccine strains, in order to allow sufficient time for the immune system to be alerted, we isolated two classes of ts mutants: first, those which immediately cease growth on transfer to the non-permissive temperature ('tights'), and second, those which continue to grow and divide for a limited time (up to four or five divisions) before growth is terminated ('coasters'). We selectively enriched for either class by adding the antibiotic immediately after temperature shift or after incubation for 2–3 hours at the non-permissive temperature.

Characterization of ts mutants

The first steps in characterizing the ts mutants were determination of cut-off temperatures, 'coaster' or 'tight' phenotypes, and reversion frequencies. Single colonies of each mutant were streaked on chocolate agar and incubated at 27, 30, 32, 34 and 36 °C. After 24 hours, growth on the primary, secondary and tertiary streaks was assessed. The temperature at which the strain could no longer form single colonies was defined as the cut-off. Growth in the primary or secondary streaks, but no single colony formation, indicated 'coasting'; no growth at all at the cut-off temperature defined 'tight' mutants.

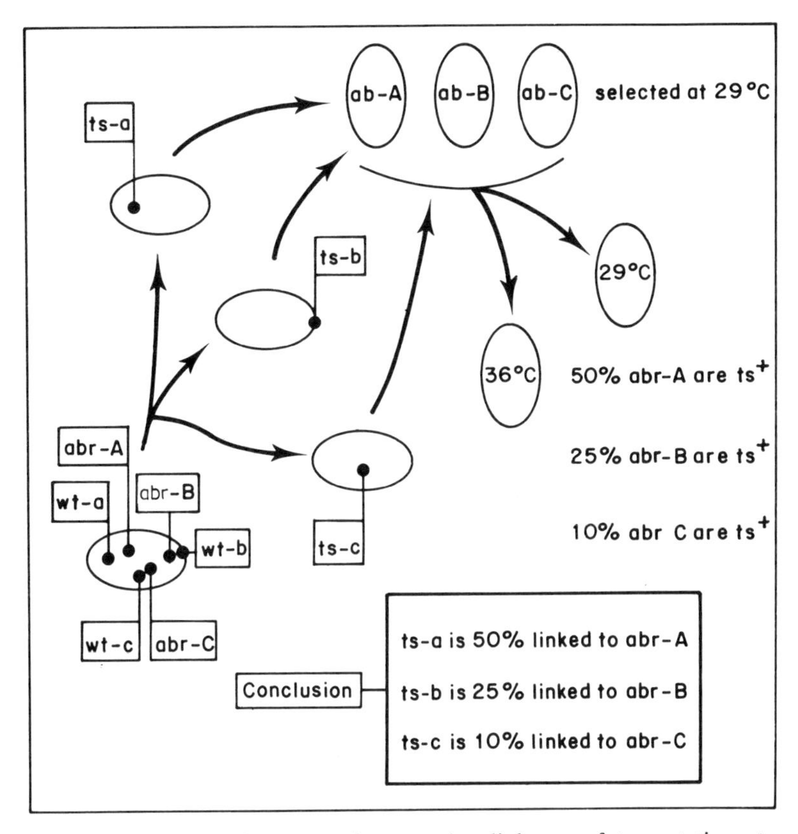

Figure 1. Outline of strategy for mapping linkages of ts mutations to selectable markers. For details of the specific steps see the text in Experimental Outline

The ability to form single colonies after several days' incubation at the non-permissive temperature indicated that the mutation was leaky, and therefore unsuitable for our work. The phenotype and cut-off temperature were confirmed in liquid cultures. Reversion frequencies were determined by incubating at least 10^9 cells on solid media at the non-permissive temperature.

Linkage determinations

Location of the ts lesions on the *H. influenzae* chromosome was accomplished by a series of transformations. The general strategy employed is outlined in Figure 1. DNA from the multiple-antibiotic-resistant strain EKNSVNal was used to transform ts derivatives of the wild-type (wt) Rd-001 and transformants selected at 29 °C on plates containing the appropriate antibiotic. Antibiotic-resistant recombinants were then streaked on duplicate plates which were incubated at the permissive and non-permissive temperatures. If, for example, a mutant acquiring the gene responsible for Sm-resistance were simultaneously 'cured' of its temperature sensitivity, then that lesion is presumably linked to the Sm-resistance gene, absent rare double recombinational events. Reciprocal experiments were also performed: DNA from ts^+ EKNSVNal was used to transform ts Rd-001 strains and the ts^+ phenotype selected. The ts^+ recombinants were scored for the acquisition of antibiotic-resistance genes by replica-plating on media containing antibiotics. Temperature-sensitive mutants of strain EKNSVNal were also mapped by a similar procedure. They were transformed with wt Rd-001 DNA and ts^+ recombinants monitored for the concomitant loss of antibiotic resistance. In the reciprocal experiment, DNA from ts EKNSVNal strains was used to transform wt Rd-001, antibiotic resistance selected at 29 °C and recombinants screened for temperature sensitivity. The plate technique developed by Juni [17] was used for all transformations. Transduction with generalized transducing phage is being used with *P. aeruginosa* and *S. typhi*.

Purification of mutant alleles

Although NG is an excellent mutagen, its tendency to induce additional mutations both closely linked and distant from the gene of interest [1, 5] can cause problems. It is therefore desirable that, once the selected mutation has been deemed suitable, it be transferred from the mutagenized 'dirty' strain to a 'clean' background. Accordingly, when the ts lesions were mapped and linkage established to antibiotic-resistance markers, the genes were transformed into an unmutagenized wt strain (Figure 2). DNA from the ts mutants generated in EKNSVNal was used to transform wt Rd-001 and the transformants plated at 29 °C on medium containing the appropriate antibiotic. Antibiotic-resistant recombinants were then screened for the presence of the ts gene. The reversion rates of the ts mutation were confirmed, as well as the growth rates of the ts transformants and their ts^+ revertants. It is important that the growth rates of ts mutants and revertants be similar at permissive temperatures so that revertants, rare as they might be, should have no advantage in batch culture. Those ts derivatives of Rd-001 whose lesions are located near an antibiotic-resistance gene were first transformed to that resistance by DNA from wt EKNSVNal, and monitored for *retention* of temperature sensitivity. The antibiotic-resistance-linked ts gene was then similarly transformed into a 'clean' wt strain. In this way both sides of the antibiotic-resistance-linked ts genes were purged of 'contaminating' mutations induced by NG treatment.

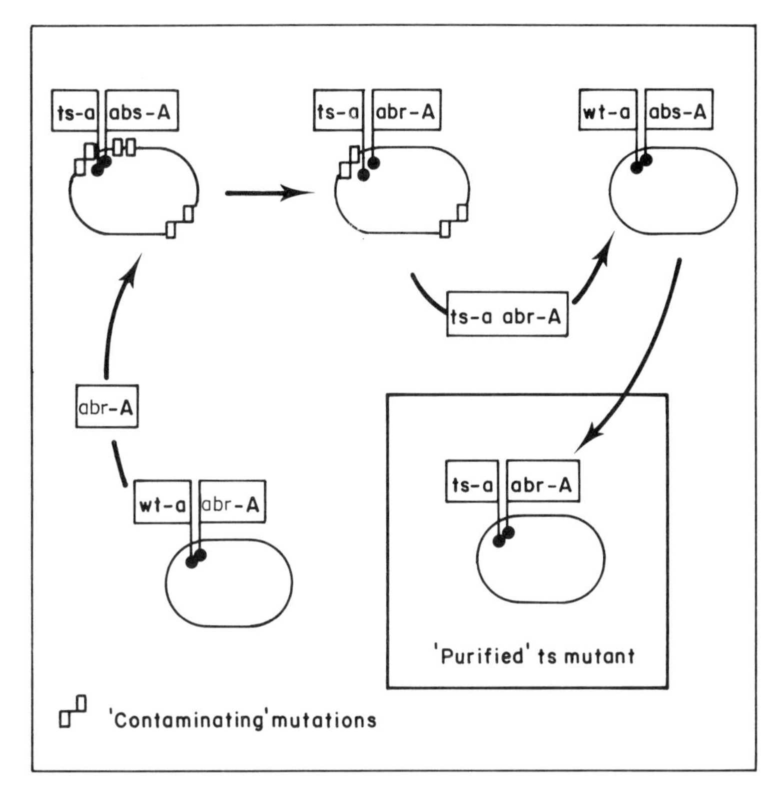

Figure 2. Outline of strategy for purification of ts mutants. For details of the specific steps see the text in Experimental Outline

Strain construction

The mutations in the 'clean' ts *H. influenzae* strains were combined by transformation, using the appropriate antibiotics for selection. Recombinants which putatively contained two ts lesions were screened for a reduction in reversion rate (Figure 3). The presence of the second ts gene was confirmed by recovering both mutations in a second transformation to a ts+ strain, and by testing the ability of DNA from these transformants to 'cure' each other, the putative double recombinant and the parental ts strains. Recombination of three ts lesions can only be confirmed by recovery of the three ts genes in separate transformations, and 'curing' experiments, because the reversion frequency of the double ts strain is already too low for accurate measurement.

Because all mutagenesis, selection and transformation experiments were done with *H. influenzae* strains derived from the unencapsulated type d, the final step in the construction was conversion to the encapsulated type. We transferred two of the ts mutations into strain Eagan, following the

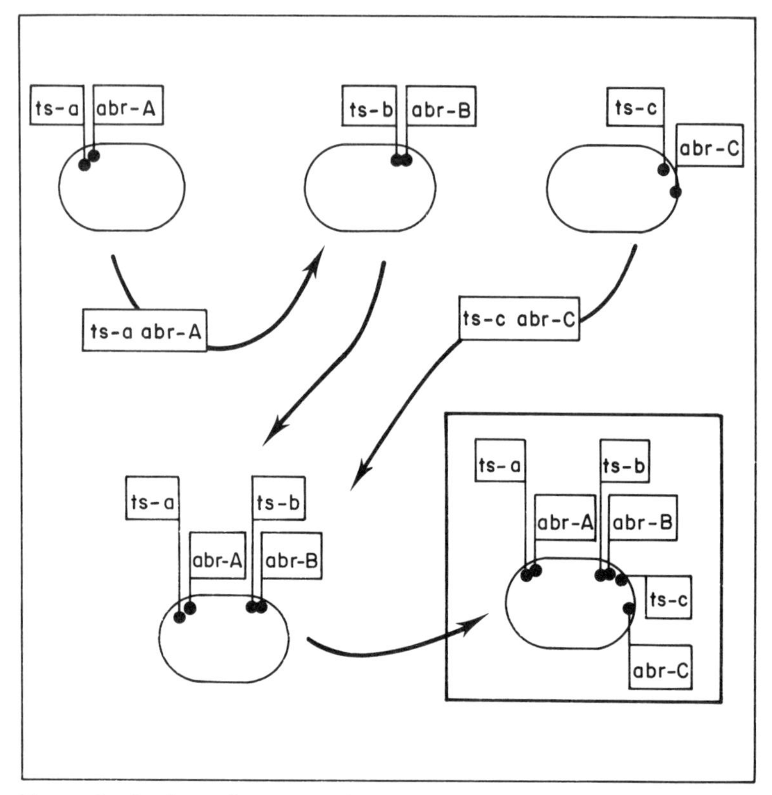

Figure 3. Outline of strategy for recombination of ts mutations. For details of the specific steps see the text in Experimental Outline

procedures described above. Retention and expression of the capsule genes in all transformants were monitored by plating on agar containing antiserum to the type b polysaccharide (the gift of Dr John Robbins).

Preliminary immunological evaluation

One encapsulated ts mutant of *H. influenzae*, containing two ts mutations, was evaluated for its ability to induce protection from wt challenge in an animal model. Sprague–Dawley rats, 6–7 days old, were exposed to an aerosolized suspension (1.5×10^9 cfu/ml) of ts *H. influenzae* in a chamber described previously[34]. Eleven days later the animals were again placed in the chamber, and exposed to an aerosol of wt *H. influenzae* (strain Eagan) and clearance of the challenge organism from the lungs was measured over 4 hours. Similar experiments were performed with DBA/2J mice to evaluate the immunogenic potential of 'tight' and 'coasting' strains of single ts mutants of *P. aeruginosa* ([34] and manuscript submitted for publication). Single ts mutants of *S. typhi* were tested in BALB/c mice using oral immunization and challenge, and intraperitoneal (ip) immunization and ip challenge with the wt suspended in 5% mucin (see Table I).

EXPERIMENTAL RESULTS

Initial ts isolates

Mutagenesis with NG and enrichment with penicillin and cefazolin resulted in the isolation of 137 ts *H. influenzae*. Of 2362 colonies screened, 137 were ts and 73 of these were chosen for further study. Similar results were obtained with *P. aeruginosa* and *S. typhi*. After temperature cut-offs were determined for the *H. influenzae* mutants, 23 were selected for the mapping studies. Linkage to antibiotic-resistance markers was firmly established for eight of the isolates.

Genetic mapping of ts *H. influenzae*

Reversion analysis, temperature cut-off experiments and preliminary mapping data indicated that several ts derivatives were suitable candidates for strain construction. Mapping experiments were repeated with these strains to confirm the linkages. The ts lesions in strains A/3, A/10, A214, C1/1, C1/4, C2/12, C2/13 and D115 were suitably linked to antibiotic-resistance markers. The Km^R-linkage of A/3, the Em^R-linkage of the C-series and the Sm^R-linkage of A214 and D115 were used to transform each of the ts mutations into Rd-001 to give 'clean' working strains for the final constructions. It should be acknowledged at this point that the antibiotics used in the feasibility study with *H. influenzae* are clinically relevant. Ideally, all linkages would be to clinically irrelevant antibiotic resistances, although it should be stressed that the resistances used in *H. influenzae* are chromosomal, recessive and not susceptible to promiscuous plasmid transfer.

Recombinant strains

Table II lists the *H. influenzae* strains containing one or more ts lesions, and their observed and calculated reversion rates. Streptomycin-resistant A214 was first transformed with A/3 DNA, Km-resistant recombinants were

Table II. Reversion rates of ts *Haemophilus influenzae*

Mutant	Observed reversion rates	Calculated reversion rates
A214	1×10^{-8}	—
A/3	6×10^{-8}	—
C/2/13	1×10^{-7}	—
A214–A/3	1×10^{-12}	6×10^{-16}
A214–A/3–C/2/13	$< 10^{-12}$	6×10^{-23}
A-17	$< 10^{-11}$	6×10^{-16}

selected and analysed for lowered reversion frequencies. Two recombinants tested yielded no colonies when plated at densities where the parental A214 gave at least 30 revertants/ml. The presence of the ts lesion linked to Km^R was confirmed by using DNA from the recombinant to transform Rd-001. Kanamycin resistance was used for selection and the recombinants screened for temperature sensitivity. The ts lesion was found in 28% of the transformants. Maintenance of the ts lesion linked to Sm^R was confirmed in a similar way and the mutation was recovered in 4% of the Sm^R-001 transformants. Strain C2/13 DNA was used to transform A214–A3, the transformants selected on plates containing erythromycin and the presence of all three ts genes confirmed by recovering them in separate transformations of Rd-001. The Sm^R-lesion was recovered in 9% of transformants, the Km^R-linked mutation in 15% and the Em^R-linked ts gene in 22% of the recipients. Although these numbers are in good agreement with the linkage data, given the qualitative nature of the transformation assay used, repeated 'curing' experiments with the 'rescued' markers suggested that one of the three ts lesions had been altered during recombination in A214–A/3–C2/13. We suspect the problem lies in the third ts mutation, from strain C2/13, the mutant derived from EKNSVNal, and the only one not subjected to double purification. We abandoned further use of this mutant for construction of the multiple ts type b. The A214 and A/3 mutations have both been transferred into strain Eagan. 'Rescue' experiments with several putative double ts Eagan recombinants have confirmed the presence of two ts mutations in strain A-17. The reversion frequency of A-17 is less than 10^{-11}, estimated from the results of cumulative platings over several years.

Growth characteristics of the mutant strains

The growth curves of the double recombinant *H. influenzae* A-17 before and after temperature shift from 29 to 36 °C are shown in Figure 4. The recombi-

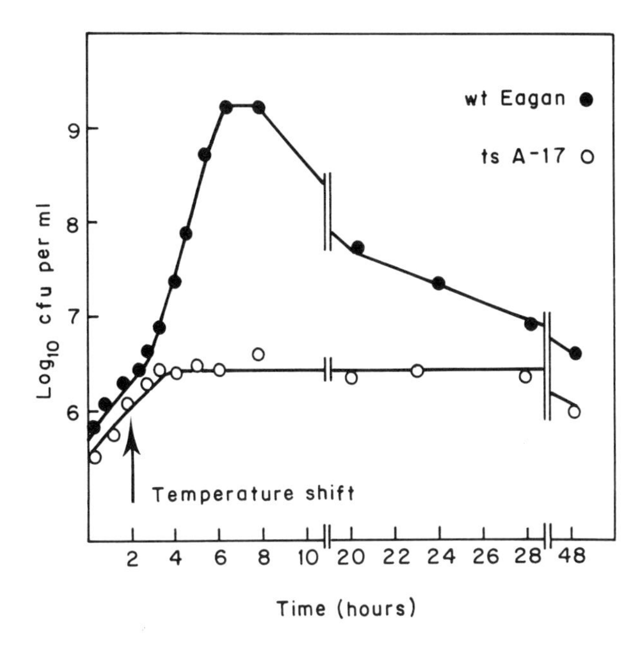

Figure 4. Growth curves of double ts and wt *H. influenzae* type b at permissive and non-permissive temperatures. Cultures of the two strains, ts A-17 and wt Eagan, were incubated at 29 °C and, at the time indicated by the arrow, the temperature was shifted to 36 °C. Samples were taken over 48 hours, diluted and plated for quantitation of colony forming units at the permissive temperature. Modified from Figure 2 in ref. [26]

nant continues to grow for two divisions after shift from 29 to 36 °C. It is significant that the mutant strain remains completely viable at 36 °C for 26 hours and, after a further 20 hours' incubation, loses only half a log in viability. One 'coasting' ts strain of *P. aeruginosa*, E/9/9, continues to divide for five divisions after temperature shift, resulting in a thirty fold increase in the number of cells [27]. Furthermore, E/9/9 remains completely viable at the non-permissive temperature for at least 48 hours, and maintains its 'coasting' phenotype *in vivo* and following reconstitution from lyophilization.

Animal studies

In a model of aerosol immunization with A-17 and aerosol challenge with the virulent strain Eagan, Sprague–Dawley rats immunized at the age of 6–7

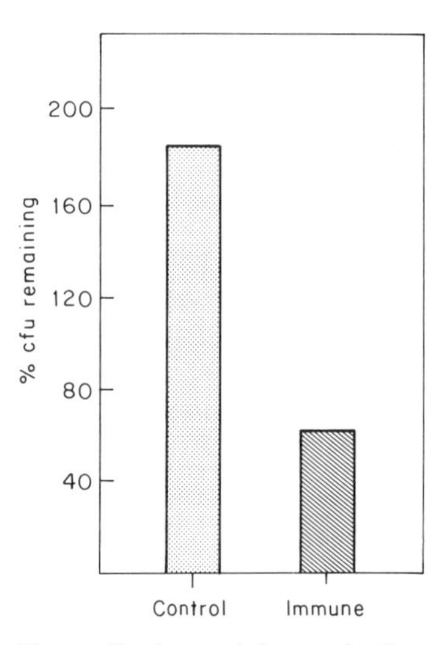

Figure 5. Aerosol immunization with a double ts mutant of *H. influenzae* enhances lung clearance of a wt challenge. Infant rats were immunized and challenged as described in Experimental Outline

days were able to clear their lungs of a challenge inoculum 11 days later, in contrast to control, saline-immunized animals, in whose lungs the organism multiplied during the 4 hours of the challenge (Figure 5). Aerosol and intranasal immunization with 'tight' and 'coasting' ts strains of *P. aeruginosa* also induce significant enhancement in lung clearance of wt challenge to DBA/2J mice, and this enhancement appears to be immunotype-specific (challenges with immunotypes 4 and 5 were not cleared as well as immunotype 1 challenges) [34, and manuscript submitted for publication]. BALB/c mice immunized orally or intraperitoneally with single ts mutants of *S. typhi* were significantly protected from oral and intraperitoneal wt challenge.

CONCLUSIONS

Haemophilus influenzae type b causes life-threatening meningitis in young children, *P. aeruginosa* is the major cause of morbidity and mortality in patients with cystic fibrosis and *S. typhi* remains a significant health problem in the underdeveloped countries of the world. Safe, effective vaccines for all these and other bacterial pathogens would go a long way towards control and even eradication of several infectious diseases.

Genetically attenuated, live vaccines are clearly superior in almost every respect to vaccine preparations based upon physical or chemical inactivation of cells or cellular products. The immunity induced by live vaccines is strong and long-lasting; administration *via* nasopharyngeal or oral routes is appropriate and simple; the cost of preparation, storage and delivery is considerably less than that required for the preparation of highly purified components; and safety can be assured by manipulation of genes – introduction of stable deletions into virulence genes, combination of multiple mutations in one strain or construction of avirulent hybrid strains carrying antigenic determinants of different pathogenic micro-organisms.

The somewhat pragmatic approach of Pasteur and the early microbiologists has now been refined, 100 years later, and with the benefits of more detailed knowledge of pathogenic mechanisms, genetic systems, immune responses and molecular biology. All that remains is the solution of relatively minor technical problems inherent in each of the approaches to the development of scientifically sound and effective, genetically attenuated live vaccines for virtually all bacterial diseases of man and animals.

ACKNOWLEDGEMENTS

The National Institute of Allergy and Infectious Diseases and the Cystic Fibrosis Foundation provided partial support for these studies.

REFERENCES

1. Adelberg, E. A., Mandel, M., and Chen, G. C. C. Optimal conditions for mutagenesis by nitrosoguanidine in *Escherichia coli* K12. *Biochem. Biophys. Res. Commun.*, **18**, 788–95 (1965).
2. Anderson, P. Antibody responses to *Haemophilus influenzae* type b and diphtheria toxin induced by conjugates of oligosaccharides of the type b capsule with the nontoxic protein CRM 197. *Infect. Immun.*, **39**, 233–8 (1983).
3. Anderson, P., Smith, D. H., Ingram, D. L., Wilkins, J., Wehrle, P. F., and Howie, V. M. Antibody to polyribophosphate of *Haemophilus influenzae* type b in infants and children: effect of immunization with polyribophosphate. *J. Infect. Dis.*, **136**, (Suppl.), S57–62 (1977).
4. Bornside, G. H. Waldemar Haffkine's cholera vaccines and the Ferran–Haffkine priority dispute. *J. Hist. Med. Allied. Sci.*, **37**, 399–422 (1982).
5. Cerda-Olmedo, E., Hanawalt, P. C., and Guerola, N. Mutagenesis of the replication point by nitrosoguanidine: map and pattern of replication of the *Escherichia coli* chromosome. *J. Mol. Biol.*, **33**, 705–19 (1968).
6. Collins, F. M. Tuberculosis. In *Bacterial Vaccines* (ed. R. Germanier), Academic Press, Orlando, Florida, 1984, pp. 373–418.
7. Davies, J. A. The response of infants to inoculation with type I pneumococcus carbohydrate. *J. Immunol.*. **33**, 1–7 (1937).

8. DuPont, H. L., Hornick, R. B., Snyder, M. J., Libonati, J. P., Formal, S. B., and Gangarosa, E. J. Immunity in shigellosis. I. Response of man to attenuated strains of *Shigella*. *J. Infect. Dis.*, **125**, 5–11 (1972).
9. Fahey, K. J., and Cooper, G. N. Oral immunization against experimental salmonellosis. I. Development of temperature-sensitive mutant vaccines. *Infect. Immun.*, **1**, 263–70 (1970).
10. Formal, S. B., Baron, L. S., Kopecko, D., Washington, O., Powell, C., and Life, C. A. Construction of a potential bivalent vaccine strain: introduction of *Shigella sonnei* form I antigen genes into the *galE S. typhi* Ty 21a typhoid vaccine strain. *Infect. Immun.*, **34**, 746–50 (1981).
11. Germanier, R., and Fürer, E. Isolation and characterization of *galE* mutant Ty 21a of *Salmonella typhi*: a candidate strain for a live, oral typhoid vaccine. *J. Infect. Dis.*, **131**, 553–8 (1975).
12. Greenberg, H., Helms, C. M., Brunner, H., and Chanock, R. M. Asymptomatic infection of adult volunteers with a temperature-sensitive mutant *Mycoplasma pneumoniae*. *Proc. Natl. Acad. Sci. USA*, **71**, 4015–19 (1974).
13. Helms, C. M., Grizzard, M. B., Prescott, B., Senterfit, L., Urmacher, S., Schiffman, G., and Chanock, R. M. Temperature-sensitive mutants of *Streptococcus pneumoniae*. I. Preparation and characterization *in vitro* of temperature-sensitive mutants of type 1 *S. pneumoniae*. *J. Infect. Dis.*, **135**, 582–92 (1977).
14. Hirschel, B., Wüthrich, R., Somaini, B., and Steffen, R. Inefficacy of the commercial live oral Ty 21a vaccine in the prevention of typhoid fever. *Eur. J. Clin. Microbiol.*, **4**, 295–8 (1985).
15. Hoiseth, S. K., and Stocker, B. A. D. Aromatic-dependent *Salmonella typhimurium* are non-virulent and effective as live vaccines. *Nature*, **291**, 238–9 (1981).
16. Honda, T., and Finkelstein, R. A. Selection and characteristics of a novel *Vibrio cholerae* mutant lacking the A (ADP-ribosylating) portion of the cholera enterotoxin. *Proc. Natl. Acad. Sci. USA*, **76**, 2052–6 (1979).
17. Juni, E. Simple genetic transformation assay for rapid diagnosis of *Moraxella osloensis*. *Appl. Microbiol.*, **27**, 16–24 (1974).
18. Kaper, J. B., and Levine, M. M. Cloned cholera enterotoxin genes in study and prevention of cholera. *Lancet*, **2**, 1162–3 (1981).
19. Levine, M. M., Woodward, W. E., Formal, S. B., Gemski, P., Dupont, H. L., Hornick, R. B., and Snyder, M. J. Studies with a new generation of oral attenuated *Shigella* vaccine: *Escherichia coli* bearing surface antigens of *Shigella flexneri*. *J. Infect. Dis.*, **136**, 577–82 (1977).
20. Levine, M. M., Dupont, H. L., Hornick, R. B., Snyder, M. J., Woodward, W., Gilman, R. H., and Libonati, J. P. Attenuated, streptomycin-dependent *Salmonella typhi* oral vaccine: potential deleterious effects of lyophilization. *J. Infect. Dis.*, **133**, 424–9 (1976).
21. Levine, M. M., Dupont, H. L., Gangarosa, E. J., Hornick, R. B., Snyder, M. J., Libonati, J. P., Glaser, K., and Formal, S. B. Shigellosis in custodial institutions. II. Clinical, immunologic and bacteriologic response of institutionalized children to oral attenuated shigella vaccines. *Am. J. Epidemiol.*, **96**, 40–9 (1972).
22. Levine, M. M., Black, R. E., Clements, M. L., Lanata, C., Sears, S., Honda, T., Young, C. R., and Finkelstein, R. A. Evaluation in humans of attenuated *Vibrio cholerae* El Tor Ogawa strain Texas Star-SR as a live oral vaccine. *Infect. Immun.*, **43**, 515–22 (1984).
23. Mäkelä, P. H., Peltola, H., Käyhty, H., Jousimies, H., Pettay, O., Ruoslahti, E., Sivonen, A., and Renkonen, O.-V. Polysaccharide vaccines of group A

Neisseria meningitidis and *Haemophilus influenzae* type b: a field trial in Finland. *J. Infect. Dis.*, **136** (Suppl.), S43–50 (1977).
24. Manning, P. A., Heuzenroeder, M. W., Yeadon, J., Leazesley, D. I., Reeves, P. R., and Rowley, D. Molecular cloning and expression in *Escherichia coli* K12 of the O antigens of the Inaba and Ogawa serotypes of the *Vibrio cholerae* O1 lipopolysaccharide and their potential for vaccine development. *Infect. Immun.*, **53**, 272–7 (1986).
25. Monto, A. S., Brandt, B. L., and Artenstein, M. S. Response of children to *Neisseria meningitidis* polysaccharide vaccines. *J. Infect. Dis.*, **127**, 394–400 (1973).
26. Morris Hooke, A., Bellanti, J. A., and Oeschger, M. P. Live attenuated bacterial vaccines: new approaches for safety and efficacy. *Lancet*, **1**, 1472–4 (1985).
27. Morris Hooke, A., Arroyo, P. J., Oeschger, M. P., and Bellanti, J. A. Temperature-sensitive mutants of *Pseudomonas aeruginosa*: isolation and preliminary immunological evaluation. *Infect. Immun.*, **38**, 136–40 (1982).
28. Parke, J. C., Schneerson, R., Robbins, J. B., and Schlesselman, J. J. Interim report of a controlled field trial of immunization with capsular polysaccharides of *Haemophilus influenzae* type b and group C *Neisseria meningitidis* in Mecklenburg County, North Carolina (March 1974–March 1976). *J. Infect. Dis.*, **136** (Suppl.), S51–6 (1977).
29. Pearson, G. D. N., and Mekalanos, J. J. Molecular cloning of *Vibrio cholerae* enterotoxin genes in *Escherichia coli* K-12. *Proc. Natl. Acad. Sci. USA*, **79**, 2976–80 (1982).
30. Pichichero, M. E., Hall, C. B., and Insel, R. A. A mucosal antibody response following systemic *Haemophilus influenzae* type b infection in children. *J. Clin. Invest.*, **67**, 1482–9 (1983).
31. Reitman, M. Infectivity and antigenicity of streptomycin-dependent *Salmonella typhosa*. *J. Infect. Dis.*, **117**, 101–7 (1967).
32. Robbins, J. D., and Robbins, J. B. Reexamination of the protective role of the capsular polysaccharide (Vi antigen) of *Salmonella typhi*. *J. Infect. Dis.*, **150**, 436–49 (1984).
33. Schneerson, R., Robbins, J. B., Egan, W., Zon, G., Sutton, A., Vann, W. F., Kaijser, B., Hanson, L. A., and Ahlstedt, S. Bacterial capsular polysaccharide conjugates. In *Seminars in Infectious Disease*. Vol. IV: *Bacterial Vaccines* (ed. J. B. Robbins, J. C. Hill and J. C. Sadoff), Thieme-Stratton, Inc., New York, 1982, pp. 311–21.
34. Sordelli, D. O., Cerquetti, M. C., Morris Hooke, A., and Bellanti, J. A. Enhancement of *Pseudomonas aeruginosa* lung clearance after local immunization with a temperature-sensitive mutant. *Infect. Immun.*, **39**, 1275–9 (1983).
35. Wahdan, M. H., Serie, C., Cerisier, Y., Sallam, S., and Germanier, R. A controlled field trial of live *Salmonella typhi* Ty21a oral vaccine against typhoid. *J. Infect. Dis.*, **145**, 292–5 (1982).

DISCUSSION – Chaired by Professor A. Capron

HANDMAN: It puzzled me that you measured serum antibodies IgM and IgG in a situation where you immunized and infected intranasally, the clearance of bacteria would have been at the level of the mucosa and not at the level of the serum. So the more useful antibodies in that situation, I would imagine, would be IgA antibodies and their level might not be the same in the serum as locally, in the lungs let's say.

HOOKE: You are absolutely right of course. The reason why we measured the serum antibody was that it was a lot easier. Also, we wanted to see if there was any breakthrough of the immunizing strains into the system. There was no detectable breakthrough. The second point is that the mechanism of the clearance of *P. aeruginosa* from the lungs is not known. Nobody really knows whether it is due to opsonizing antibody; certainly granulocytes are necessary. Serum IgG may break through into the lungs with the inflammation induced by *P. aeruginosa*. We are, of course, looking at mucosal antibody in a different model, because the ultimate aim, naturally, would be intranasal immunization and the induction of protective (not blocking) IgA.

ADA: This is along the same lines. We have recently developed an ELISA plaque technique for looking at antibody-secreting cells in the lung following influenza virus infection. Curiously, this had not been done before. You could use the same technology to look at the existence and persistence of antibody-secreting cells to a bacterial antigen. You could determine how long you had memory or long-lived antibody-producing cells in the lung itself.

HOOKE: Exactly. It is certainly the direction we are going in.

EASMON: Since you did measure IgG and IgM, can I ask if it was opsonic?

HOOKE: We have not done those experiments yet, but certainly they have to be done.

Towards Better Carbohydrate Vaccines
Edited by R. Bell and G. Torrigiani

Published by John Wiley & Sons Ltd

14

Studies on carbohydrate antigens of bacterial pathogens

JOHN B. ROBBINS, RACHEL SCHNEERSON AND SHOUSUN CHEN SZU
National Institute of Child Health and Human Development, National Institutes of Health, Bethesda, MD, USA
WILLIAM EGAN AND WILLIE F. VANN
Office of Biologics Research and Review, Food and Drug Administration, Bethesda, MD, USA
WALTER W. KARAKAWA
Department of Biochemistry, Pennsylvania State University, University Park, PA, USA

INTRODUCTION

Carbohydrates, notably polysaccharides (PS), are important pathogenic and protective antigens of bacteria that cause invasive diseases of humans [3, 5, 18, 49, 50, 52]. We report our recent studies into the immunological and physico-chemical properties of PS from capsulated bacterial pathogens: *Streptococcus pneumoniae* (pneumococci), *Neisseria meningitidis* (meningococci) and *Staphylococcus aureus* (staphylococci). In addition, we report that ultrasonic irradiation (UI) can be used to depolymerize PS into preparations of defined and homogeneous molecular weight that retain the structure of their repeating units.

PNEUMOCOCCAL CELL-WALL POLYSACCHARIDE (Cw-ps) ANTIBODIES ARE NOT PROTECTIVE

Pneumococcal infections continue to cause considerable morbidity in both industrialized and Third World nations [3, 12, 22, 47]. Pneumococcal vaccine, composed of 23 of the most frequently encountered capsular polysaccharide (CPS) types in patients, has deficiencies limiting its universal use: (a) although effective in older children and adults, the vaccine fails to induce protective levels of antibodies in infants and young children and in patients with immunodeficiencies (those with the highest attack rates of pneumococcal diseases) [3, 12, 39, 47, 54]; (2) a small fraction of pneumococcal diseases are caused by CPS types not in the vaccine [3, 5, 12, 39, 51]. These limitations have prompted a search for a vaccine which would be more immunogenic and exert a more comprehensive coverage of pneumococci.

Briles *et al.*, showed that phosphorylcholine-specific (PC) antibodies protected mice against intravenous challenge with several pneumococcal types [7–9, 66]. The fine specificity of the PC-antibodies, as characterized by their idiotype, subclass and the isotype composition, was related to the protective effect [8, 9]. Further, C-reactive protein, a serum protein which binds PC, was shown to confer protection against pneumococcal infections in the mouse [42]. The Cw-ps, present in all pneumococci, was the most likely candidate for this protective antigen [2, 9, 56, 60, 67]. The Cw-ps is a linear copolymer composed of a pentasaccharide repeating unit with PC linked to its galactose [29], has a low molecular weight and is a poor immunogen in healthy adults [56, 57].

Cell-wall polysaccharide was covalently bound to bovine serum albumin (BSA), a model carrier protein, with the heterobifunctional coupling agent, *N*-succinimidyl 3-(2-pyridyldithio-propionate) (SPDP) in order to increase its immunogenicity [10, 61]. The resultant Cw-ps–BSA conjugate was reactive with monoclonal PC-specific antibodies. The Cw-ps–BSA conjugate, incorporated into Freund's adjuvant, was injected twice into rabbits. Another rabbit antiserum, with high levels of antibodies reactive with Cw-ps and with PC specificity was prepared by Dr Jørgen Henrichsen, WHO Collaborating Centre for Reference and Research on Pneumococci, Statens Seruminstituut, Copenhagen, by intravenous injections of a mutant strain of pneumococcus, SRC-2, which has a capsule-like structure composed of the Cw-ps [6, 60]. These two antisera were fractionated into globulins by precipitation with 50% saturated ammonium sulphate, in order to remove non-immunoglobulin PC-binding proteins [45].

Anti-Cw-ps antibodies were quantified in both globulin preparations by the quantitative precipitin reaction using purified Cw-ps as the antigen. The Cw-ps conjugate elicited antibodies to the backbone of the polysaccharide only as addition of PC did not inhibit the precipitation of the Cw-ps to the immune globulin. Addition of PC, in contrast, reduced the precipitation with Cw-ps with the SRC-2 globulin by about 15%.

No change in the LD_{50} of type 3 or type 6A pneumococci, injected IP into mice, was exerted by passive immunization with the Cw-ps–BSA-induced antibodies. Passive immunization with the SRC-2 globulin conferred protection against both pneumococcal types, albeit at a lower level than that reported for type-specific antibodies [60]. Adsorption of the SRC-2 globulin with Cw-ps, moreover, did not affect its protective activity. Active immunization, induced by intraperitoneal injection of the Cw-ps–BSA conjugate, also failed to protect mice against lethal challenge 2 weeks later with either type 3 or type 6A pneumococci. These data provide evidence that the protective actions against lethal infection by capsulated pneumococci in the mouse model conferred by some PC-antibodies are not mediated by antibodies to the Cw-ps. Holmberg *et al.* arrived at the same conclusion; that antibodies to the Cw-ps were not protective, based upon a seroepidemiological study of pneumococcal pneumonia in a community [25]. The non-capsular component(s) of pneumococci that are reactive with the protective PC-specific antibodies have not been identified. Another PC-containing oligosaccharide, the Forssman or F-antigen, was shown not to induce protective immunity against pneumococcal infection in the mouse [2].

It should be noted that the IP route of challenge of mice with pneumococci was found to be a reliable method for assaying both the virulence of pneumococci and the protective effect of rabbit type-specific antibodies prepared for passive immunization of patients [60, 61]. In this assay, less than 1 μg of anti-CPS antibody per mouse conferred type-specific protection. Considerably higher amounts of non-capsular antibodies are required to induce a comparable level of protection against challenge with capsulated pneumococci in this method. These findings should be considered when data for protection conferred by antibody of a single specificity in animal models are extrapolated to clinical immunity.

ULTRASONIC IRRADIATION (UI) OF BACTERIAL POLYSACCHARIDES

The immunogenicity of PS is related to their molecular weight. There is a direct relation between the immunogenicity and molecular weight of purified PS [18, 26, 31, 41]. This relation has been used to standardize CPS vaccines in order to predict reliably their immunogenicity [64]. Makela *et al.* showed a complex relation between the immunogenicity and molecular weight of dextrans bound to albumins [40]. Conjugates prepared with dextrans of intermediate molecular weights (*circa* 40 000 daltons) elicited higher levels of anti-dextran antibodies than did conjugates prepared with dextrans of either higher or lower molecular weight. These, and other experiments, have stimulated interest in studying PS of lower and more homogeneous molecular weight distribution than the parent molecule.

The molecular weight of biopolymers, including PS, may be reduced into fragments that retain biological activity by several techniques including acid and akaline hydrolysis, enzymatic digestion, thermal denaturation or chemical degradation. These treatments usually produce products in low yields, more heterogeneous than the parent molecule, and which may have modified chemical structures.

Shearing stress, such as UI, has been shown to depolymerize macromolecules including DNA and PS. Martin *et al.* showed that UI of Vi CPS reduced its molecular weight, immunogenicity and protective action against *Salmonella typhi* infection in mice [41]. Curiously, in spite of the long and successful application of UI to the study of DNA, there is still no detailed understanding of the mechanism(s) of its depolymerizing action.

Because of our interest in studying bacterial polysaccharides of different molecular weights, the depolymerization exerted by UI on representative compounds, including dextran (neutral), *Haemophilus influenzae* type b (Hib) and pneumococcus (Pn) type 6A and type 6B (acidic with phosphodiester linkage) and Pn type 9N (acidic with uronic acid) PS, was studied [59]. Prolonged UI depolymerized all these PS to a finite, similar and homogeneous molecular weight distribution of about 50 000 daltons. The rate of depolymerization depended upon the concentration and viscosity of the PS. Addition of glycerol increased the viscosity of the solvent; the rate of depolymerization was increased and the limit product had a lower molecular weight. Both the phosphodiester and glycosidic linkages of the Hib were cleaved by UI. This was shown by the equal ratios of monophosphate terminal residues (^{31}P n.m.r. spectroscopy) and reducing end groups (Park–Johnson reaction) in the final product. Rupture of carbon–carbon bonds within the monosaccharides was not detected.

We compared the depolymerization induced by thermal energy and by UI of the constitutionally related Pn type 6A and type 6B CPS. Thermal depolymerization of type 6B CPS occurred by random cleavage of the linkages within the repeating unit [69]. In contrast, thermal depolymerization of type 6A was largely due to cleavage of the phosphodiester bond. Type 6A, which has a more labile phosphodiester bond, was depolymerized about 10^3 times faster than type 6B. In contrast, UI depolymerized type 6A and type 6B at the same rate and by random cleavage of all linkages.

Our explanation for these results, including the finite and similar molecular weights of all the PS achieved by prolonged UI, is that the mechanical torque necessary to cleave the linkages is dependent upon the length of the PS. When the molecular weight of the PS is reduced to about 50 000 daltons, the rigidity of the shortened chain length increases so that mechanical torque generated by UI was unable to induce further cleavage. Studies of PS structure, conformation and interaction with ligands can be facilitated by homogeneous and partially depolymerized products. For example, the molecular weight of native Vi CPS (>4 × 10^6 daltons) was too high for resolution by gel filtration on 2B Sepharose and the linewidths of the ^{13}C n.m.r. signals were broad (~25 Hz). Ultrasonic irradiation of the Vi resulted in a homogeneous polymer of about 78 000 daltons. This depolymerized Vi could now be dissolved at 20 mg/ml which allowed accumulation ^{13}C n.m.r. signals that showed a reduced linewidth of ~14 Hz and an improved signal-to-noise level.

Ultrasonic irradiation is a reproducible, convenient, non-destructive method for preparing fragments that have both the same repeating unit and a more homogeneous molecular weight distribution than the native PS. The process only disrupts the linkages between the monosaccharides.

CROSS-REACTIVITY BETWEEN THE CAPSULAR POLYSACCHARIDES OF MENINGOCOCCUS GROUP A AND *ESCHERICHIA COLI* K93 AND K51

As Fothergill and Wright first showed for Hib, there is an age-related development of serum bactericidal antibodies that is inversely related to the age incidence of invasive diseases due to capsulated bacteria [3, 5, 16–18, 50]. In many instances the acquisition of these bactericidal (mostly anti-CPS) antibodies has been shown to be due to an interaction between the host and non-pathogenic cross-reacting bacteria of the respiratory and gastrointestinal flora [52]. That the acquisition of CPS antibodies could be stimulated by cross-reacting and not the homologous antigen was convincingly illustrated by the case of meningococcus Group A, the causative organism of epidemic meningitis [17, 18]. Group A diseases have a different epidemiology from those caused by the other pathogenic capsular groups of meningococci. Meningitis due to Group A meningococci occurs with high frequency on a seasonal basis in central Africa or as epidemics, lasting 1 or 2 years, throughout the world [66]. Yet, in central Africa with its high endemicity and sporadic epidemics, asymptomatic carriage of Group A meningococci is about 1–2% [23]. Group A meningococci have been only rarely detected in the USA for the past 40 years [49], either as isolates from cases of meningitis or from asymptomatic carriers. Yet, in all these settings, high endemicity, sporadic epidemics or in the virtual absence of the homologous organism, most adults have protective levels of Group A CPS antibodies. Until recently, only certain strains of *Bacillus pumilis* and *Streptococcus faecium*, two species of bacteria infrequently encountered in humans, have been found to cross-react with the Group A meningococcal CPS.

Guirgis *et al.* discovered strains of *E. coli* in stools of patients and of their families that yielded immunospecific haloes of precipitation when cultivated on Group A meningococcal antiserum-agar during a study of bacterial meningitis in Egypt, 1977–78 [23]. Drs Ida and Frits Ørskov, WHO Collaborating Centre for Research and Reference on *Escherichia*, Copenhagen, identified the cross-reacting antigens as the K93 and K51 CPS of *E. coli*. These two CPS were also detected in surveys of stool and blood isolates in the Clinical Center of the NIH, Bethesda, USA, schoolchildren in Copenhagen and in the WHO Reference collection. None of the cross-reactive *E. coli* had detectable ST, LT or Shiga-like toxins. The K93 strains from Egypt were of either of the *O*-107 : K93 : H27 or the *O*107 : K93 : SP serotype and may be considered as descendants of a single bacterium or as a clone [44]. The purified K93 CPS and K51 CPS did not cross react with each other. *Escherichia coli* strains of each capsular type were injected intravenously into rabbits and elicited precipitating and bactericidal antibodies to Group A meningococci. The K93 CPS precipitated 47% and the K51 CPS precipitated 25% of Group A meningococcal CPS antibodies from hyperimmune equine serum. The bactericidal activity against Group A meningococcal organisms was reduced from the equine antiserum by adsorption with either of the two cross-reacting *E. coli* CPS. The epidemiological, serological and biochemical characterization of strains bearing these two K types suggest that these *E. coli* could serve as a stimulus for the wide prevalence of 'natural' Group A meningococcal CPS antibodies.

The structures of the Group A meningococcal and the two cross-reacting *E. coli* CPS have been elucidated [4, 18]. The Group A CPS is a pseudo-randomly *O*acetylated α-1 $\rightarrow$ 6-linked homopolymer of D-ManNAc-1-PO_4- (about 70% of the C_3 are *O*-acetylated). The K51 CPS is a linear copolymer of $\rightarrow$3)-GlcNAc-1-(PO_4- (*O*-acetylated at the C_6 position). This compositionally and structurally related PS removed only 25% of the Group A CPS antibodies. We were surprised to find that the K93 CPS, which precipitated 47% of Group A antibodies, had no obvious resemblance to the Group A meningococcal CPS. K93 CPS was found to be a $\rightarrow$3)-β-D-Gal *f*-(1 $\rightarrow$ 4)-β-GlcUA *p*-(1-, with the C5 and C6 of galactose being *O*-acetylated [53]. The K93 composition and linkages were found to be identical to the *E. coli* K53; the latter is *O*-acetylated in the C2 position of galactose and does not cross-react with the Group A meningococcal CPS. De-*O*-acetylation of K93 removed its cross-reactivity with the Group A CPS [4].

These findings provide another illustration that the three-dimensional structure, and not the composition *per se*, of PS (and presumably of all antigens) accounts for their immunological reactivity. Studies to characterize the three-dimensional structure of the cross-reactive PS are under way.

Immunization of both infants and adults with Group A meningococcal capsular polysaccharide vaccine induces protective levels of serum antibodies [18]. Yet our current Group A meningococcal CPS vaccine has three deficiences which could be solved with this information about cross-reacting antigens and other developments in PS chemistry; (1) two injections of Group A meningococcal PS vaccine are required in infants and children up to 18 months to induce protective immunity; (2) the duration of Group A vaccine-induced immunity is not long [18]. Levels of vaccine-induced antibodies and protection decline in 1–2 years in children and in about 3–5 years in adults [19–22, 38, 46, 48]; (3) the immunogenicity of the Group A vaccine is reduced in infants and children in Africa whose general health and nutritional status is not optimal (malaria is particularly immunosuppressive against Group A meningococcal CPS vaccine) [20–22, 48]. The immunogenicity of the Group A CPS has been increased by binding it covalently to a carrier protein, tetanus toxoid [28]. The repertoire of B lymphocytes producing Group A antibodies, especially in infants and young children, might be increased by immunization with compositionally different but structurally related PS. We are studying the immunologic properties of PS–protein conjugates of meningococcal Group A alone and in combination with the two *E. coli* cross-reacting CPS in order to evaluate their potential for vaccination of infants and young children.

NEWLY DISCOVERED CAPSULAR POLYSACCHARIDES OF STAPHYLOCOCCUS AUREUS

Staphylococcus aureus causes several diseases in humans. The pathogenesis of some of these diseases, such as 'toxic shock syndrome' and 'scalded skin syndrome', have been related to activity of exoproteins secreted by this bacterial species. The pathogenesis of and immunity to bacteriaemic diseases caused by *S. aureus*, a major cause of hospital-acquired infections with considerable morbidity and mortality, remains obscure.

Capsular polysaccharides were isolated from *S. aureus*, strains 'Smith', 'M' and 'Dp', and their structures elucidated; all contained an aminouronic acid in their repeat unit [24, 34, 35, 65]. Strains bearing these CPS are usually mucoid and are easily distinguished from other *S. aureus*. Several groups have provided evidence that these CPS exert anti-opsonic activity similar to that observed with other gram-positive capsulated bacterial pathogens. Phagocytosis of these capsulated strains by peripheral blood polymorphonuclear leucocytes (PMNs) was enhanced by antibody and complement [11, 36, 62]. Strains bearing these CPS types, however, have only rarely been isolated from the blood of patients [1, 34] and cannot be considered as pathogenic.

Karakawa *et al.* collected strains of *S. aureus* from patients and prepared monospecific hyperimmune capsular typing antisera [1, 32–37, 43]. Techniques used for other capsulated bacterial pathogens were modified for the isolation and for the identification of the CPS types from these isolates. Serological methods were developed to identify whether isolates of *S. aureus* were capsulated. A capsular typing scheme was proposed with individual strains designated as representatives of eight CPS types [34, 37]. With these monospecific capsular typing antisera, it was found that two CPS, type 5 and type 8, comprised about 70% of bacteraemic isolates from patients in the USA, Sweden and Israel [1, 15, 16]. Several phage types were associated with type 5 and some with type 8 CPS. The phage type 80/81, associated with the severe outbreaks of bacteraemic *S. aureus* disease in nurseries for new-borns during the 1950s, was associated with CPS type 8. The phage type 95 was found on type 8 and phage type 94/96 was found only on type 5 *S. aureus* strains. In contrast to the mucoid appearance of strains bearing CPS types 1–3, the colonial morphology of types 4–8 is not unique. The capsules of type 5 and type 8 have been visualized by electron microscopy [55].

Monoclonal and polyclonal antibodies, specific for types 5 and 8 CPS, were isolated and characterized [43]. Precipitin analyses with these antisera revealed two antigenic determinants on the type 8 CPS. The native antigenic structure of the type 8 CPS is conferred by an *O*-acetyl moiety. One of the monoclonal type 8 antibodies reacted with a de-*O*-acetylated type 8 CPS. These antisera facilitated opsonophagocytosis of *S. aureus* strains of the homologous CPS type. The antibody reactive with the native type 8 CPS had a higher specific activity in this bioassay than the monoclonal and polyclonal antisera that reacted with the de-*O*-acetylated type 8 CPS. Similarly, type 5 CPS antibodies exhibited type-specific opsonphagocytosis.

Recently, three additional CPS types have been recognized. With these 11 capsular antisera, it has been possible to identify CPS of about 90% of bacteraemic *S. aureus* isolates. Most of the remaining blood isolates were capsulated, as measured by their failure to react with antisera elicited by non-capsulated strains; capsulated strains are not agglutinated with antisera to non-capsular structures. This 'covering up' of non-capsular structures by the CPS has been noted in *E. coli* and *Salmonellae*.

We propose, by analogy with other capsulated bacterial pathogens, that the newly described CPS confer the property of invasiveness to *S. aureus* [3, 5, 13, 18, 27, 30, 49, 52, 53, 58, 63]. The evidence for this proposal is as follows.

1. Almost all strains isolated from the blood of patients with bacteraemia are capsulated. Capsulated and non-capsulated strains, however, are found from superficial sites such as the skin and nasopharynx.
2. Non-capsulated strains are opsonized by PMNs in the presence of normal sera. Capsulated strains required anti-CPS antibodies and complement for maximal phagocytosis (CPS 'shield' *S. aureus* strains from non-immune resistance mechanisms).
3. Although 11 CPS types have been identified to date, only some have been

associated with bacteraemia. Strains of the newly discovered CPS type 5 and type 8 account for about 70% of *S. aureus* isolates from patients with bacteraemia.

4. Preliminary findings indicate that patients who recover from *S. aureus* bacteraemia synthesize anti-CPS antibodies specific for the infecting type.

If our hypothesis and this preliminary evidence are valid, then active or passive immunity to CPS, in conjunction with antibiotics and other supportive therapy, could be used to prevent and/or treat *S. aureus* bacteraemia. We plan to synthesize type 5 and type 8 CPS–protein conjugates in order to prepare hyperimmune plasma for a clinical study, as has been done with anti-*E. coli* antibodies in order to evaluate this hypothesis [68].

SUMMARY

We have reviewed some of our studies into the physico-chemical and immunological properties of bacterial PS. The potential of the Cw-ps of pneumococci as a species-specific protective antigen was investigated: information was provided which made it doubtful that this structure could induce protective immunity. Two *E. coli* CPS were discovered to cross react with meningococcus Group A CPS, the protective antigen of epidemic meningitis. We plan to study whether vaccines composed of protein conjugates of these CPS could augment the serum antibody response to Group A meningococcal CPS. The concept that the pathogenesis of and immunity to bacteraemia caused by *S. aureus* are similar to those of other capsulated bacteria causing invasive diseases, including hospital-acquired infections, continues to gain credence. Finally, an established but incompletely characterized technique of depolymerizing macomolecules, UI, has been shown to have potential for preparing PS in a more homogeneous form with an unchanged composition and structure in high yields. Basic information and practical solutions for health problems may evolve from investigations of polysaccharides of pathogenic bacteria.

ACKNOWLEDGEMENTS

We are grateful to Dr Charles U. Lowe, NIH, for his review of this manuscript and for his helpful comments and suggestions.

REFERENCES

1. Arbeit, R. D., Karakawa, W. W., Vann, W. F., and Robbins, J. B. Predominance of two newly described capsular polysaccharide types among clinical isolates of *Staphylococcus aureus*. *Diag. Microbiol. Infect.*, **2**, 85–91 (1984).

2. Au, C. C., and Eisenstein, T. K. Evaluation of the role of the pneumococcal Forssman antigen (F-polysaccharide) in the cross-serotype protection induced by pneumococcal subcellular preparations. *Infect. Immun.*, **31**, 169–73 (1981).
3. Austrian, R. Pneumococcal infections. In *Bacterial Vaccines* (ed. R. Germanier), Academic Press, New York, 1984, pp. 257–85.
4. Bax, A., Summers, M. F., Guirgis, N., Schneerson, R., Robbins, J. B., Ørskov, F., Ørskov, I., Vann, W. F., and Egan, W. Structural studies of the *Escherichia coli* K93 and K53 capsular polysaccharides. *Carb. Res.*, in press (1986).
5. Bishop, C. T., and Jennings, H. J. Immunology of polysaccharides. In *The Polysaccharides*, Vol. 1 (ed. G. O. Aspinall), Academic Press, New York, 1982, pp. 291–330.
6. Bornstein, D. L., Schiffman, G., Bernheimer, H. F., and Austrian, R. Capsulation of pneumococcus with soluble C-like (C_s) polysaccharide. I. Biological and genetic properties of (C_s) pneumococcal strains. *J. Exper. Med.*, **128**, 1385–400 (1968).
7. Briles, D. E., Clafin, L. J., Shroer, K., Forman, C., Basta, P., Lehmeyer, J., and Benjamin, W. H. Jr The use of hybridoma antibodies to examine antibody-mediated antimicrobial activities. In *Monoclonal Antibodies and T-cell Hybridomas. Perspectives and Technical Advances* (ed. G. J. Hammerling, U. Hammerling and J. F. Kearney), Elsevier/North-Holland Biomedical Press, New York, 1981, pp. 285–90.
8. Briles, D. E., Clafin, J. L., Shroer, K., and Forman, C. Mouse IgG3 antibodies are highly protective against infection with *Streptococcus pneumoniae. Nature*, **294**, 88–90 (1981).
9. Briles, D. E., Forman, C., Hudak, S., and Claflin, J. L. Anti-phosphorylcholine antibodies of the T15 idiotype are optimally protective against *Streptococcus pneumoniae. J. Exp. Med.*, **156**, 1177–85 (1982).
10. Carlsson, J., Drevin, H., and Axen, R. Protein thiolation and reversible protein-protein conjugation. *Eur. J. Biochem.*, **173**, 723–37 (1978).
11. Christina, M. J. E., Vandenbroucke-Grauls, H. M., Thussen, W. M., and Verhoef, J. Interaction between human polymorphonuclear leukocytes and *Staphylococcus aureus* in the presence and absence of opsonins. *Immunol.*, **52**, 427–35 (1984).
12. Douglas, R. M., and Kerby-Eaton, E. *Acute Respiratory Infections in Childhood*, 1985. Proceedings of an International Workshop, Sydney, August 1984.
13. Ehrenworth, L., and Baer, H. The pathogenicity of *Klebsiella pneumoniae* for mice – the relationship to the quantity and rate of production of type-specific capsular polysaccharide. *J. Bacteriol.*, **72**, 713–17 (1956).
14. Fournier, J.-M., Hannon, K., Moreau, M., Karakawa, W. W., and Vann, W. F. Isolation of type 5 capsular polysaccharide from *Staphylococcus aureus. Infect. Immun.*, in press (1987).
15. Fournier, J. M., Vann, W. F., and Karakawa, W. W. Purification and characterization of *Staphylococcus aureus* type 8 capsular polysaccharide. *Infect. Immun.*, **45**, 87–93 (1984).
16. Fothergill, L. D., and Wright, J. Influenzal meningitis: relation of age incidence to the bactericidal power of blood against the causal organism. *J. Immunol.*, **24**, 273–84 (1933).
17. Goldschneider, I., Gotschlich, E. C., and Artenstein, M. S. Human immunity to the meningococcus. II. Development of natural immunity. *J. Exp. Med.*, **129**, 1327–48 (1969).

18. Gotschlich, E. C. Meningococcal meningitis. In *Bacterial Vaccines* (ed. R. Germanier), Academic Press, New York, 1984, pp. 237–52.
19. Gotschlich, E. C., Rey, M., Sanborn, W. R., Triau, R., and Cvjetanovic, B. The immunological responses observed in field studies in Africa with Group A meningococcal vaccines. *Prog. in Immunobiological Stand.*, **129**, 485–91 (1972).
20. Greenwood, A. M., Greenwood, B. M., Bradley, A. K., Ball, P. A. J., and Giles, H. M. Enhancement of the immune response to meningococcal polysaccharide vaccine in a malaria endemic area by administration of chloroquine. *Ann. Trop. Med. Parasit.*, **75**, 261–3 (1981).
21. Greenwood, B. M., Whittle, H. C., Bradley, A. K., Fayet, M. T., and Giles, H. M. The duration of the antibody response to meningococcal vaccination in an African village. *Trans. Royal Soc. Trop. Med. Hyg.*, **74**, 756-80 (1980).
22. Greenwood, B. M. Selective primary health care: strategies for control of disease in the developing world. XIII. Acute bacterial meningitis. *Rev. Infect. Dis.*,**6**, S374–89 (1984).
23. Guirgis, N., Schneerson, R., Bax, A., Egan, W., Robbins, J. B., Ørskov, I., and Ørskov, F. *Escherichia coli* K51 and K93 capsular polysaccharides cross-reactive with Group A meningococcal polysaccharide. Immunochemical, structural and epidemiological studies. *J. Exp. Med.*, **162**, 1837–62 (1985).
24. Hanessian, S., and Haskell, T. H. Structural studies on staphylococcal polysaccharides. *J. Biol. Chem.*, **239**, 2758–64 (1964).
25. Holmberg, A., Krook, A., and Sjogren, A.-M. Determination of antibodies to pneumococcal C-polysaccharide in patients with community-acquired pneumonia. *J. Clin. Microbiol.*, **22**, 808–14 (1983).
26. Howard, J. G., and Courtenay, B. M. Influence of molecular structure on the tolerogenicity of bacterial dextrans. *Immunol.*, **29**, 599–610 (1975).
27. Howard, C. J., and Glynn, A. A. The virulence for mice of strains of *Escherichia coli* related to the effects of K antigens on their resistance to phagocytosis and killing by complement. *Immunol.*, **20**, 767–80 (1977).
28. Jennings, H., and Lugowski, C. Immunochemistry of Groups A, B and C meningococcal polysaccharide tetanus toxoid conjugates. *J. Immunol.*, **127**, 104–8 (1981).
29. Jennings, H. J., Lugowski, C., and Young, N. M. Structure of the complex polysaccharide C-substance from *Streptococcus pneumoniae* type 1. *Biochem.*, **19**, 4712–19 (1980).
30. Joiner, K. A., Brown, E. J., and Frank, M. M. Complement and bacteria. *Ann. Rev. Immunol.*, **2**, 461–91 (1984).
31. Kabat, E. A., and Bezer, A. E. The effect of variation in molecular weight on the antigenicity of dextran in man. *Arch. Biochem. Biophys.*, **78**, 306–10 (1958).
32. Karakawa, W. W., and Kane, J. A. Characterization of the surface antigens of *Staphylococcus aureus*, strain K-93M. *J. Immunol.*, **108**, 1199–208 (1972).
33. Karakawa, W. W., and Kane, J. A. Immunochemical analysis of a Smith-like antigen isolated from two human strains of *Staphylococcus aureus*. *J. Immunol.*, **115**, 564–8 (1975).
34. Karakawa, W. W., and Vann, W. F. Capsular polysaccharides of *Staphylococcus aureus*. *Semin. Infect. Dis.*, **4**, 285–93 (1982).
35. Karakawa, W. W., and Young, D. A. Immunochemical study of diverse surface antigens of a *Staphylococcus aureus* isolate from an osteomyelitis patient and their role in phagocytosis. *J. Clin. Microbiol.*, **9**, 399–408 (1979).
36. Karakawa, W. W., Young, D. A., and Kane, J. A. Structural analysis of the cellular constituents of a fresh clinical isolate of *Staphylococcus aureus* and their

role in interaction between the organisms and polymorphonuclear leukocytes and serum factors. *Infect. Immun.*, **21**, 496–505 (1978).

37. Karakawa, W. W., Fournier, J. M., Vann, W. F., Arbeit, R., Schneerson, R., and Robbins, J. B. Methods for the serological typing of the capsular polysaccharides of *Staphylococcus aureus. J. Clin. Microbiol.*, **22**, 445–7 (1985).
38. Lepow, M. L., Goldschneider, I., Gold, R., Randolph, M., and Gotschlich, E. C. Persistence of antibody following immunization of children with Groups A and C meningococcal polysaccharide vaccines. *Pediat.*, **60**, 673–80 (1977).
39. Makela, P. H., Herva, E., Sibakov, M., Henrichsen, J., Luotonen, J., Leinonen, M., Timonen, M., Koskela, M., Pukander, J., Gronroos, P., Pontynen, S., and Karma, P. Pneumococcal vaccine and otitis media. *Lancet*, **ii**, 547–51 (1980).
40. Makela, O., Peterfly, F., Outschoorn, J. G., Richter, A. W. and Seppala, I. Immunogenic properties of alpha(1–6) dextran, its protein conjugates and conjugates of its breakdown products in mice. *Scand. J. Immunol.*, **19**, 541–50 (1984).
41. Martin, D. G., Jarvis, F. G. and Milner, K. C. Physicochemical and biological properties of sonically treated Vi antigen. *J. Bact.*, **94**, 1411–16 (1967).
42. Mold, C., Nakayama, S., Holzer, T. J., Gewurz, H., and Clos, T. W. C-reactive protein is protective against *Streptococcus pneumoniae* infection in mice. *J. Exp. Med.*, **154**, 1703–8 (1981).
43. Nelles, M. J., Newlander, C. A., Karakawa, W. W., Vann, W. F. and Arbeit, R. D. Reactivity of type-specific monoclonal antibodies with *Staphylococcus aureus* clinical isolates and purified capsular polysaccharide. *Infect. Immun.*, **49**, 14–18 (1985).
44. Ørskov, F., Ørskov, I., Evans, D. J. Jr, Sack, R. B., Sack, D. A., and Wadstrom, T. Special *Escherichia coli* serotypes among enterotoxingenic strains from diarrhea in adults and children. *Med. Microbiol. Immunol.*, **162**, 73–80 (1976).
45. Oliveira, E. B., Gotschlich, E. C., and Liu, T.-Y. Comparative studies on the binding properties of human and rabbit C-reactive proteins. *J. Immunol.*, **124**, 1396–402 (1980).
46. Peltola, H. Meningococcal disease: still with us. *Rev. Infect. Dis.*, **5**, 71–9 (1983).
47. Public Health Service Advisory Committee Recommendation on Immunization Practices. Pneumococcal polysaccharide vaccine. *Morbidity and Mortality Weekly Report*, **30**, 410–12, 417–19 (1981).
48. Reingold, A. L., Broome, C. V., Hightower, A. W., Ajello, G. W., Bolan, G. A., Adamsbaum, C., Jones, E. E., Philips, C., Tiendrebeogo, H., and Yada, A. Meningococal polysaccharide A vaccine: evidence of age-specific differences in the duration of clinical protection following vaccination. *Lancet*, **ii**, 114–18 (1985).
49. Robbins, J. B. Vaccines for the prevention of encapsulated bacterial diseases: current status, problems and prospects for the future. *Immunochem.*, **15**, 839–54 (1978).
50. Robbins, J. B., Schneerson, R., and Pittman, M. *Haemophilus influenzae* type b infections. In *Bacterial Vaccines* (ed. R. Germanier), Academic Press, New York, 1984, pp. 245–290.
51. Robbins, J. B., Austrian, R., Lee, C.-J. Rastogi, S. C., Schiffman, G., Henrichsen, J., Makela, P. H., Broome, C. V., Facklam, R. R., Tiesjema, R. H., and Parke, J. C. Jr Considerations for formulating the second-generation pneumococcal vaccine with emphasis on the cross-reactive types within groups. *J. Infect. Dis.*, **148**, 1136–59 (1983).
52. Robbins, J. B., Schneerson, R., Egan, W. B., Vann, W. F., and Liu, D. T. Virulence properties of bacterial capsular polysaccharides – unanswered ques-

tions. In *The Molecular Basis of Microbial Pathogenicity* (ed. H. Smith, J. J. Skehel and M. J. Turner), Dahlem Konferenzen, 22–26 October 1980. Verlag Chemie GmbH, Weinheim, 1980, pp. 115–32.

53. Roberts, R. B. The relationship between Group A and Group C meningococcal polysaccharides and serum opsonins in man. *J. Exp. Med.*, **131**, 499–513 (1970).
54. Siber, G. R., Weitzman, S. A., Aisenberg, A. C., Weinstein, H. J., and Schiffman, G. Impaired antibody response to pneumococcal vaccine after treatment for Hodgkin's disease. *New Engl. J. Med.*, **299**, 442–8 (1978).
55. Sompolinsky, D., Samra, Z., Karakawa, W. W., Vann, W. F., Schneerson, R., and Malik, Z. Encapsulation and capsular types in isolates of *Staphylococcus aureus* from different sources and relationship to phage types. *J. Clin. Microbiol.*, **22**, 828–34 (1985).
56. Skov Sørensen, U. B., and Henrichsen, J. C-polysaccharide, the common pneumococcal antigen. *Acta Microbiol. Path. Scand. Sect. C.* in press (1986).
57. Skov Sørensen, U. B., and Henrichsen, J. C-polysaccharide, the common pneumococcal antigen. *Acta Microbiol. Path. Scand. Sect. C.*, in press (1986).
57. Skov Sørensen, U. B., and Henrichsen, J. C-polysaccharide in a pneumococcal vaccine. *Acta Path. Microbiol. Scand. Sect. C.*, **92**, 351–6 (1984).
58. Sutton, A., Schneerson, R., Kendall-Morris, S., and Robbins, J. B. Differential complement resistance mediates virulence of *Haemophilus influenzae* type b. *Infect. Immun.*, **35**, 95–104 (1982).
59. Szu, S. C., Zon, G., Schneerson, R., and Robbins, J. B. Characterization of the depolymerization of bacterial polysaccharides induced by ultrasonic irradiation. *Carb. Res.*, **155**, 7–20 (1986).
60. Szu, S. C., Clarke, S., and Robbins, J. B. Protection against pneumococcal infection in mice conferred by phosphocholine-binding antibodies: specificity of phosphocholine binding and relation to several types. *Infect. Immun.*, **39**, 993–9 (1983).
61. Szu, S. C., Schneerson, R., and Robbins, J. B. Rabbit anti-cell wall polysaccharide antibodies fail to protect mice against lethal challenge with encapsulated pneumococci. *Infect. Immun.*, **54,** 448–55 (1986).
62. Verbrugh, H. A., Peterson, P. K. Bach-Yen, T., Sisson, S. P., and Kim, Y. Opsonization of encapsulated *Staphylococcus aureus*: the role of specific antibody and complement. *J. Immunol.*, **129**, 1681–7 (1982).
63. Wood, W. B. Jr, and Smith, M. B. Surface phagocytosis—its relation to the mechanism of recovery in acute pneumonia caused by encapsulated bacteria. *Trans. Assoc. Am. Phys.*, **60**, 77–81 (1947).
64. World Health Organization Expert Committee on Biological Standardization. *Technical Report Series 610. World Health Organization, Geneva, Switzerland, 1977.*
65. Wu, T. C. M., and Park, J. T. Chemical characterization of a new surface antigenic polysaccharide from a mutant of *Staphylococcus aureus. J. Bacteriol.*, **108**, 874–84 (1971).
66. Yother, J., Forman, C., Gray, B. M., and Briles, D. E. Protection of mice from infection with *Streptococcus pneumoniae* by anti-phosphocholine antibody. *Infect. Immun.*, **36**, 184–8 (1982).
67. Yurchak, A. M., and Austrian, R. Serologic and genetic relationships between pneumococci and other respiratory streptococci. *Trans. Assoc. Amer. Phy.*, **79**, 368–75 (1966).
68. Ziegler, E. J., McCutchan, A., Fierer, J., Glauser, M. P., Sadoff, J. C., Douglas, H., and Braude, A. I. Treatment of gram-negative bacteremia and shock with

human antiserum to a mutant *Escherichia coli. New Engl. J.Med.* **307**, 1225–30 (1982).
69. Zon, G., Szu, S. C., Egan, W., Robbins, J. D., and Robbins, J. B. Hydrolytic stability of pneumococcal Group 6 (Type 6A, 6B) capsular polysaccharides. *Infect. Immun.*, **37**, 89–103 (1982).

DISCUSSION – Chaired by Professor A. Capron

EASMON: I am very interested in the data on these different capsular types of staphylococci and I have got a number of questions that I would like to put to you. Do you know anything about the mechanism of the capsule action in preventing the opsonic effect of cell-wall antibodies? Is it related to the mechanism already shown by Brian Wilkinson for the heavily capsulated types 1–3?

ROBBINS: We haven't studied that. I think the most likely answer is that it resembles in many ways the action of the Vi antigen which blocks the agglutinability of anti-LPS antibodies to *Salmonella typhi*. It explains why the Vi capsule was discovered comparatively recently in the history of *Salmonella*. The blocking action of the Vi and the *S. aureus* capsular polysaccharide is steric. I have no other explanation of it. The capsulated strains resist opsonization by white blood cells; in the presence of antibody and complement, phagocytosis and intracellular killing of *S. aureus* is enhanced. Now remember staph disease is not like meningococcus Group A disease, if you have meningococcus Group A in your nose and you don't have antibody, it is likely that you are going to get meningitis. We are covered with capsulated and non-capsulated *S. aureus*; the mechanism of disease is different, *S. aureus* isolated from the blood are invariably capsulated. So we think it does have a pathogenic mechanism. But I can't give you the kind of details that you want yet. This work is in its earliest stage.

EASMON: Could I follow that by asking, is there any idea of the prevalence of anticapsular antibody to these particular types in the population? Carrying out opsonic studies on a wide variety of *S. aureus* strains, many of which have been derived from blood, it has certainly been our impression that you can get near-optimum opsonization and phagocytosis with a wide range of sera from normal adults.

ROBBINS: The first answer is that these capsules are not stable, and are best grown on phosphate-poor media. I suggest that you try Columbia agar; it gives optimum expression of the capsules. The second answer is that we have no data on the prevalence of antibodies to the two capsular types. Many people have these levels, maybe Dr Schneerson would like to comment.

SCHNEERSON: We don't have data about the prevalence of *S. aureus* in the general population, we do have preliminary data that patients recovering have a marked increase in capsular antibodies.

EASMON: So, again, phenotypic variation may be a factor with these organisms?

ROBBINS: I think we don't know anything else about the surface proteins or other things about the staph. Dr Kabat showed that the teicolic acids of staphylococcus differ from strain to strain in their *N*-acetyl-glucosamine linkages, so there are probably other differences in staph.

KABAT: Dr Robbins, have you done anything to sort out which of the determinants in the *E. coli*s are related to the cross-reaction with the meningococcal polysaccharides? For example, you could reduce the uronic acid to see what happens; you could de-acetylate etc., so that, by several of these procedures, you could pin down the reactivity.

ROBBINS: Dr Kabat, the *O*-acetyl on the C5 and the C6 is randomly acetylated. If these *O*-acetyls are removed its reactivity with meningococcus Group A is lost. If that *O*-acetyl is on C2, it doesn't react with meningococcus Group A (K53). So the *O*-acetyl must allow for a critical determinant. Let me tell you how critical it must be. The K93 polysaccharide precipitates half the antibodies of meningococcus Group A antiserum and immunization makes excellent meningococcus Group A bacteriocidal antibody but, if it is not there, the cross-reaction is gone. It is all wrapped up into the configuration conferred by that *O*-acetyl. We haven't worked with the K51 yet.

KABAT: It would be very interesting to see how much residual reactivity you had due to the acetyl when you got rid of the charge.

MAKELA: We certainly want to try and break polysaccharides with your method. Is any normal ultrasound source sufficient or does one need a very expensive machine for that?

ROBBINS: There is no way of measuring the output of a sonicator. These results were obtained with two sonicators. There is a technical problem and that is that, during the ultrasonication, the probe actually disintegrates and small amounts of metal get into your sample. They can be removed by filtration.

SUTHERLAND: There are, of course, some studies from David Brandt in Irvine in California, some years ago, on the use of ultrasonics. One feature I find rather surprising is that you say that is random breakage and yet you are getting apparently a very uniform molecular weight. This does seem a slight contradiction, could you try and clarify it for me?

ROBBINS: Maybe I didn't make myself clear. The breaking of the linkages seems random because the same number of linkages are broken in the final product, that is, there doesn't seem to be one linkage favoured. The uniformity of the product at the end, I think, is due to the physical property of the polysaccharide that permits it to be broken, that is, when it gets too small it no longer has a torque on it. I am not a physicist, as you can see, but the explanation seems reasonable. I was surprised that, when you increase the solvent viscosity, the rate of breaking was increased in the final product even though, at a limit, was smaller but, of course, the rate of breaking when you measure the viscosity of the polysaccharide is just the opposite – the more viscous the polysaccharide the longer the breaking. The physicist, Dr Szu, says that in the presence of high solvent viscosity, the moment on the polysaccharide itself increases so it is more susceptible to breaking; it is almost as if you put the polysaccharide in a vice and now your breaking can be more effective. I hope I have answered your question.

HANDMAN: In the case of the pneumococcal vaccines, is there anything special in the adjuvant that they are given with or in the way that they are injected, so that in fact you induce good mucosal immunity?

ROBBINS: Pneumococcus vaccine is given as a saline solution and secretory IgA antibody to the polysaccharides is only induced in a fraction of the vaccine recipients. Protection against pneumococcal disease can be afforded by serum antibody; secretory antibody is not the only mechanism by which immunity can be afforded. I think that the most effective immunity induced by pneumococcal vaccine is against bacteraemia and its complications. But Dr Helena Mäkelä showed that you can prevent otitis media with pneumococcal vaccine in infants and children, provided the types can induce antibody. Unfortunately, the types that the infants respond least to are the ones that cause the most disease.

KABAT: How much dialysable material do you find after the ultrasonic treatment?

ROBBINS: We never looked. But on a weight basis we get most of what we started with.

KABAT: What I am trying to get at is the method of ultrasonic degradation. If there were a preferential splitting at the ends, it would tend to narrow the size range. If there were preferential splitting at the longer ends, that might be the reason that you got . . .

ROBBINS: It might be. With the *H. influenzae* type b we could account for all the new groups, and they all increased proportionately. That's why we say it is random. Our measurements may not be accurate to say that it is 100% random, but no linkages were spared. Now with the pneumococcus 6B and A, that have such different properties of thermal, alkaline and acid susceptibility, again there was no difference; it broke the same way.

GEYSEN: If, as you believe, each of the bonds is equally susceptible as the polymer A, you don't believe that there is a preferential linkage bond that is broken, one would predict that the length that you will reduce it down to ought to be the function of the frequency. In other words, it ought to be related to the wavelength of the ultrasonic oscillations so that, if you change the frequency, you would predict on that basis, if all bonds are equally susceptible or at least they're not favoured, that you will change the actual size that you will reduce it down to.

ROBBINS: We're going to do it. All we did was turn the power up!

GEYSEN: Another comment. In fact, you can measure the energy input of an ultrasonic bath, you literally measure the power input.
ROBBINS: We asked the representatives of the factory if we could somehow monitor the ultracentrifugation with something that we could give a number to, so much shaking, so many vibrations, and they said they couldn't. They said there was uniformity in each instrument.
GEYSEN: We had a bath and had to tune it in terms of the volume that it holds to get the actual power transferred. That's very important. We in fact stripped the protein and the antibodies off that plastic pin using ultrasonic treatment. We monitor the power input . . .
ROBBINS: Your idea of altering the frequency is good idea.
JENNINGS: In fact only 70 per cent. of the mannosamines are *O*-acetylated at position 3 and it seems to be completely true in any strain or any growth medium that you use. One of the question I was going to ask is that, if you made an antisera to the de-*O*-acetylated type A, and then you removed the acetate from the K93, would they still cross react?
ROBBINS: We haven't done it. If you de-*O*-acetylate the K93, it no longer reacts with meningococcus Group A sera. Now, *vice versa*, we have not done. The K93 sera will precipitate with the Group A meningococcus, but we do not have the de-*O*-acetylated Group A polysaccharide.
JENNINGS: It may be that the critical factor would be the three-dimensional type relationship between the *O* acetyl and the acid group.
ROBBINS: We were surprised when Bill and Ed Bax proposed the structure. It doesn't even look like Group A meningococcus polysaccharide. This structure was verified from three or four other K93 strains. The interesting relation between the K93 and the K53 is that antiserum to K93 reacts very nicely with 53 and *vice versa*. But K53 serum does not react with meningococcus Group A polysaccharide and the de-*O*-acetylated K93 does not react with the Group A serum.
JENNINGS: A very unusual example of a cross-reaction, and one of the things that crossed my mind when you told me about this structure was the fact it was fortunate that Michael Heidelberger didn't identify this example earlier in his career, otherwise he would have been very confused.

Towards Better Carbohydrate Vaccines
Edited by R. Bell and G. Torrigiani

Published by John Wiley & Sons Ltd

15

Streptococci: prospects for vaccines

J. Rotta
Institute of Hygiene and Epidemiology, 10042 PRAHA 10, Czechoslovakia

The genus *Streptococcus* includes a large number of species with diverse biological properties. While some streptococcal species are typical pathogens for man or animals, others are opportunistic pathogens provoking infections in the immunocompromised host or causing clinically apparent affections in specific situations only [70].

The disease caused by streptococci occur with a variety of clinical patterns. The upper respiratory tract infections rank among the most frequent bacterial infections in the moderate climatic zone. The data reported over the last two or three decades indicate that these illnesses are also common in the subtropical and tropical areas. Moreover, the incidence and prevalence of the sequelae of Group A streptococcal infection, such as rheumatic fever and rheumatic heart disease, are several times higher than in Europe, the United States of America and Japan [65]. It can be stated that the streptococcal disease complex is of worldwide health importance.

The control of streptococcal infections and their sequelae (rheumatic fever, rheumatic heart disease and acute glomerulonephritis) is based on conventional procedures elaborated in the past half-century. It consists of early and accurate diagnosis confirmed by microbiological examination and of efficient treatment or prevention by antibiotics [56].

The circulation of pathogenic streptococci in the population cannot effectively be reduced. It has to be assumed that the world population will be exposed to streptococci over many decades to come. Moreover, it cannot be

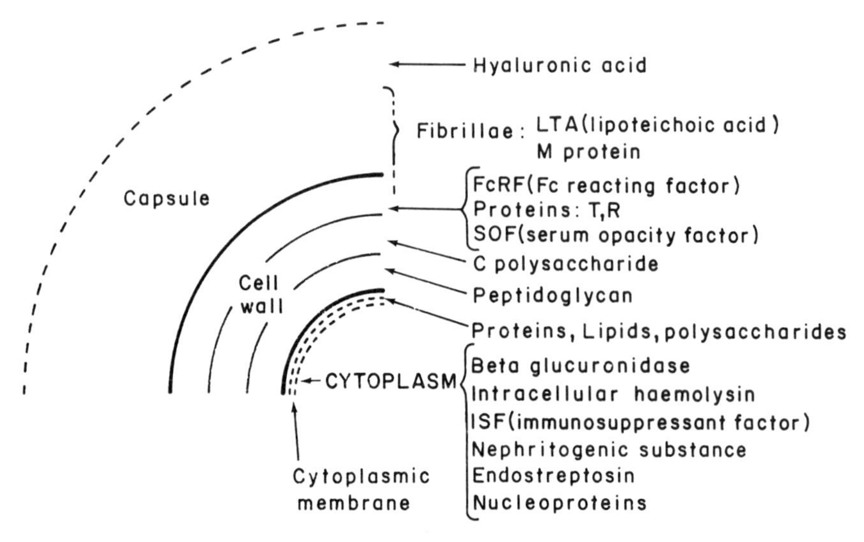

Figure 1. Scheme of Group A streptococcus cell

guaranteed that resistance to the antibiotics used at present (namely to penicillin) will not develop in the future. These facts are the stimulus for the search for new, alternative approaches to the control of streptococcal infections.

A vaccine against the most important streptococcal pathogens is most frequently considered for control in the future. The other possible control approaches, for example the blockage of adherence of streptococci to epithelial cells or the induction of non-specific resistance to streptococcal infection, are rather subjects of theoretical discussion and pilot experiments at laboratory level only.

The infections caused by *Group A streptococci* are the most important streptococcal illnesses, not only because of the frequency but also because of the risk from the sequelae, such as rheumatic fever and acute glomerulonephritis.

The research on a Group A streptococcal vaccine consisting of the M proteins dates back several decades [26]. Only in recent years were studies launched to cover the major aspects of the problem, i.e. the identification of the chemical structure of the M protein molecule and the complete characterization of its biological properties [12, 13, 32, 45].

The virulence factor in Group A streptococcus is the M protein located on the surface of the cell wall (Figure 1). It protects the streptococcus from phagocytosis. This antigen is also the type-specific substance (at present more than 70 M types are known) and, in turn, the immunity to Group A streptococcal infection is type specific. The antibody to M protein neutralizes its antiphagocytic effect.

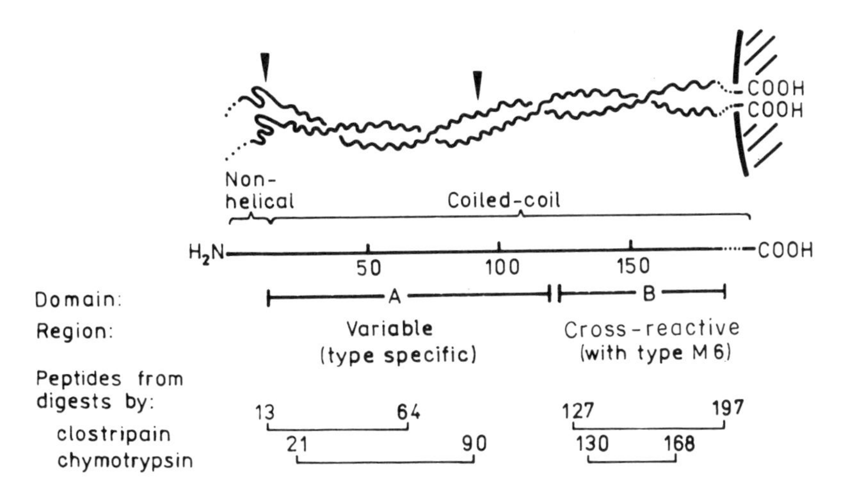

Figure 2. Type 5 M protein. Scheme of peptic fragment Pep M5 (N-terminal half of the molecule). Peptides used for identification of immunological properties of domains A and B (based on data by Fischetti and co-workers, 1986 (32))

The M protein molecule has a two-chain, α-helical coiled-coil structure, with the exception of the non-helical N-terminal 12-residue segment (Figure 2). This structure is determined by the occurrence of a seven-residue periodicity in the distribution of non-polar and charged amino-acid residues. The length of the single M protein molecule representing each fibre is about 500 Å; the carboxyl terminal region of the M protein molecule is located within the cell wall [46, 53]. In the M5 type, a complete amino-acid sequence of biologically active 197 residue fragment of M protein was determined [45].

The M protein usually has more epitopes located in various parts of the molecule [12]. Furthermore, the M protein of some types (e.g. of type 5) may contain one or more epitopes cross-reactive with sarcolemmal membrane proteins of human myocardium [22]. Finally, different serotypes may share common antigenic determinant(s) responsible for the immunological cross-reactivity [31]. For example, the pepsin-derived N-terminal half of the Group A streptococcal type 5 M protein cross reacts with the type 6 M protein. Two different domains, A and B, were identified by using peptides isolated

Pep M24 protein CNBr cleaved peptides:	Amino-terminal regions											
	1	2	3	... 14	15	16	17	18	19	20	21	22
CB3	Asn	Phe	Ser	... Glu	Ala	Glu	Lys	Ala	Ala	Leu	?	Ala
CB4	Asn	Phe	Ser	... Glu	Ala	Glu	Lys	Ala	Ala	Leu	Glu	Ala
CB5	Asn	Phe	Ser	... Glu	Ala	Glu	Lys	Ala	Ala	Leu	Glu	Ala
CB6	Asn	Phe	Ser	... Glu	Ala	Glu	Lys	Ala	Ala	Leu	Glu	Ala
CB7	Asn	Phe	Ser	... Glu	Ala	Glu	Lys	Ala	Ala	Leu	Ala	Ala
Group A streptococcus	- GlcNAc	-	MurNAc -		Ala	Glu	Lys	Ala	Ala	Ala		
peptidoglycan												
(two chains)	- GlcNAc	-	MurNAc -		Ala	Glu	Lys	Ala	Ala	Ala -		

Figure 3. Similarity of amino-acid sequence in M24 protein and peptidoglycan molecules. Identical amino-acid sequence. (Based on data by Beachey and co-workers [14])

from the clostripain and chymotrypsin digests of this peptic type 5 M protein fragment [46]. While domain A is a variable region containing the epitope(s) specific for type 5 streptococcus only, domain B contains antigenic epitope(s) cross-reacting with type 6.

Valuable data on the structure of type 24 M protein were obtained by employing limited digestion with pepsin. An extract from M24 streptococci was prepared, purified and cleaved with cyanogen bromide (at the place of methionyl residues). Each of the seven cyanogen bromide peptides obtained possessed the type-specific determinant that inhibited opsonic antibodies in anti-M24 type-specific serum. The precipitating antigen was present in the larger CB1 and CB2 peptides (88 and 90 amino-acid residues) but it was absent in the five smaller peptides CB3–CB7 (from 34 to 45 amino-acid residues). The amino-acid sequences of CB1 and CB2 were identical to each other – up to the 27th amino acid and of the CB3–CB7 – up to the 20th amino acid. This finding indicates that the M24 molecule is composed of repeating covalent structures [12]. Interestingly, there is some similarity between the amino-acid sequence of the M24 protein segment and the peptidoglycan molecule (Figure 3).

Both the CB6 and the CB7 peptides, when covalently conjugated with a polylysine carrier, became highly immunogenic, stimulating type-specific opsonic, bactericidal and precipitating antibody against type 24 streptococci. Cross-absorption experiments revealed that the peptides isolated by cyanogen bromide cleavage share some anti-opsonic determinants. In addition, they contain anti-opsonic distinct determinants. It is, therefore, evident that the M protein possesses several distinct anti-opsonic determinants of known primary structure [11, 13].

Pepsin extracted and purified M24 protein produced in human volunteers (two to four subcutaneous injections of 100–200 μg, at intervals of 2 weeks) an immune response detectable by type-specific (opsonizing and mouse-protecting) antibodies and cellular immunity (skin test). Heart-reactive antibodies were not present [14].

As mentioned above, the complete amino-acid sequence of a biologically active 197 residue of a peptic fragment of M5 protein was identified. The fragment represents nearly a half of the native M protein molecule, it interacts with opsonic antibodies and produces these antibodies in rabbits. The 197-residue fragment contains some nearly identical repeating sequences, namely four 7-residue segments and two 10-residue segments. There is some homology in partial sequences of the M proteins types 6 and 24 [45, 47].

In type M5, which is known to be frequently isolated from infections leading to rheumatic fever, one protective antigenic determinant has been found to be cross-reactive with human heart tissue. Antibody from a rabbit immunized with peptide fragment of M5 protein prepared by pepsin cross reacted with sarcolemmal membranes of human heart and opsonized not only type 5 but also type 19 streptococci, which are also rheumatogenic. It could be absorbed by carcolemmal membranes and M5 or M19 streptococci, but not by other types of streptococci. This also documents that the heart cross-reactive determinant of type 5 is cross-protective [21].

Recently, a complete nucleotide sequence of type 6M protein has been reported. A 42 amino-acid signal peptide presumably located in the cell wall with the membrane anchor sequence at the carboxyl-terminal end of the M protein were identified [32].

A large body of information has been obtained on synthetic peptides corresponding to particular native peptides isolated from the M protein molecules.

Dodecapeptide was synthesized, starting at residue 18 and ending at residue 29 of the CB7 peptide of type 24M protein. In rabbits, it produced an immune response with antibody type-specific, opsonizing and not cross reacting with the human heart tissue [11]. Similarly, a synthetic peptide of a larger number of amino acids identical with CB3 in structure, containing 35 amino-acid residues was immunogenic. None of the antibodies reacted with the human heart tissue.

Two peptides representing fragments of the M5 protein were chemically synthesized; the first one corresponding to the region 1–20 amino acids (S1-M5) of the purified native M5 molecule prepared by pepsin extraction, and the second one corresponding to the region 20–40 amino acids (S2-M5). Neither of the synthetic peptides was able to absorb heart-reactive antibody. Only the S1-M5 contained a type-specific antigenic determinant as measured by inhibition in ELISA test. Only S1–M5 also produced a type-specific, opsonic and non-heart cross-reactive antibody if covalently linked to tetanus toxoid and injected in to rabbits [23].

If the vaccine is made from synthetic subunits of M proteins it is obvious that the synthetic peptides are to be used with suitable carriers and immunostimulating materials. Although hundreds of synthetic immunostimulating substances have been prepared so far [3, 66], many of them derived from the bacterial peptidoglycan after its biological activity was recognized [57], a fully suitable substance is not yet available.

In vitro recombinant DNA technology was another successful approach employed for the better understanding of the structure of the M protein molecule. The structural gene for the type 6 streptococcal M protein was cloned into *Escherichia coli*. The M protein produced by *E. coli* accumulated in the periplasmic space. Its amino-acid composition was nearly identical to that isolated from streptococci. The purified *E. coli* M6 protein removed opsonic antibodies from both the human and the rabbit sera, and led to the production of opsonic antibodies in rabbits [62].

The results achieved with native as well as with synthetic peptides corresponding to particular fragments of the native M protein molecule are encouraging for vaccine trials in a selected population at high risk, such as in individuals with rheumatic heart disease. Many points have to be ascertained before these trials, namely the safety of the vaccine and the duration of immunity induced by the vaccine.

Although all the information currently available represents a solid basis for research aiming at preparing a safe and effective vaccine against Group A streptococcal infections, more work and data are required before the ultimate goal is reached.

The pathogenicity of Lancefield *Group B streptococcus* for man was documented in 1938 [27]. It took three or four decades to obtain a larger body of information on the virulence factor of the micro-organism, the nature of the protective antibody, the carriership rates of the germ in humans, the clinical patterns of Group B streptococcal disease, the age-groups mostly affected, the mode of microbe transfer in the population, the morbidity and mortality in various environmental conditions and on the prospects for more efficient control in the individuals at risk [34, 55]. The size of the health problem caused by Group B streptococci is not negligible in Europe, the United States of America and in Japan, and it is assumed to be also of importance in other parts of the world.

The only prospect known at present for improved control of Group B streptococcal infection is the introduction of a vaccine for active immunization or of a hyperimmune serum for passive protection. A dilemma, however, exists whether or not to proceed along these lines. It emanates from a rather high prevalence of Group B streptococci in the population (e.g. the carriership on the vaginal mucosa) on the one hand and from a low incidence of serious Group B infections (e.g. of perinatal and infant diseases in Europe) in the other. Apart from this there are several other questions: whom to vaccinate (provided vaccine is available), when to apply the vaccine, how to identify the individuals at risk, etc. Nevertheless, fundamental research has resulted in several achievements which could enable the use of vaccine in particular situations in the future.

The virulence factor as well as the type-specific substance in Group B streptococci is the capsular polysaccharide. In turn, the immunity is type specific, since the protective IgG antibody is directed to the capsular polysaccharides. Of the Group B types Ia, Ib, II, III, IV and V, type III is the most common, causing two-thirds of neonatal and infant infections [6].

Every pregnant woman carrying Group B streptococci on the vaginal mucosa is a potential source of infection to the neonate if placental transfer of IgG antibody at a protective level had not occurred in the neonate [17, 67]. There are differences in the transfer of antibody to particular types. Type III antibody is the least transferable. It is likely that, in infection with type III, an amount of more than 2 mg of antibody per ml of serum confers considerable immunity to protect the infected infant [7].

The chemical structure of capsular type polysaccharides Ia, Ib, II and III has been identified [20, 35, 36, 40]. This was achieved by use of materials isolated from the capsules at neutral pH, since the conventional extraction techniques by acid treatment led to hydrolysis of the molecule, in particular of the terminal sialic acid [9, 37, 39]. By Lancefield's classical extraction procedure [41], the type polysaccharides revealed the content of galactose, glucose and 2-acetamido-2-deoxyglucose in D form. The native antigens contained in terminal position [20, 35, 36] acid-labile sialic acid residues. The molar ratios of the four sugars in the case of the types Ia, Ib and III polysaccharides were determined 2 : 1 : 1 : 1, in type II polysaccharide 3 : 2 : 1 : 1. The scheme of the molecules based on data by Jennings *et al.* [35–38] is depicted in Figure 4. It shows that types Ia and Ib only differ by the β-1,4 linkage and the β-1,3 linkage in the side-chain, respectively. The molecule of antigen II is structurally more complex. That of type III is characterized by an α-2 $\rightarrow$ 6-linked terminal sialic acid. In type III, the core has no sialic acid. The molecule is chemically identical with the pneumococcal type 14 polysaccharide. Serologically both polysaccharides strongly cross react.

The purified polysaccharides are immunogenic for man, as revealed in volunteers [8]. The antibody response varies according to particular types (highest after type II, poorest after type Ia); previous exposure of the individual to the homologous Group B streptococcus type strongly stimulates antibody production. The study of the naturally acquired and vaccine-induced antibody to the most important type III has revealed that, 4 weeks after immunization, sera from adults predominantly contained IgG. In contrast,

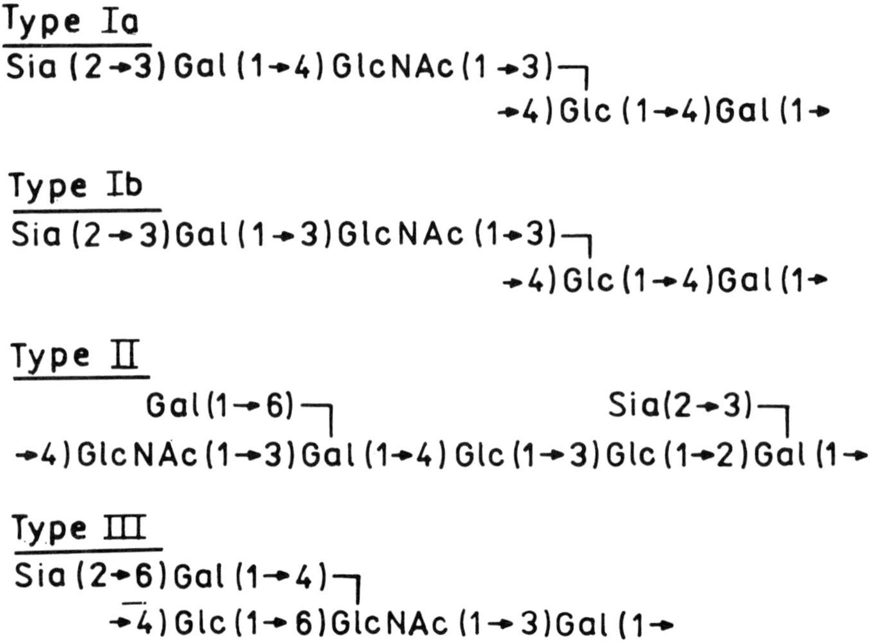

Type Ia

Sia (2→3) Gal (1→4) GlcNAc (1→3)┐
→4) Glc (1→4) Gal (1→

Type Ib

Sia (2→3) Gal (1→3) GlcNAc (1→3)┐
→4) Glc (1→4) Gal (1→

Type II

Gal (1→6)┐ Sia(2→3)┐
→4) GlcNAc (1→3) Gal (1→4) Glc (1→3) Glc (1→2) Gal (1→

Type III

Sia (2→6) Gal (1→4)┐
→4) Glc (1→6) GlcNAc (1→3) Gal (1→

Figure 4. Scheme of Group B streptococcal-type polysaccharides. Sia = *N*-acetylneuraminic acid. All saccharide units have D-configuration and are in pyranose form. Saccharides are joined by β-bonds, except sialic acid (by α-bond). (Based on data by Jennings *et al.* [35].)

early convalescent sera of neonates with type III infection responding by antibody contained significantly more IgM antibody. This indicates that immunization of pregnant women could be efficacious in the prevention of invasive neonatal type III infection [24]. The immunization with polysaccharides of types Ia, II and III led to IgG antibody response transferable *per placentam*. The antibody was opsonizing and presumably protective, as revealed in model infection on neonatal rats pretreated with sera of human volunteers vaccinated with type III polysaccharide [19].

A number of points remain to be better or further clarified, for example genetic regulation of the antibody response, the modification of the answer by linkage of polysaccharides to proteins, the role of Gm allotypes in adults, provision of more information on the adequate strategy of immunologically active and passive methods for prevention of Group B streptococcal neonatal infections, the assessment of the safety of the vaccine if administered at the beginning of the third trimester of pregnancy, persistence of sufficient antibody level in neonates and others.

Serious neonatal infections, although rather infrequent, are uncontrollable by measures available at present and justify the research of novel methods for control of streptococcal Group B infection.

The consistent presence of *Streptococcus sanguis* and *S. mutans* in dental plaque and the cariogenicity of *S. mutans* in experimental animals indicate the potential association of these streptococci with human dental caries [15, 42, 48]. Research was launched into the cellular components and extracellular products of both microbes with the aim of elaborating a vaccine for active immunization against dental caries in man. Conclusive data were obtained on the antigenic components [25, 51, 58] and on their role in model experimental caries in animals [59, 60].

The value of the data on the antigenic components of *S. sanguis* is weakened by the taxonomic uncertainty of this streptococcal species and by some confusion regarding the reference strains used for the elaboration of the identification scheme. The major antigen seems to be the Group H specific substance which is a glycerol teichoic acid. There are at least four other antigens cellularly located but their nature is not too well known [54]. Much remains to be clarified regarding the biological properties of this streptococcus and the factors involved in the host–parasite interaction.

Streptococcus mutans has been extensively studied. The antigenic components of eight serological types, a–h, have been described so far [30, 63]. Each contains a type-specific cell-wall polysaccharide, the major components being glucose, galactose and rhamnose. The first two types, a and b, also contain *N*-acetyl-glucosamine and *N*-acetyl-galactosamine. The extracellular products of *S. mutans* comprise several types of polysaccharides playing a role in the colonization of hard tissue surfaces in the mouth. They are either glucans formed by glucosyltransferase or fructans synthesized by fructosyltransferase. The chemical composition and the amount of water-soluble or water-insoluble glucans vary according to individual types.

A series of experiments aimed at documentation of possible immunization effect by *S. mutans* vaccine against dental caries has been performed in the last decade [18, 43, 61]. Whole bacteria, cell walls, crude cell fractions and materials containing glucosyltransferases were mostly used. The model experiments considered closest to human conditions were carried out on monkeys (*Macaca fascicularis*). Whole cells or disrupted cells gave protection from caries in animals maintained on a caries-promoting diet [16]. Materials containing glucosyltransferases increased susceptibility rather than providing immunity. The vaccine applied intra-oral submucosally was more effective than if administered subcutaneously. Some evidence has been provided that the vaccine made of serotype c of *S. mutans* could be of substantial value in prevention of caries, since this type is largely distributed in urban populations and it also possesses antigens common to other serotypes.

Later experiments carried out on rabbits or monkeys by using vaccines composed of semi-purified proteins isolated from cell walls of *S. mutans* by extraction with SDS at 100 °C, revealed that the levels of antibodies to two protein antigens only (A and C) were in correlation with dental caries protection while the antibody to antigen B was not.

No antibody to antigen D could be detected. Moreover, antigen B cross reacted with human heart tissue [53]. However, as recently reported, antibodies to serotypes c and g ribosomal vaccines do not react with either human heart or renal antigens [29], and are therefore unlikely to produce any deleterious effect on the tissues concerned. An attempt to vaccinate perorally with formalin-killed, freeze-dried *S. mutans* cells in capsules has failed, as far as antibody production is concerned. Nevertheless, it positively affected the levels and duration of colonization of teeth by *S. mutans* experimentally administered on to cleaned teeth [18].

It is evident that more information on the dental caries problem in relation to the role of *S. mutans* in the pathogenesis and on its antigenic components is required before the prospect of a vaccine can be foreseen.

The *S. pneumoniae* vaccine is the only one so far prepared against infections by pathogens belonging to the genus *Streptococcus*. At present, it is commercially available and used for control of diseases caused by pneumococci. The prerequisite for its elaboration was the recognition of the type-specific capsular polysaccharide which is the factor of virulence. It is called SSS (specific soluble substance). The antibodies to this polysaccharide are responsible for immunity [5] which, in turn, is type-specific. The species-specific substance consists of a ribitol teichoic acid with choline phosphate.

The proposal for the composition of the vaccine, which is polyvalent, was made possible by monitoring and mapping of the prevailing types responsible for the most serious pneumococcal diseases (pneumonia and meningitis) in various parts of the world. So far, 83 capsular types have been identified.

The vaccines, consisting of various numbers of type polysaccharides, were prepared and used in field trials. At first, 4-, 6- or 12-valent vaccines were used. Since 1974, the 14- and 23-valent (second generation) pneumococcal vaccines have been used [54]. The particular types for the vaccines were identified on the basis of clinical and epidemiological studies.

Recently a WHO co-operative study was carried out to find out the prevailing types in various parts of the world, in particular in developing countries, with the aim of proposing a revision of the vaccine composition so that it could be used more widely. About 5000 strains were typed, of these 59% were isolated from blood and 19% from CSF.

The technology of vaccine preparation consists of prolonged incubation of the germ in soy broth, centrifugation to separate the debris and chromatographic isolation of the polysaccharide from the supernatant fluid. The ultimate goal is to purify the polysaccharide sufficiently, to make the vaccine as polyvalent as possible by covering the prevailing types and to obtain optimum antibody response to a maximum number of types.

With the vaccines so far prepared, relatively good safety was documented. The polysaccharides in the vaccines are so-called T cell-independent antigens, producing good antibody response in individuals above 2 years of age. A recommendation was made to explore the possibility of conjugating the polysaccharides with suitable proteins so that they could be used even in the youngest children.

The indications for vaccination are the elderly population at risk [69], in particular if hospitalized [50, 64], and splenectomized individuals. In splenectomized persons, the antibody levels are lower and decline faster than in the controls [1, 28]. A pneumococcal vaccination programme directed at high-risk in- and out-patients was claimed to be effective [44]. In splenectomized children, vaccination should not be considered as the only preventive measure. It was shown in these children, that with 14-valent vaccine, a higher titre than a two-fold antibody increase was recorded in 60% of all single type antibodies resulting in protection (at least 300 mg antibody N/ml) against 55% of types only, which predominantly occur in serious infections in childhood [52]. The level of 250–300 mg N/ml is considered protective [69]. It was noticed that a decline of serum antibody occurs after vaccination and that there are highly significant differences in the decline related to the particular types in the vaccine [28]. A lower antibody response by IgM in splenectomized individuals as compared with healthy (control) persons was also reported, but in both groups vaccination induced a significant IgM and IgG responses [2]. There are data indicating that the best prevention of serious infections in adults following splenectomy is a combination of both pneumococcal vaccine and penicillin [71]. Pneumococcal vaccination was also shown to lead to a good antibody response in patients with sickle cell anaemia at or after 2 years of age and to suppress the incidence of pneumococcal infections in these individuals [68].

There are some questions to be answered before the pneumococcal vaccination is made fully satisfactory, for example selection of the right types, the duration of antibody levels after vaccination, differences in the antigenicity of polysaccharides of particular types, low or no antibody increase after a booster dose [49], side (local) reactions after revaccination and others. All these points should be a stimulus to further research.

A large body of information is already available to cope successfully with a vaccine programme against infections by the most important pathogenic streptococci. More data, however, are required. The impact on health of infections caused by streptococci fully justifies the work carried out at present or planned for the future.

REFERENCES

1. Aaberge, I. S., and Heier, H. E. Long-term effect of pneumococcal polysaccharide vaccination on serum IgM and IgG antibody levels in individuals splenectomized for trauma. *Acta Pathol. Microbiol. Immunol. Scand.*, **92**, 363–9 (1984).
2. Aaberge, I. S., Heier, H. E. and Hem, E. IgM and IgG response to pneumococcal polysaccharide vaccine in normal individuals and individuals splenectomized due to trauma. *Acta Pathol. Microbiol. Immunol. Scand.*, **92**, 11–16 (1984).
3. Adam, A., and Lederer, E. Muramyl peptides: immunomodulators, sleep factors, and vitamins. *Medicinal Research Reviews*, **4**, 111–52 (1984).
4. Appelbaum, B., and Rosan, B. Antigens of *Streptococcus sanguis*: purification and characterization of the b antigen. *Infection and Immunity*, **19**, 896–904 (1978).
5. Austrian, R. The current status of polyvalent pneumococcal vaccine. *Clin. Ther.*, **6**, 572–5 (1984).
6. Baker, C. J., and Edwards, M. S. Group B streptococcal infections. In *Infectious Diseases of the Fetus and Newborn Infant*, 2nd edn (ed. J. D. Remington and J. O. Klein), W. B. Saunders, Philadelphia, 1983, pp. 820–81.
7. Baker, C. J., Edwards, M. S. and Kasper, D. L. Role of antibody to native type III polysaccharide of group B streptococcus in infant infection. *Pediatrics*, **68**, 544–9 (1981).
8. Baker, C. J., and Kasper, D. L. Group B streptococcal vaccines. *Reviews of Infectious Diseases*, **7**, 458–67 (1985).
9. Baker, C. J., Kasper, D. L. and Davis, C. E. Immunochemical characterization of the 'native' type III polysaccharide of group B streptococcus. *J. Exp. Med.*, **143**, 258–70 (1976).
10. Beachey, E. H., Seyer, J. M., Dale, J. B. and Hasty, D. L. Repeating covalent structure and protective immunogenicity of native and synthetic polypeptide fragments of type 24 streptococcal M protein. *J. Biol. Chem.*, **258**, 13250–7 (1983).
11. Beachey, E. H., Stollerman, G. H., Johnson, R. H., Ofek, I. and Bisno, A. L. Human immune response to immunization with a structurally defined polypeptide fragment of streptococcal M protein. *J. Exp. Med.*, **150**, 862–77 (1979).
12. Beachey, E. H., Seyer, J. M., Dale, J. B., Simpson, W. A. and Kang, E. H. Type-specific protective immunity evoked by synthetic peptide of streptococcus pyogenes M protein. *Nature*, **292**, 457–9 (1981).
13. Beachey, E. H., Seyer, J. M. and Kang, E. H. Repeating covalent structure of streptococcal M protein. *Proc. Natl. Acad. Sci. USA*, **75**, 3163–7 (1978).
14. Beachey, E. H., Seyer, J. M., and Kang, E. H. Primary structure of protective antigens of type 24 streptococcal M protein. *J. Biol. Chem.*, **255**, 6284–9 (1980).
15. Beighton, D., and Hayday, H. The stability of *Streptococcus mutans* populations in the dental plaque of monkeys (*Macaca fascicularis*). *Journal of Applied Bacteriology*, **52**, 191–200 (1982).
16. Bowen, W. H., Cohen, B, Cole, M. F., and Colman, G. Immunisation against dental caries. *British Dental Journal*, **139**, 45–58 (1975).
17. Christensen, K. K., Christensen, P., Dahlander, K., Faxelius, G., Jacobson, B. and Svenningsen, N. Quantitation of serum antibodies to surface antigens of group B streptococci types Ia, Ib and III: low antibody levels in mothers of neonatally infected infants. *Scand. J. Infect. Dis.*, **12**, 105–10 (1980).
18. Cole, M. F., Emilson, C. G., and Hsu, S. D. Effect of peroral immunization of humans with *Streptococcus mutans* on induction of salivary and serum antibodies and inhibition of experimental infection. *Infect. Immun.*, **46**, 703–9 (1984).

19. De Cueninck, B. J., Eiserstein, T. K., McIntosh, T. S., Shockman, G. D., and Swenson, R. M. Type-specific protection of neonatal rats from lethal group B streptococcal infection by immune sera obtained from human volunteers vaccinated with type III–specific polysaccharide. *Infect. Immun.*, **37**, 961–5 (1982).
20. De Cueninck, B. J., Greber, T. F., Eisenstein, T. K., Swenson, R. M. and Shockman, F. D. Isolation, chemical composition and molecular size of extracellular type II and type Ia polysaccharides of group B streptococci. *Infect. Immun.*, **41**, 527–34 (1983).
21. Dale, J. B., and Beachey, E. H. Protective antigenic determinant of streptococcal M protein shared with sarcolemmal membrane protein of human heart. *J. Exp. Med.*, **156**, 1165–76 (1982).
22. Dale, J. B., and Beachey, E. H. Multiple, heart-cross-reactive epitopes of streptococcal M proteins. *J. Exp. Med.*, **161**, 113–22 (1985).
23. Dale, J. B., Seyer, J. M. and Beachey, E. H. Type-specific immunogenicity of a chemically synthesized peptide fragment of type 5 streptococcal M protein. *J. Exp. Med.*, **158**, 1727–32 (1983).
24. Edwards, M. S., Fuselier, P. A., Rench, M. A., Kasper, D. L., and Baker, C. J. Class specificity of naturally acquired and vaccine-induced antibody to type III group B streptococcal capsular polysaccharide – determination of a radioimmunoprecipitin assay. *Infect. Immun.*, **44**, 257–61 (1984).
25. Ferretti, J. J., Shea, C. and Humphrey, M. W. Cross-reactivity of *Streptococcus mutans* antigens and human heart tissue. *Infection and Immunity*, **30**, 69–73 (1980).
26. Fox, E. N. M Proteins of group A streptococci. *Bacteriological Reviews*, **38**, 57–86 (1974).
27. Fry, R. M. Fatal infections by haemolytic streptococcus group B. *Lancet*, **1**, 199–201 (1938).
28. Giebink, G. S., Le, C. T. and Schiffman, G. Decline of serum antibody in splenectomized children after vaccination with pneumococcal capsular polysaccharides. *J. Pediatr.*, **105**, 576–82 (1984).
29. Gregory, R. L., Schechmeister, I. L. and Brubaker, J. C. Lack of cross-reactivity of antibodies to ribosomal preparations from *Streptococcus mutans* with human heart and kidney antigens. *Infect. Immun.*, **46**, 42–7 (1984).
30. Hamada, S., Mitzuno, J. and Kotani, S. Serological properties of cellular and extracellular glycerol teichoic acid antigens of *Streptococcus mutans*. *Microbios*, **25**, 155–66 (1979).
31. Havlíček, J., Kühnemund, O., Šrámek, J., and Pokorný, J. Cross reactions between M types of streptococcus pyogenes. In *Basic Concepts of Streptococci and Streptococcal Diseases* (ed. S. E. Holm and P. Christensen), Reedbooks, Chertsey, 1982, p. 82.
32. Hollingshead, S. K., Fischetti, V. A. and Scott, J. R. Complete nucleotide sequence of type 6 M protein of the group A streptococcus. *J. Biol. Chem.*, **261**, 1677–86 (1986).
33. Hughes, M., Machardy, S. M., Sheppard, A. J. and Woods, N. C. Evidence for an immunological relationship between *Streptococcus mutans* and human cardiac tissue. *Infection and Immunity*, **27**, 567–88 (1980).
34. Jelínková, J. Group B streptococci in the human population. *Current Topics in Microbiology and Immunology*, **76**, 127–65 (1977).
35. Jennings, H. J., Katzenellenbogen, E., Lugowski, C. and Kasper, D. L. Structure of native polysaccharide antigens of type Ia and type Ib group B streptococcus. *Biochemistry*, **22**, 1258–64 (1983).

36. Jennings, H. J., Lugowski, C. and Kasper, D. L. Conformational aspects critical to the immunospecificity of the type III group B streptococcal polysaccharide. *Biochemistry*, **20**, 4511–18 (1981).
37. Jennings, H. J., Rosell, K. G. and Kasper, D. L. Structure and serology of the native polysaccharide antigen of type Ia group B streptococcus. *Proc. Natl. Acad. Sci. USA*, **77**, 2931–5 (1980).
38. Jennings, H. J., Rosell, K. G., Katzenellenbogen, E. and Kasper, D. L. Structural determination of the capsular polysaccharide antigen of type II group B streptococcus. *J. Biol. Chem.*, **258**, 1793–8 (1983).
39. Kane, J. A., and Karakawa, W. W. Multiple polysaccharide antigens of group B streptococcus, type Ia: emphasis on a sialic acid type-specific polysaccharide. *J. Immunol.*, **118**, 2155–60 (1977).
40. Kasper, D. L., Baker, C. J., Galdes, B., Katzenellenbogen, E., and Jennings, H. J. Immunochemical analysis and immunogenicity of the type II group B streptococcal capsular polysaccharide. *J. Clin. Invest.*, **72**, 260–9 (1983).
41. Lancefield, R. C. Cellular antigens of group B streptococci. In *Streptococci and Streptococcal Diseases: Recognition, Understanding, and Management* (ed. L. W. Wanamaker and J. M. Matsen), Academic Press, New York, 1972, pp. 57–65.
42. Lehner, T., Challacombe, S. J., Wilton, and Caldwell, J. Cellular and humoral immune responses in vaccination against dental caries in monkeys. *Nature*, **264**, 69–72 (1976).
43. Lehner, T., Russell, M. W. and Caldwell, J. Immunisation with a purified protein from *Streptococcus mutans* against dental caries in rhesus monkeys. *Lancet*, 1, 995–6 (1980).
44. Magnussen, C. R., Valenti, W. M. and Mushtin, A. I. Pneumococcal vaccine strategy. Feasibility of a vaccination program directed at hospitalized and ambulatory patients. *Arch. Intern. Med.*, **144**, 1755–7 (1984).
45. Manjula, B. N., Acharya, A. S., Mische, S. M., Fairwell, T. and Fischetti, V. A. The complete amino acid sequence of a biologically active 197-residue fragment of M protein isolated from type 5 group A streptococci. *J. Biol. Chem.*, **259**, 3686–93 (1984).
46. Manjula, B. N., Acharya, A. S., Mische, S. M., Fairwell, T. and Fischetti, V. A. Antigenic domains of the streptococcal pep. M 5 protein; localization of epitopes cross-reactive with type 6 M protein and identification of a hypervariable region of the M molecule. *J. Exp. Med.*, **163**, 129–38 (1986).
47. Manjula, B. N., Acharya, A. S., Mische, S. M., Fairwell, T. and Fischetti, V. A. Primary structure of streptococcal pep. M 5 protein: absence of extensive sequence repeats. *Proc. Natl. Acad. Sci. USA*, **80**, 5475–9 (1983).
48. McGhee, J. R., and Michalek, S. M. Immunobiology of dental caries: microbial aspects and local immunity. *Annual Review of Microbiology*, **35**, 595–638 (1981).
49. Mufson, M. A., Kvause, H. E. and Schiffman, G. Reactivity and antibody responses of volunteers given two or three doses of pneumococcal vaccine. *Proc. Soc. Exp. Biol. Med.*, **177**, 220–5 (1984).
50. Murphy, T. F., and Fine, B. C. Bacteremic pneumococcal pneumonia in the elderly. *Am. J. Nephrol.*, **4**, 32–7 (1984).
51. Peach, S. L., and Russell, R. R. B. Antigens of *Streptococcus mutans* cell walls. In *Basic Concepts of Streptococci and Streptococcal Diseases* (ed. S. E. Holm and P. Christensen), Reedbooks, Chertsey, 1982, pp. 114–16.
52. Pedersen, F. K., Henrichsen, J. and Schiffman, G. Antibody response to vaccination with pneumococcal capsular polysaccharides in splenectomized children. *Acta Paediatr. Scand.*, **71**, 451–5 (1982).

53. Phillips, G. N. Jr, Flicker, P. F., Cohen, C. and Manjula, B. N. Streptococcal M protein: alfa Helical coiled-coil structure and arrangement on the cell surface. *Proc. Natl. Acad. Sci. USA*, **78**, 4689–93 (1981).
54. Robbins, J. B. Considerations for formulating the second-generation pneumococcal capsular polysaccharide vaccine with emphasis on the cross-reactive types within groups. *J. Infect. Dis.*, **148**, 1136–59 (1983).
55. Ross, P. W. Group B streptococcus – profile of an organism. *J. Med. Microbiol.*, **18**, 139–66 (1984).
56. Rotta, J., and Facklam, R. R. *Manual of Microbiological Diagnostic Methods for Streptococcal Infections and their Sequelae.* WHO/BAC/80.1, 1980.
57. Rotta, J., Prendergast, T. J., Kavakawa, W. W., Harmon, C. K. and Krause, R. M. Enhanced resistance to streptococcal infection induced in mice by cell wall mucopeptide. *J. Exp. Med.*, **122**, 877–90 (1965).
58. Russell, M. W., Bergmeier, L. A., Zanders, E. D. and Lehner, T. *et al.* Protein antigens of streptococcus mutans: purification and properties of a double antigen and its protease-resistant component. *Infection and Immunity*, **28,** 486–93 (1980).
59. Russell, R. R. B., and Colman, G. Immunization of monkeys (*Macaca fascicularis*) with purified *Streptococcus mutans* glucosyltransferase. *Archives of Oral Biology*, **26**, 23–8 (1981).
60. Russell, R. R. B., Peach, S. L., Colman, G. and Cohen, B. Immunisation of monkeys (*Macaca fascicularis*) with antigens purified from *Streptococcus mutans. British Dental Journal*, **152**, 81–4 (1982).
61. Russell, R. R. B., Peach, S., Colman, G. and Cohen, B. Antibody responses to antigens of *Streptococcus mutans* in monkeys (*Macaca fascicularis*) immunized against dental caries. *J. Gen. Microb.*, **129**, 865–75 (1983).
62. Scott, J. R., and Fischetti, V. A. Expression of streptococcal M protein in *Escherichia coli. Science*, **221**, 758–60 (1983).
63. Scully, C. M., and Lehner, T. Bacterial and strain specificities in opsonization, phagocytosis and killing of *Streptococcus mutans. Clin. Exp. Immunol.*, **35**, 128–32 (1979).
64. Shapiro, E. D., and Clemens, J. D. A controlled evaluation of the protective efficacy of pneumococcal vaccine for patients a high risk of serious pneumococcal infections. *Ann. Intern. Med.*, **101**, 325–30 (1984).
65. Strasser, T., and Rotta, J. The control of rheumatic fever and rheumatic heart disease: an outline of WHO activities. *WHO Chronicle*, **27**, 49–54 (1973).
66. Takada, H., and Kotani, S. Immunopharmacological activities of synthetic muramyl-peptides. In *Immunology of the Bacterial Cell Envelope* (ed. D. E. S. Stewart-Tull and M. Davies) John Wiley and Sons Ltd, 1985, pp. 119–52.
67. Vogel, L. C., Boyer, K. M., Gadzala, C. H. and Gotoff, S. P. Prevalence of type-specific group B streptococcal antibody in pregnant women. *J. Pediatr.*, **96**, 1047–51 (1980).
68. Weintrus, P. S., Schiffman, G. and Addiego, J. E. Jr. Long-term follow-up and booster immunization with polyvalent pneumococcal polysaccharide in patients with sickle cell anemia. *J. Pediatr. (St Louis)*, **105**, 261–3 (1984).
69. Wiedermann, G. Pneumokokkenimpfung in der Geriatrie (Pneumococcal vaccination in elderly people). *Fortschr. Med.*, **102**, 333–5 (1984).
70. World Health Organization *Bull. Wld Hlth Org.*, **56**, 887–912 (1978). Recent advances in rheumatic fever control and future prospects: a WHO memorandum.
71. Zarrabi, M. H., and Rosner, F. Serious infections in adults following splenectomy for trauma. *Arch. Intern. Med.*, **144**, 1421–4 (1984).

DISCUSSION – Chaired by Professor A. Capron

ROBBINS: Czechoslovakia has about 11 million people?
ROTTA: Total population is 15 million.
ROBBINS: How many cases of neonatal meningitis due to Group B streptococcus occur each year in Czechoslovakia?
ROTTA: As I have indicated, rather very few. We do not have the accurate figures for the whole country and I can only refer to the data derived from few prospective studies. We have about two deaths due to Group B streptococcal septicaemia with meningitis per 1000 live births. We have good information that about 10% of the women are carriers of Group B streptococcus on the vaginal mucosa. Therefore if the vaccine were made available – whom to vaccinate? The data from the USA indicate more cases of fatal Group B streptococcus infection in new-borns than do the data from the UK or other countries in Europe. I am sure that you have a good information system, but I do not have an explanation for the difference in the incidence of the fatal septicaemia in new-borns.
CAPRON: Is anything known about studies to be made of structures with parasites concerning the adhesive structures of bacteria to epithelial or endothelial cells? I am referring mainly to what is called adhesiotopes which, for instance, concern such structures as fribronectin receptors. I understand from the literature that such a type of structure has now been described in bacteria such as streptococci. Do we know anything about the possible function of these possible fribronectin receptors and so on for the adhesion of bacteria, to epithelial cells, for instance?
ROTTA: Yes, the Group A streptoeoccus has the receptor for fibronectin and this receptor is the lipoteichoic acid in the fibrillae. Another important factor in Group A streptococcus is the receptor for fibrinogen. Whether it is intimately linked to the M protein or a part of the M protein molecule we do not know with certainty. It obviously plays a role in the pathogenesis of the disease; using the fibrinogen in the immunoabsorbent column, we can isolate the M protein.

Part IV: Carbohydrates as Immunogens

Towards Better Carbohydrate Vaccines
Edited by R. Bell and G. Torrigiani

Published by John Wiley & Sons Ltd

16

T cell-independent responses to polysaccharides: their nature and delayed ontogeny

JAMES G. HOWARD
The Wellcome Trust, London, UK

The concept of 'thymus-independent' (TI) antigens arose from the observation that neonatally thymectomized mice retained the capacity to give unimpaired humoral responses to large polymeric molecules [4, 17] and this was later found to be the case with 'nude' (nu/nu) animals. The most important of these antigens biologically are bacterial polysaccharides, although similar features have been observed and studied with polymers of D-amino acids and synthetic substances such as polyacrylamide and polyvinyl pyrrolidone. These are all large molecules with a high density of repeating epitopes and subject to very slow degradation leading to their prolonged persistence *in vivo*. They induce immune responses which bypass the conventional requirement for T-cell help. Mel Cohn has upheld the theoretical view that T cells are necessary but on a minuscule scale, so far undetected. In practice, the characteristic features of responses to TI antigens are so dissimilar from those to 'thymus-dependent' (TD) antigens that they are most usefully considered in a category apart. A brief summary of this distinctive profile is presented here based on results obtained in mice by numerous scientists working with a variety of different antigens. Generalities are stressed at the expense of exceptions. One important practical distinction between responses to TI and TD antigens is that wholly *in vitro* systems for studying the former have been largely unsuccessful despite numerous attempts. A notable but somewhat unrepresentative exception has been the IgA response to α1 → 3 dextran [36].

A classification of TI antigens into TI-1 and TI-2 was proposed by Mosier and his colleagues nearly 10 years ago [31]. TI-2 antigens do not induce responses in CBA/N mice (an X-chromosome-linked defect) or in early post-natal life and are virtually devoid of polyclonal activating activity. Most bacterial polysaccharides studied are of this type, except lipopolysaccharide (endotoxin) 0 antigens which are TI-1 and possess the opposite features. Nossal and Pike [32] have argued against rigorous application of this distinction on collective evidence that TI-1 and TI-2 antigens form a continuous spectrum rather than two sharp nodal groups.

HUMORAL RESPONSES TO TI ANTIGENS

Immunogenicity and specificity of polysaccharides

A relatively large multideterminant polymer is necessary to induce a response, as shown by progressive depolymerization studies. In the case of α1 → 6 dextran, immunogenicity is lost between 70 and 20 kd, with β2 → 6 levan below 15 kd and with type III pneumococcal polysaccharide (S3) between 31 and 4 kd [15, 16, 19, 24].

Responses to different sugar linkages on the same polymer are immunologically specific and function independently with regard to immunogenicity and tolerogenicity (e.g. α1 → 3 and α1 → 6-linked glucose in dextran B1355) [14].

B-cell receptors 'see' different sizes of epitope on the same homopolymer leading to responses with tri- up to hexa- or hepta-saccharide components. This was originally studied serologically by Kabat with dextran and SIII oligosaccharide inhibition studies. Similar results have been obtained subsequently with antibody secreting cells. The larger the epitope involved the better is the avidity of the corresponding antibody.

Persistence of antibody secretion

After an initial peak following primary immunization, antibody levels plateau at a lower level and diminish very gradually over many weeks or months. In most instances the plateau reveals regular cyclical rises and falls when frequent assays are made [8]. TI-2 antigens give responses in nu/nu athymic mice of increased magnitude which decline more slowly than in their euthymic counterparts. There is evidence that this is due to absence of the normal regulatory T cell-dependent auto-anti-idiotypic response [35]. Loss of the cyclical plateau in 'nude' mice has been attributed to the same cause [21], although this has been questioned as an exclusive explanation [10]. Auto-anti-idiotypic regulation assumes importance in responses to polysaccharides in view of their restricted heterogeneity and frequent dominant idiotypes. There is usually little or no avidity maturation detectable [37].

Isotype restriction and lack of sequential switch

Thymus-independent antigens induce predominantly IgM responses, with a variable minority of non-IgM components whose presence and isotype is influenced by the inbred strain of mouse used. IgG_3 is commonly, but not exclusively, induced by polysaccharides [28] and IgA less frequently so [20]. Others are also recorded. Different epitopes on the same polymer can give rise to distinct isotype responses independently [33]. No sequential isotype switching sequence is observed in contrast to a response to TD antigens. The kinetics of IgM and non-IgM plaque-forming cell components are coincident, implying that there is direct induction to non-IgM secretion [3, 20, 26]. Non-IgM formation is largely T-cell dependent and is not found in nu/nu mice [18, 20, 26]. This T-cell involvement is not MHC restricted and probably involves the release of B-cell growth and differentiation factors. Evidence suggests it is triggered by idiotypic determinants on B or accessory cells rather than by the antigen itself.

Antigen competition

Thymus-independent antigens do not indulge in antigenic competition with one another, nor are they influenced by the potential competition induced by TD antigens. In fact, responses to them may even be somewhat augmented by simultaneous injection with particulate TD antigens such as heterologous erythrocytes [39]. This freedom from the constraints of competition has permitted the use of multi-type polysaccharide vaccines (e.g. pneumococcus).

Refractoriness to adjuvants

A wide experience has accumulated that responses to TI antigens are difficult to augment with conventional adjuvant additives. A lot of negative data remain unpublished. A notable recorded exception has been killed *Coryne-bacterium* parvum which amplified responses to both DNP–levan [9] and S3

[11], whereas both complete Freund's adjuvant and *Bordetella pertussis* were without effect.

POLYSACCHARIDE ANTIGENS AND T CELLS

Binding

There is no convincing direct evidence available which demonstrates the specific binding of polysaccharides (or other TI antigens) to T cells.

Memory

Consistent failure to induce significant T-cell memory responses has been experienced even with cell transfer techniques. Response to a secondary challenge is at best of only slightly higher magnitude than the primary, while avidity remains relatively low. In contrast, B-cell memory has been induced with meningococcus B polysaccharide [29] and elicited with S3 [6], but in each case a TD conjugate was required for elicitation and induction respectively.

Cell-mediated immunity

A classical feature is the complete absence of delayed-type hypersensitivity (DTH) induction and expression with polysaccharide antigens. (One documented exception concerned DTH induced in guinea-pigs with S2 + complete Freund's adjuvant, but this has never been confirmed or studied further.)

Suppressor and amplifier T cells

Extensive studies have been made of the involvement of regulatory-T cells in responses to S3 [2], but relatively little with other TI-2 antigens, except polyvinyl pyrrolidone. Evidence is based largely on *in vivo* effects on S3 responses following anti-lymphocyte serum treatment of euthymic but not athymic mice, or following thymectomy. Reversal could be obtained by thymocyte transfer. Suppressive effects were inferred in 'low-dose' tolerance and post-immunization refractoriness, while amplifying effects distinct from classical help involved the use of Concanavalin A. Attempts at cell transfer were for long unsuccessful, but success has at last been achieved with cells taken within 24 hours of priming [1, 7]. These regulatory functions have not been associated as yet with any particular T-cell subset(s) nor has a direct S3/T-cell interaction been demonstrated. The generality, amplitude and implication of these observations for responses to polysaccharides as a whole remain conjectural.

TOLERANCE

Doses of 0.1–1 mg of most polysaccharides (about 100 × the optimum immunogenic dose) induce a state of profound specific unresponsiveness (synonymous with paralysis or high-dose zone tolerance). Tolerogenicity is lost in parallel with immunogenicity (dextran B512 and S3) on depolymerization [15, 16], but low molecular weight non-immunogenic fractions of levan retain some tolerogenicity [27]. Multivalency is a requisite and oligosaccharides do not tolerize. Some evidence suggests that susceptibility of B cells to tolerance increases with the size of epitope recognized [14, 37]. Two different epitopes on the same polysaccharide can induce immunity to one and tolerance to the other at the same time (e.g. dextran B1355) [14].

The characteristic neonatal susceptibility to TD antigens does not extend to polysaccharides. On a body-weight basis, new-born mice are no more susceptible to tolerization by them than are adults [13, 34]. The mechanism involved is unknown, except that a requirement exists for multipoint binding to B-cell Ig receptors. Nothing is known about the subsequent cellular and molecular events. Polysaccharide tolerance is of very long duration. In the presence of residual antigen *in vivo*, periods in excess of 1 year are usually found [12]. Spontaneous recovery occurs similarly in intact and thymectomized mice, as predictable on the basis of helper-T cell independence. Full recovery in the absence of antigen can be studied by cell transfer into irradiated recipients and takes 10–12 weeks – a period commensurate with B-cell regeneration from stem cells.

DELAYED ONTOGENY

The onset of full responsiveness to polysaccharide TI-2 antigens in mice is strikingly delayed in the post-natal period in comparison with LPS and other TI-1 antigens, to which adult levels are attained (like TD antigens) within 1–2 weeks. Responses to TI-2 antigens are only first detectable at age 2–3 weeks, but full development is not reached until 4 weeks (S3 and $\alpha 1 \rightarrow 3$ dextran) or much later still with levan and $\alpha 1 \rightarrow 6$ dextran (7 and 13 weeks respectively) [5, 13, 30, 38]. The relative unresponsive state at 2 weeks is a transferable property of spleen cells injected into irradiated recipients [13]. Normal adult bone marrow cells also show the same delayed ontogenic acquisition of responsiveness to TI-2 antigens when similarly transferred [14]. The ontogeny of adult-type heterogeneous affinity responses to these antigens is also slow (3–4 weeks) in comparison with TD antigens and is a T cell-independent process [22]. Responsiveness to TI-2 antigens has been associated with Lyb 5^{+} B cells which show parallel delayed ontogeny and are relatively T-cell independent [25]. Treatment *in vivo* with anti-Lyb 5.1 serum blocks the capacity to respond to these antigens. Nevertheless, recent studies with dextran B512 have demonstrated that the presence of specific B-cell precursors is constant throughout development [23]. Hence, the delay in their capacity to respond seems likely to have some regulatory or maturation basis. Available data suggest that the 2–3 month post-natal development period in mice corresponds to 2 years of age in man.

SHORTCOMINGS OF POLYSACCHARIDES AS PROPHYLACTIC IMMUNOGENS

The detailed studies which have been made in mice highlight a number of features, as follows, which need to be circumvented if they are relevant to human immunization.

1. They are frequently poor immunogens – antibody concentrations rarely exceed 0.1 mg/ml in mice. Meningococcus B polysaccharide is an extreme example.
2. Restriction of isotypes induced.
3. Lack of affinity maturation.
4. Lack of T-cell memory.
5. Inefficacy of conventional adjuvants.
6. Delayed ontogeny of responsiveness.

The sole advantage over immunization with TD antigens is the lack of polysaccharide involvement in antigenic competition.

The use of carbohydrate conjugates or anti-idiotypes as immunogens could reverse these six 'againsts' and one 'for'.

REFERENCES

Note: The bibliography cited does not provide comprehensive substantiation for all the points made in this overview.

1. Baker, P. J., Amsbaugh, D. F., Stashak, P. W., Caldes, G., and Prescott, B. Direct evidence for the involvement of T suppressor cells in the expression of low-dose paralysis to type III pneumococcal polysaccharide. *J. Immunol.*, **128,** 1059 (1982).
2. Baker, P. J., and Prescott, B. Regulation of the antibody response to pneumoc-

occal polysaccharides by thymus-derived (T) cells: mode of action of suppressor and amplifier T cells. In *Developments in Immunology* (ed Rudbach and Baker), Elsevier, 1979, Vol. 2, p. 67.
3. Barthold, D. R., Prescott, B., Stashak, P. W., Amsbaugh, D. G., and Baker, P. J. Regulation of the antibody response to type III pneumococcal polysaccharide. III. Role of regulatory T cells in the development of an IgG and IgA antibody response. *J. Immunol.*, **112,** 1042 (1974).
4. Basten, A., and Howard, J. G. Thymus independence. In *Contemporary Topics in Immunobiology* (ed. A. J. S. Davies), Plenum, New York, 1973, Vol. 2, p. 265.
5. Bona, C., Lieberman, R., Chen, C. C., Mond, J., House, S., Green, I., and Paul, W. E. Immune response to levan. I. Genetics and ontogeny of anti-levan and anti-insulin antibody response and expression of cross-reactive idiotype. *J. Immunol.*, **120,** 1436 (1978).
6. Braley-Mullen, H. Secondary IgG responses to type III pneumococcal polysaccharide. I. Kinetics and antigen requirements. *J. Immunol.*, **115,** 1194 (1975).
7. Braley-Mullen, H. Direct demonstration of specific suppressor T cells in mice tolerant to type III pneumococcal polysaccharide: two-step requirement for development of detectable suppressor cells. *J. Immunol.*, **125,** 1849 (1980).
8. Britton, S., and Möller, G. Regulation of antibody synthesis to *Escherichia coli* endotoxin. I. Suppressive effect of endogenously produced and passively transferred antibodies. *J. Immunol.*, **100,** 1326 (1968).
9. Del Guercio, P. Effects of adjuvants on the antibody response to a hapten on a thymus-independent carrier. *Nature New Biol.*, **238,** 213 (1972).
10. Hiernaux, J. R., Chiang, J., Baker, P. J., Delisi, C., and Prescott, B. Lack of involvement of auto-anti-idiotypic antibody in the regulation of oscillations and tolerance in the antibody response to levan. *Cell. Immunol.*, **67,** 334 (1982).
11. Howard, J. G., Christie, G. H., and Scott, M. T. Biological effects of *Corynebacterium parvum*. IV. Adjuvant and inhibitory effects on B lymphocytes. *Cell. Immunol.*, **7,** 290 (1973).
12. Howard, J. G., Courtenay, B. M., and Hale, C. Lack of effect of thymectomy on spontaneous recovery from tolerance to levan. *Eur. J. Immunol.*, **6,** 837 (1976).
13. Howard, J. G., and Hale, C. Lack of neonatal susceptibility to induction of tolerance by polysaccharide antigens. *Eur. J. Immunol.*, **6,** 486 (1976).
14. Howard, J. G., Moreno, C., Hale, C., and Vicari, G. Influence of molecular structure on the tolerogenicity of bacterial dextrans. IV. Epitope size recognition and genetic resistance to $\alpha 1 \rightarrow 3$ glucosyl tolerance induction by dextran B1355. *Eur. J. Immunol.*, **7,** 431 (1977).
15. Howard, J. G., Vicari, G., and Courtenay, B. M. Influence of molecular structure on the tolerogenicity of bacterial dextrans. I. The $\alpha 1 \rightarrow 6$ linked epitope of dextran B512. *Immunology*, **29,** 585 (1975).
16. Howard, J. G., Zola, H., Christie, G. H., and Courtenay, B. M. Studies on immunological paralysis. V. The influence of molecular weight on the immunogenicity, tolerogenicity and antibody-neutralising activity of type III pneumococcal polysaccharide. *Immunology*, **21,** 535 (1971).
17. Humphrey, J. H., Parrott, D. M. V., and East, J. Studies on globulin and antibody production in mice thymectomised at birth. *Immunology*, **7,** 419 (1964).
18. Ivars, F., Nyberg, G., Holmberg, D., and Coutinho, A. Immune response to bacterial dextrans. II. T cell control of antibody isotypes. *J. Exp. Med.*, **158,** 1498 (1983).

19. Kabat, E. A., and Bezer, A. E. The effect of variation in molecular weight on the antigenicity of dextran in man. *Arch. Biochem.*, **78,** 306 (1958).
20. Kagnoff, M. F. IgA anti-dextran B1355 responses. *J. Immunol.*, **122,** 866 (1979).
21. Kelsoe, G., Isaak, D., and Cerny, J. Thymic requirement for cyclical idiotypic and reciprocal anti-idiotypic immune responses to a T-independent antigen. *J. Exp. Med.*, **151,** 289 (1980).
22. Lewin, M. L., and Siskind, G. W. Ontogeny of B-lymphocyte function. XIII. Kinetics of maturation of neonatal B lymphocytes to produce a heterogeneous antibody response to a T-independent antigen. *Cell. Immunol.*, **60,** 234 (1981).
23. Lundkvist, I., Holmberg, D., Ivars, F., and Coutinho, A. The immune response to bacterial dextrans. III. Ontogenic development and strain distribution of specific clonal precursors. *Eur. J. Immunol.*, **16,** 957 (1986).
24. Miranda, J. J., Zola, H., and Howard, J. G. Studies on immunological paralysis. X. Cellular characteristics of the induction and loss of tolerance to levan (polyfructose). *Immunology*, **23,** 843 (1972).
25. Mond, J. J. Use of the T lymphocyte regulated type 2 antigens for the analysis of responsiveness of Lyb-5^+ and Lyb-5^- B lymphocytes to T lymphocyte derived factors. *Immunol. Rev.*, **64,** 99 (1982).
26. Mongini, P. K. A., Stein, K. E., and Paul, W. E. T cell regulation of IgG subclass antibody production in response to T-independent antigens. *J. Exp. Med.*, **153,** 1 (1981).
27. Moreno, C., Courtenay, B. M., and Howard, J. G. Molecular size and structure in relation to the tolerogenicity of small fructosans (levans). *Immunochemistry*, **13,** 429 (1976).
28. Moreno, C., and Esdaile, J. Immunoglobulin isotype in the murine response to polysaccharide antigens. *Eur. J. Immunol.*, **13,** 262 (1983).
29. Moreno, C., Lifely, M. R., and Esdaile, J. Immunity and protection of mice against *Neisseria meningitidis* group B by vaccination, using polysaccharide complexed with outer membrane proteins: a comparison with purified B polysaccharide. *Infect. Immun.*, **47,** 527 (1985).
30. Morse, H. C., Prescott, B., Cross, S. S., Stashak, P. W. and Baker, P. J. Regulation of the antibody response to type III pneumococcal polysaccharide. V. Ontogeny of factors influencing the magnitude of the plaque-forming cell response. *J. Immunol.*, **116,** 279 (1976).
31. Mosier, D. E., Mond, J. J., and Goldings, E. A. The ontogeny of thymic independent antibody responses *in vitro* in normal mice and mice with an X-linked B cell defect. *J. Immunol.*, **119,** 1874 (1977).
32. Nossal, G. J. V., and Pike, B. L. A re-appraisal of 'T-independent' antigens. II. Studies on single hapten-specific B cells from neonatal CBA/H or CBA/N mice fail to support classification into TI-1 and TI-2 categories. *J. Immunol.*, **132,** 1696 (1984).
33. Sarvas, H. O., Aaltonen, L. M., Peterfy, F., Seppala, I. J. T., and Makela, O. IgG subclass distributions in anti-hapten and anti-polysaccharide antibodies induced by haptenated polysaccharides. *Eur. J. Immunol.*, **13,** 409 (1983).
34. Siskind, G. W., Paterson, P. Y., and Thomas, L. Induction of unresponsiveness and immunity in newborn and adult mice with pneumococcal polysaccharide. *J. Immunol.*, **90,** 929 (1963).
35. Schrater, A. F., Goidl, E. A., Thorbecke, J., and Siskind, G. W. Production of auto-anti-idiotypic antibody during the normal immune response to TNP-ficoll. III. Absence in nu/nu mice: evidence for T-cell dependence of the anti-idiotypic-antibody response. *J. Exp. Med.*, **150,** 808 (1979).

36. Trefts, P. E., Rivier, D. A., and Kagnoff, M. F. T cell-dependent IgA anti-polysaccharide response *in vitro*. *Nature*, **292,** 163 (1981).
37. Vicari, G., and Courtenay, B. M. Restricted avidity of the IgM antibody response to dextran B512 in mice: studies on inhibition of specific plaque-forming cells by oligosaccharides. *Immunochemistry*, **14,** 253 (1977).
38. Wood, C., Fernandez, C., and Möller, G. Ontogenic development of the suppressed secondary response to native dextran. *Scand. J. Immunol.*, **16,** 287 (1982).
39. Wood, C., Fernandez, C., and Möller, G. Potentiation of the PFC response to thymus-independent antigens by heterologous erythrocytes. *Scand. J. Immunol.*, **16,** 293 (1982).

DISCUSSION – Chaired by Professor G. L. Ada

KABAT: Dr Howard, I am afraid that I have been fighting a losing battle, but I am going into battle again. What you call $\alpha 1 \rightarrow 3$ dextran, is not $\alpha 1 \rightarrow 3$, it is an alternating $\alpha 1 \rightarrow 3$, $\alpha 1 \rightarrow 6$ dextran which is highly branched. So you cannot get any $\alpha 1 \rightarrow 3$ determinants and $\alpha 1 \rightarrow 6$ determinants, no matter how you think about it. The best you can accomplish is to have an $\alpha 1 \rightarrow 6$ terminal, followed by an $\alpha 1 \rightarrow 3$, followed by an $\alpha 1 \rightarrow 6$, followed by an $\alpha 1 \rightarrow 3$. Or an $\alpha 1 \rightarrow 3$ terminal, followed by an alpha $1 \rightarrow 6$ etc., depending on the nature of the branching. You have to rethink some of those data, and it would be very helpful to do this in terms of the structure because, if you have the immunodominant portion of some of the antibody being $\alpha 1 \rightarrow 3$ and the immunodominant portion of another fraction of the antibody being $\alpha 1 \rightarrow 6$, then this could be applied for your populations. This would be rather important. I have been calling attention to this for a long while and everybody still speaks of $\alpha 1 \rightarrow 3$.

HOWARD: We used $\alpha 1 \rightarrow 3$, as a short designation for plaque-forming cells that could be inhibited specifically by incorporation in the gel of oligosaccharides of the nigerose series. The others, the $\alpha 1 \rightarrow 6$, were inhibited by oligosaccharides of the isomaltose series. In view of your more recent data that $\alpha 1 \rightarrow 3$ and $\alpha 1 \rightarrow 6$ linkages form mixed epitopes our nigerose inhibitable PFCs could be called '$\alpha 1 \rightarrow 3$ dominant' for short.

KABAT: The nigerose oligosaccharides are relatively poor inhibitors compared to the alternating ones. At that time, alternating $\alpha 1 \rightarrow 3$ $\alpha 1 \rightarrow 6$ oligosaccharides were not available.

HOWARD: Well, they worked quite well in these old experiments.

KABAT: Well, lots of things work, but not for the right reasons.

HOWARD: The specificities are distinct, and behave independently *vis-à-vis* induction of immunity and tolerance.

KABAT: I am only trying to get you to revise your phrasing, in terms of the latest structural information. The specificities are distinct but not for the reasons we thought were correct at the time.

ROBBINS: One other comment. Most of the work, as you say, has been done with pneumococcus type 3. I just want to point out that pneumococcus type 3 is the most unusual capsule of polysaccharide in its immunological behaviour that has been studied in humans. It is the one polysaccharide that induces virtually an adult immune response in new-borns. The others have not been studied sufficiently so that much of what you are saying, at least in reference to polysaccharides from bacterial pathogens, relies on one bacterial polysaccharide atypical in a way.

HOWARD: There was a certain amount of earlier work of the kind discussed with S2, at NYU, and we switched over to the use of levan and dextrans because of the problems peculiar to S3. I think that there have also been a few things done with the *Klebsiella* polysaccharides.

ROBBINS: *Klebsiella* polysaccharides have not been studied extensively in humans. There are species differences in immunological reactivity to polysaccharides between the man and the mouse.

MOSIER: I wanted to amplify on the answer to Dr Robbins's question about B-cell memory to responses. We have no evidence for any B-cell memory in pure B-cell mice, made by reconstituting immunodeficient *scid* mice, with cell-sorter purified B cells. A second immunization results simply in elicitation of the same number of TNP specific precursors as one immunization with TNP–Ficoll, a model polysaccharide antigen. The presence of T cells has absolutely no influence on the magnitude of that response. So, at least for this model antigen system, there is no B-cell priming. What one engenders is a very long-lived population of B cells.

ROBBINS: How do you define memory? How do you define B-cell memory, what is the definition of it?

MOSIER: Memory implies distinguishing features between a primary and secondary response. One has no trouble in distinguishing a primary and secondary anti-protein response, but I know of no criteria by which you can distinguish a primary and secondary thymus-independent response.

ADA: Possibly one mechanism would be that you find a higher frequency of precursor cells but, as you cannot get an *in vitro* response, that is rather difficult to test directly. That would be the most direct way.

ROBBINS: So, therefore, a primary response without B-cell memory is when you inject an animal that has no demonstrable precursor cells?

ADA: No, you get an increased frequency per 10^6 cells. Instead of having, say, $10/10^6$ cells, you have a $100/10^6$ cells. That is what you have with T-cell memory.

ROBBINS: I have always had trouble understanding, it has never been related to a cell type or a function. It really refers to what you measure in the serum or what you measure in the plaque-forming cell system.

ADA: No. The estimation is done by limit dilution analysis so that one well will contain the progeny of only one cell dilution. One, in effect, measures the production of clones.

Could I ask a question? You did show apparently, Dr Howard, a high and low responder strain. BALB/c, I think, was the high responder and CBA the low responder. Is that due to MAC effects?

HOWARD: No, it is attributable to a germ-line gene for the $\alpha 1 \rightarrow 3$ dominant response in BALB/c which is linked to the lambda chain.

CAPRON: Regarding this essential problem of absence of evidence of specific binding to T cells. I wonder if you are aware Dr Howard, or somebody in the audience, of work which appeared about six or seven months ago in the *Journal of Clinical Investigation*, from a French (Parisian) group, working on *Candida albicans manans*, showing, I think, rather clear evidence of T-cell binding of the antigen, the restriction in presention by macrophages to the DR/Q1A. Have you seen this paper? It seems to be the first example, as long as it is confirmed?

HOWARD: Yes, but we do need other examples of this kind of thing, if it is going to hold up as a generality.

Towards Better Carbohydrate Vaccines
Edited by R. Bell and G. Torrigiani

Published by John Wiley & Sons Ltd

17

Subclass composition of human IgG antibodies to *Haemophilus influenzae* type b polysaccharide

OLLI MÄKELÄ, NINA RAUTONEN, ILKKA SEPPÄLÄ, JUHANI ESKOLA AND HELENA KÄYHTY
Department of Bacteriology and Immunology, University of Helsinki and the National Public Health Institute, Helsinki, Finland

SUMMARY

Six volunteers were immunized with *Haemophilus influenzae* type b polysaccharide (Hib). Blood samples were taken before the immunization, and 14 and 28 days after. The magnitude of the antibody response and its isotype composition were studied with special emphasis on the subclass composition of IgG antibodies. Three vaccinees responded well (more than a fivefold increase in antibody concentration) to the immunogen, and also the amount of IgG antibodies increased more than fivefold in these individuals. More than 80% of the IgG antibodies in all post-vaccination blood samples consisted of IgG_1 or IgG_2; proportions of IgG_3 and IgG_4 were small. The ratio of IgG_1 to IgG_2 antibodies varied greatly. In one vaccinee 91% of IgG antibodies were IgG_2, whereas in another vaccinee 72% were IgG_1. In the third individual, the two subclasses were almost equally represented. These findings were concordant with those we had previously made about antibodies to the meningococcal A polysaccharide [7], and suggest that IgG antibodies to polysaccharides are not always restricted to IgG_2 in normal human beings.
While IgG_1 is the predominant subclass of human IgG antibodies to protein

antigens, to viruses and to at least some bacterial antigens [1, 4, 9, 10, 12, 14], IgG_2 has a major share in antibodies to polysaccharides. Some authors have found IgG polysaccharide antibodies to be predominantly IgG_2 [2, 5, 8, 15]. Others have found IgG_1 and IgG_2 in almost equal proportions in the responses of adults to meningococcal type A polysaccharide (MenA) [7]. Hammarström *et al.* [2] found that, while adults produced IgG_2-rich antibodies to pneumococcal type 6, polysaccharide antibodies of children had much more IgG_1. The different findings might be caused by different measuring techniques or different immunization schedules. On the other hand, some polysaccharides may induce predominantly IgG_2 (and IgM) antibodies, while others induce considerable amounts of IgG_1 antibodies.

Human and murine IgG_1 seem to be analogous subclasses in that both are strongly represented in responses to protein antigens and in responses that are associated with a good immunological memory [4, 9, 11–13]. Since long-lasting memory is an aim of vaccination, we want to know whether some polysaccharide vaccines induce plenty of IgG_1 antibodies but others do not. For this purpose we are studying the subclass composition of antibodies to Hib.

MATERIALS AND METHODS

Blood samples were taken from six healthy young adults who were then injected intramuscularly with 25 μg of Hib (Lederle lot 7-1391-131A). Blood samples were taken 14 and 28 days after vaccination.

Blood samples were also taken from 34 other individuals who were then vaccinated with a tetravalent meningococcal polysaccharide vaccine. Blood samples were taken again on day 14. Most data on their responses have been published [7]. Antibodies to MenA or Hib were measured with solid-phase RIA which gives antibody concentrations of different immunoglobulin classes and subclasses in equal units. The MenA assay has been described [7] and it gives concentrations in weight units. The Hib assay was conducted in an analogous way with four exceptions:

1. Tubes were coated with 0.005% polysaccharide whereas, in the case of MenA, the coating concentration was 0.01%.
2. Monoclonal anti-IgG_2 antibody HP6014 [3, 6] was used in the Hib assay.
3. Blank values (BSA-buffer substituted vaccinee serum) were subtracted from the sample counts in the Hib antibody assay, as described in the published MenA antibody assay, but in the Hib assay, background values were also subtracted. Background values were obtained by omitting the antigen (Hib) from a parallel set of tubes and they are caused by non-specific binding of human immunoglobulins on to plastic which cannot be completely blocked by BSA saturation. The final sample count (specific

count) in the Hib assay was: measured counts − blank − (background − blank of background).

4. No standard serum was used in the Hib antibody assay, and the concentrations are given in arbitrary units. The unit is approximately the same for all isotypes [12] and the isotype composition of Hib antibodies can therefore be determined.

RESULTS AND DISCUSSION

Of the six individuals immunized with the Hib vaccine, three exhibited a strong response in all immunoglobulin classes (nos. 1, 3 and 4, Table I). Vaccinee no. 2 had a high concentration of antibodies before vaccination, and no response was observed. Antibodies of vaccinees nos. 5 and 6 remained low all the time. In two vaccinees the response had almost peaked by day 14. In vaccinee no. 1 the antibody concentration continued to increase from day 14 to day 28 (Table I).

The subclass composition of IgG antibodies could be calculated reliably in three vaccinees (nos. 1, 3 and 4). IgG_3 and IgG_4 did not contribute much in any of them. IgG_1 and/or IgG_2 accounted for more than 85% of IgG antibodies in all three individuals. IgG_1 was the main subclass in vaccinee no. 1 (70–80% of all IgG antibodies) IgG_2 in vaccinee no. 3 (more than 90% of IgG antibodies), and the two subclasses had almost equal proportions in vaccinee no. 4 (Table I).

These limited data gain weight when the IgG subclass composition of Hib antibodies is compared with the composition of IgG antibodies to the MenA (Figure 1). The main subclasses in MenA antibodies were IgG_1 and IgG_2. Again, some individuals produced predominantly IgG_1 antibodies, others predominantly IgG_2 antibodies and still others the two subclasses in approximately equal proportions. Together, the two series of data suggest that not nearly all human antipolysaccharide responses are restricted to the IgG_2 subclass.

ACKNOWLEDGEMENT

This work was supported by the Sigrid Juselius Foundation.

REFERENCES

1. Van der Giessen, M., and Groeneboer-Kempers, O. The subclasses of human IgG antibodies against tetanus toxoid. *Clin. exp. Immunol.*, **25**, 117–21 (1976).

Table I. Concentration of antibodies to the *Hemophilus influenzae* type b polysaccharide in six vaccinees. The unit is arbitrary but the same throughout the table. Day 0 – pre-vaccination sample, day 14 and day 28 are samples, 14 and 28 days after vaccination

Vaccinee	and time of sample (day)	Antibody concentration in IgG_1	IgG_2	IgG_3	IgG_4	Sum[a]	Antibody concentration in IgG	IgA	IgM	Sum[b]	Total concentration of antibodies determined with anti-L-chain
No. 1	0	160	<100	105	<115	<480	300	140	1 800	2 240	4 000
	14	2 000	300	225	<115	2 525	2 500	1 450	3 600	7 550	8 000
	28	2 000	400	150	230	2 780	4 500	1 350	2 700	8 550	20 000
No. 2	0	<100	<100	115	<115	<430	400	120	1 500	2 020	3 000
	14	<100	<100	115	<115	<430	400	400	1 250	2 050	4 000
	28	<100	<100	<74	<115	<389	150	270	1 600	2 020	4 000
No. 3	0	<100	200	150	<115	<565	800	480	1 250	2 250	4 000
	14	1 100	20 000	225	230	21 555	20 000	14 000	1 800	35 800	24 000
	28	1 400	20 000	225	230	21 855	22 000	14 000	3 600	39 600	24 000
No. 4	0	<100	<100	<74	<115	<389	<100	<80	<90	<270	<100
	14	850	1 400	<74	<115	2 250	2 100	640	810	3 550	2 100
	28	800	1 200	<74	<115	2 000	4 000	560	720	5 280	4 000
No. 5	0	<100	<100	<74	<115	<389	<100	<80	<90	<270	<100
	14	<100	150	<74	<115	<439	500	<80	<90	500	<100[c]
	28	<100	160	<74	<115	<449	800	<80	<90	500	<100[c]
No. 6	0	<100	<100	<74	<115	<389	<100	<80	<90	<270	<100
	14	<100	<100	<74	<115	<389	200	160	140	500	<100[c]
	28	<100	<100	<74	<115	<389	200	160	160	520	200[c]

[a] The sum of antibodies detected in the subclass assays. It should theoretically be equal to the concentration detected in the IgG antibody assay.
[b] The sum of concentrations detected in IgG, IgA and IgM antibody assays, it should be equal to the concentration in the last column.
[c] The background values (non-specific binding of Ig) were high in these cases.

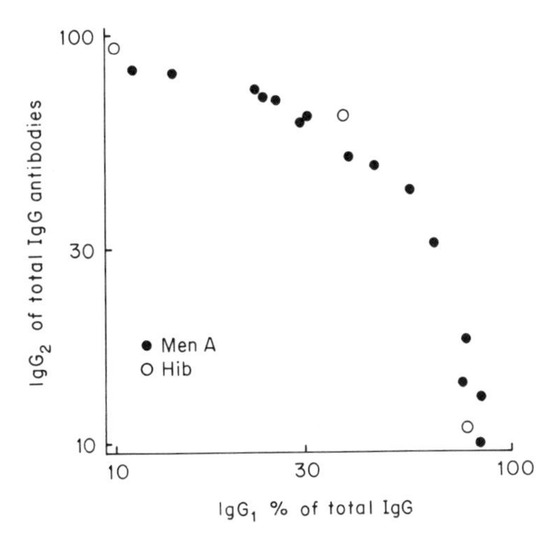

Figure 1. Proportions of IgG_1 and IgG_2 (%) of all detected IgG antibodies to meningococcal type A polysaccharide (black dots, data from ref. [7], or *Haemophilus* type b polysaccharide (circles, vaccinees 1, 3 and 4, Table I)

2. Hammarström, L., Persson, M. A. A., and Smith, C. I. E. Immunoglobulin subclass distribution of human anti-carbohydrate antibodies: aberrant pattern in IgA-deficient donors. *Immunology*, **54**, 821–6 (1985).
3. Jefferis, R., Reimer, C. B., Skvaril, F., de Lange, G., Ling, N. R., Lowe, J., Walker, M. R., Vaermans, J. P., Magnusson, C. G., Kubagawa, H., Cooper, M., Vardtal, F., Vandvik, B., Haaijman, J. J., Mäkelä, O., Sarnesto, A., Lando, Z., Gergely, J., and Radl, J. Evaluation of monoclonal antibodies having specificity for human IgG sub-classes: results of an IUIS/WHO collaborative study. *Immunology Lett.*, **10**, 223–52 (1985).
4. Julkunen, I., Hovi, T., Seppälä, I., and Mäkelä, O. Immunoglobulin G subclass antibody responses in influenza A and parainfluenza type 1 virus infections. *Clin. exp. Immunol.*, **60**, 130–8 (1985).
5. Matter, L., Wilhelm, J. A., Angehrn, W., Skvaril, F., and Schopfer, K. Selective antibody deficiency and recurrent pneumococcal bacteremia in a patient with Sjögren's syndrome, hyperimmunoglobulinemia G, and deficiencies of IgG2 and IgG4. *N. Engl. J. Med.*, **312**, 1039–42 (1985).
6. Papadea, C., Check, I. J., and Reimer, C. B. Monoclonal antibody-based solid-phase immunoenzymometric assays for quantifying human immunoglobulin G and its subclasses in serum. *Clin. Chem.*, **31**, 1940–5 (1985).
7. Rautonen, N., Pelkonen, J., Sipinen, S., Käyhty, H., and Mäkelä, O. Isotype concentrations of human antibodies to group A meningococcal polysaccharide. *J. Immunol.*, in press (1986).
8. Riesen, W. F., Skvaril, F., and Braun, D. G. Natural infection of man with group A streptococci. *Scand. J. Immunol.*, **5**, 383–90 (1976).
9. Sarnesto, A., Ranta, S., Väänänen, P., and Mäkelä, O. Proportions of Ig classes and subclasses in rubella antibodies. *Scand. J. Immunol.*, **21**, 275–82 (1985).

10. Sarnesto, A., Julkunen, I., and Mäkelä, O. Proportions of Ig classes and subclasses in mumps antibodies. *Scand. J. Immunol.*, **22**, 345–50 (1985).
11. Sarvas, H. O., Seppälä, I. J. T., Tähtinen, T., Peterfy, F., and Mäkelä, O. Mouse IgG antibodies have subclass associated affinity differences. *Mol. Immunol.*, **20**, 239–46 (1983).
12. Seppälä, I. J. T., Rautonen, N., Sarnesto, A., Mattila, P. S., and Mäkelä, O. The percentages of six immunoglobulin isotypes in human antibodies to tetanus toxoid: standardization of isotypespecific second antibodies in solid-phase assay. *Eur. J. Immunol.*, **14**, 868–75 (1984).
13. Seppälä, I., Pelkonen, J., and Mäkelä, O. Isotypes of antibodies induced by plain dextran or a dextran–protein conjugate. *Eur. J. Immunol.*, **15**, 827–33 (1985).
14. Stevens, R., Dichek, D., Keld, B., and Heiner, D. IgG1 is the predominant subclass of in Vivo and in Vitro produced anti-tetanus toxoid antibodies and also serves as the membrane IgG molecule for delivering inhibitory signals to anti-tetanus toxoid antibody-producing B cells. *J. Clin. Immunol.*, **3**, 65–9 (1983).
15. Yount, W. J., Dorner, M. M., Kunkel, H. G., and Kabat, E. A. Studies on human antibodies. VI. Selective variations in subgroup composition and genetic markers. *J. exp. Med.*, **127**, 633–46 (1968).

DISCUSSION – Chaired by Professor G. L. Ada

ADA: Can I just ask for clarification? The conjugate contained chicken serum albumin (CSA) as the conjugate?

MÄKELÄ: That was the conjugate used in the mouse experiment, not in the human experiment.

ADA: What was the human conjugate?

MÄKELÄ: Diphtheria toxoid.

ADA: To which people had been immunized previously?

MÄKELÄ: Yes.

ADA: So they had immunological memory?

MÄKELÄ: Yes.

ROBBINS: Is it your conclusion, Dr Mäkelä, that the differences in the antibodies induced by the conjugate compared to the polysaccharide are really quantitative not qualitative? That is, there are more antibodies induced by the conjugate, but they have the same overall distribution with respect to subclass and isotype?

MÄKELÄ: I think there is a statistically significant difference. Again, its a borderline case – 60% of the antibodies induced by the polysaccharide are IgG.

ROBBINS: We come to the same conclusion. Briefly, I have tried to compare in the literature where a comparison can be made, where adults were immunized with the polysaccharide or with the conjugate. When you compare the fold increase, which is probably the most reliable way of contrasting the antibody data, the conjugates in the adults are considerably more immunogenic than the polysaccharide. A conjugate prepared by Connaught, which uses the adipic acid hydrazide method, differs from our materials in two ways that are worth while mentioning: (1) in our experiments we derivatize the polysaccharide and then attach the derivative to the protein. The Connaught method uses the method we first proposed, and that was to derivatize the protein and then attach the activated polysaccharide. We find that the second method makes for a more immunogenic carrier, because it is difficult not to over-derivatize the carrier; (2) Connaught has a patent in which they heat the polysaccharide before they conjugate it to the protein but it results in a slightly lower molecular weight polysaccharide. The second point, that the individuals are already sensitized to the carrier protein, might be an explanation for why you do not demonstrate booster effects in adults. That is, you may not be able to recruit a booster response within a month to someone who already has been immunized several times with the carrier protein.

MÄKELÄ: That may be an explanation. On the other hand, when we immunized mice with the dextran protein conjugate we saw a good secondary response with conjugate that had a small polysaccharide moiety and little or no secondary response when the conjugate had a large polysaccharide moiety.

ROBBINS: The method Connaught used was on the first description. We looked to see what is the immune response of adult humans with multiple injections of toxoids, and the booster responses after three or four injections in adults don't always follow what you would expect in young animals that had not seen the carrier protein before. But the fact remains that, when you inject adults with these conjugates, you don't get a booster response either to the polysaccharide and not much to the carrier protein. It may be a phenomenon that we haven't studied in adult humans who have been immunized years before.

ADA: A discussion about carriers should follow the papers we will have tomorrow. Are there any other questions about the isotype restrictions?

SÖDERSTRÖM: Dr Mäkelä, have you done any experiments where you looked at the booster effects of the micro-organisms following priming with the conjugate?

MÄKELÄ: We have not studied booster effects at all in human beings.

MORENO: I just wanted to add that, in my modest experience with IgG isotype distribution in mice, immunization with different purified polysaccharides tends to indicate that the example of dextran is B1355, in which there is tremendous predominance of IgG_3 antibodies, is not necessarily followed by meningococcal polysaccharide Group C, at least in CBA mice (C. Moreno and J. Esdaile, *Eur. J. Immunol.*, **13**, 262–4 (1983)). Here the distribution of isotypes varies enormously from mouse to mouse and you can find antibodies to all IgG subclasses but IgG_3. Moreover, I think the pattern shows a tremendous variability in relation to dose of antigen used. So, although the original observation is correct, and I don't doubt it for a minute, it is difficult to generalize from that experience.

ROBBINS: I have a suggestion: the variability in individuals with respect to their subclass distribution *might* be explained by differences in the fine specificities of antibodies on the antigen to which individuals make antibodies; that is, it might be epitope-specific. This could be studied with *H. influenzae* type b and meningococcus Group C polysaccharides by seeing if the serum previously absorbed with the cross-reacting polysaccharides gives the same subclass distribution. It might be that various epitopes induced differences in subclass restriction. So what you are measuring with the subclasses may be individuals that make varying proportions of antibodies to epitopes on the polysaccharides.

ADA: Are you saying that cells of different Ig subclasses respond better to some epitopes than to others; for example, a IgG responds better to this type of epitope than does a IgG_2 cell?

ROBBINS: Yes. I think that is a possibility to explain the variability, and it can be studied by absorption of the serum with cross-reacting polysaccharides which can remove antibodies to one of the epitopes.

ADA: Does anybody have any evidence for this?

ROBBINS: I just said it's a possibility to explain the variability, that is all.

MÄKELÄ: The individuals that appeared on my slide were different, each symbol represented a different individual, but some of the people who had been vaccinated with the *Haemophilus* b were also vaccinated with meningococcal vaccine. I did not have the meningococcal data at the time the slide was prepared, but we now have the data from fifteen or so individuals and there are a few whose *Haemophilus* antibodies are predominantly gamma 2 and whose MenA antibodies are predominantly gamma 1 or *vice versa*. But the total number of such individuals is five or so.

ROBBINS: Dr Mäkelä, have you had an opportunity to look at the subclass distribution of *H. influenzae* type b antibodies in adults who have been sick with the disease and recovered?

MÄKELÄ: No.

GRIFFISS: We have developed some data that relate to this question with Dr Söderström. We vaccinated a group of seventeen IgA-deficient individuals with A and C meningococcal capsules and studied them along with seventeen vaccinated controls. The IgA-deficient individuals fell into three different groups. The smallest group responded with a normal amount of antibody and with a normal isotype distribution of that antibody; the only defect was the absence of IgA. The next larger group responded with significantly more antibody than the controls and showed a loss of IgG isotype restriction; that is, the controls responded with only one or two IgG isotypes, usually IgG_1 and IgG_2, whereas the IgA-deficient individuals responded with three or all four IgG isotypes. They also tended to be far out on the distribution for total serum IgG_1. The third and largest group of IgA-deficient individuals didn't respond at all to either polysaccharide. An obvious interpretation is that IgA deficiency marks for three different levels of immune dysregulation. Another interpretation that is particularly interesting, is that there is an active restriction in the immunoglobulin isotypes with which an individual responds, and that that restriction is lost in some of these IgA-deficient individuals. It is certainly clear that there is active restriction of the isotype response to these polysaccharides.

MÄKELÄ: Did you see considerable amounts of gamma 3 and gamma 4 in these deficient individuals?

GRIFFISS: IgG_4 is particularly hard to measure, but if you accept the limitations of the assays, IgG_3 and IgG_4 were predominant parts of the response in the IgA-deficient individuals who did respond.

MÄKELÄ: Could you compare the concentrations of the different subtypes?

GRIFFISS: We have difficulty doing that because of competition among the subclasses for the antigen. In situations where all four isotypes are present, there is a lot of competition; with normal individuals who have a predominant isotype or perhaps two isotypes, there is less competition. Dr Söderström and I were not discussing ways of making the quantitation more accurate, using the level of saturation binding and then the decay part of the curve. If we integrate those two, we may be able to extract more useful data.

MÄKELÄ: But, apart from the competition, you have to correct for the affinity differences between the second antibody. Did you do that?

GRIFFISS: We were using second antibodies recommended by WHO; we did not correct for affinity differences.

MÄKELÄ: Then you cannot tell what proportions the different subclasses have.

GRIFFISS: That's right, and we make no effort to do so. The data are that an individual either did or did not respond with that subclass.

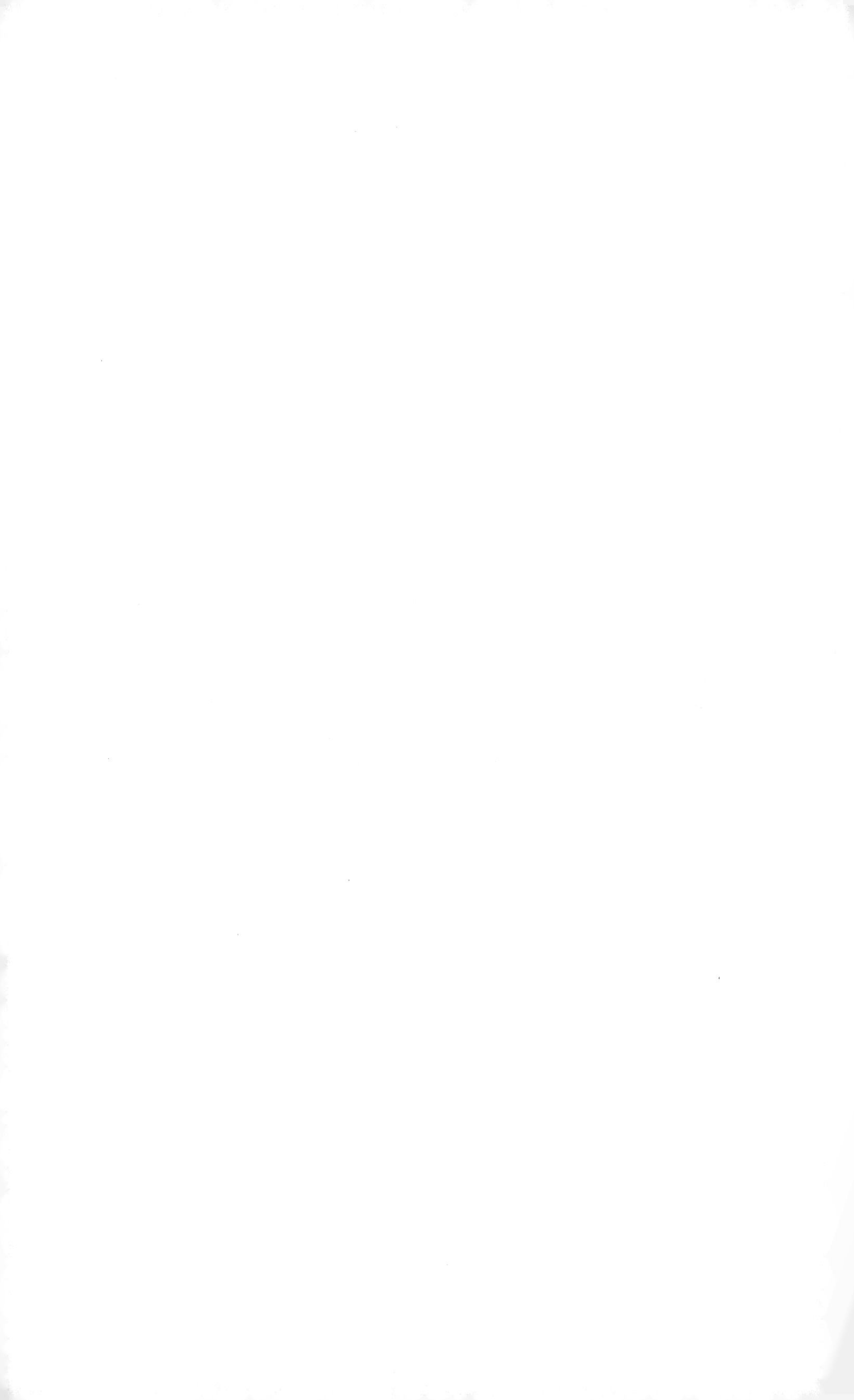

Towards Better Carbohydrate Vaccines
Edited by R. Bell and G. Torrigiani

Published by John Wiley & Sons Ltd

18

The physiology of B lymphocytes capable of generating anti-polysaccharide antibody responses

DONALD E. MOSIER AND ANN J. FEENEY
Division of Immunology, Medical Biology Institute, 11077 North Torrey Pines Road, La Jolla, CA 92037, USA
PEGGY SCHERLE
Immunology Graduate Program, University of Pennsylvania, Philadelphia, PA, 19104, USA

INTRODUCTION

Not all B lymphocytes are created equal, and the B cells that generate anti-polysaccharide antibody responses have a set of characteristics that distinguish them from B cells responding to protein antigens. An understanding of the characteristics of B-lymphocyte subsets is important for the goal of enhancing potentially protective anti-polysaccharide responses in humans. That goal can be achieved by only two routes; increasing the amount of antibody made by the B-cell subset that normally responds to polysaccharides, or convincing B cells that are normally unresponsive to participate in anti-polysaccharide antibody production. As will be reviewed here, both of these routes currently offer some promise for improving the response of humans to polysaccharide antigens, but there also are some major problems associated with each approach.

This chapter will concentrate on the characteristics of mouse B lymphocytes that respond to defined haptens coupled either to protein or polysaccharide molecules, and thus will define the two subsets actually or potentially involved in these model anti-polysaccharide responses. The role of T cells in anti-polysaccharide response will be discussed, and the potential disadvantages of conjugate bacterial polysaccharide–protein vaccines will be emphasized. Finally, some suggestions for augmenting anti-polysaccharide responses will be given.

EXPERIMENTAL SYSTEM

We have studied the antibody response of inbred strains of mice to the small haptenic determinants trinitrophenyl (TNP) or phosphorylcholine (PC) coupled to protein carriers such as keyhole limpet haemocyanin (KLH) or to polysaccharide carriers such as Ficoll (an ether cross-linked polysucrose of 400 kD mean molecular weight), lipopolysaccharide (LPS) from *Escherichia coli*, or unidentified polysaccharide and protein components which comprise the capsular cell wall of *Brucella abortus*. The response to hapten determinants on polysaccharides obeys the same rules as antibody responses against the polysaccharide carrier [39], and has the advantage that the same pool of hapten-binding B lymphocytes are at least potentially responsive to both the hapten–protein and hapten–polysaccharide conjugate. Phosphorylcholine is a natural component of bacterial polysaccharides, and we have used the R36a strain of *Streptococcus pneumoniae* as an immunogen which elicits a PC-specific antibody response. These studies have been presented [15, 17, 30, 31, 34–36, 38, 41, 52, 55] and reviewed [37, 39, 40] previously.

The anti-hapten antibody response to the above antigens has been characterized with respect to the number of antibody-forming cells, the amount of antibody in serum or culture medium, the isotype distribution [43] and the clonal heterogeneity of the response. The antibodies formed in response to TNP immunization are typically heterogeneous, with the products of many clones of B cells contributing to the response. The response to TNP–Ficoll is less heterogeneous than that to TNP–KLH, and anti-TNP antibodies utilizing the lambda light chain are frequent. In contrast, the primary antibody response to PC on either protein or polysaccharide carriers is quite homogeneous with upwards of 90% of antibodies sharing the same germline-encoded heavy chain and light chain variable (V) regions which together comprise the characteristic T15 idiotypic marker [16, 48, 54]. Only two other germline-encoded anti-PC antibodies are commonly identified; these share the T15 heavy chain V region but use different kappa light chain V regions. These antibodies are named after the prototypic PC-binding myeloma proteins MOPC 603 and McPC 511/167 that utilize the 603 and 511/167 light chain V regions respectively [14]. Anti-idiotypic reagents that identify the T15, 603 and 511/167 antibodies can thus subdivide the anti-PC response into its three component parts. Secondary antibody responses to PC–protein conjugates may contain in addition new antibodies that recognize PC-related determinants much better than PC and are not related to T15, 603 or 511/167 [12, 17].

The antibody responses to TNP–KLH or PC–KLH differ in isotype distribution from the antibodies formed in response to TNP–Ficoll or R36a. IgG_1 antibodies predominate in the response to hapten–protein conjugates, whereas the hapten–polysaccharide directed antibodies are predominately of the IgM and IgG_3 isotypes. Mouse IgG_3 is the equivalent of human IgG_2, and the IgG_3 dominance of anti-polysaccharide responses in the mouse parallels the IgG_2 dominance of human antibodies to polysaccharides [6].

ONTOGENY OF ANTI-POLYSACCHARIDE RESPONSES

The ability to generate most anti-polysaccharide antibody responses is acquired relatively late during the ontogeny of the immune system. The ability to respond to TNP–Ficoll, for instance, appears at 10–14 days of age in mice, 2 weeks after the first B cell capable of generating anti-TNP responses are first identified [24, 35]. The response to PC does not appear until 7 days of age in mice, and the ability to respond to other polysaccharides such as levan and dextran is even more delayed [8, 49]. The inability of neonatal humans to respond to bacterial polysaccharides is well demonstrated [4] and is of major clinical importance.

Only one class of polysaccharide antigens seems able to stimulate antibody responses in early neonates, and these antigens also are able to elicit responses in x-linked immunodeficient (*xid*) mice. The antigens, which share the property of being mitogenic for normal B lymphocytes, include TNP–lipopolysaccharide (TNP–LPS) and TNP–*B. abortus*. This class of T-independent antigen has been designated by us as TI-1, in contrast to TI-2 antigens like TNP–Ficoll that stimulate neither neonatal nor *xid* antibody responses [37]. The distinction between TI-1 and TI-2 antigens is important because most bacterial polysaccharides are non-mitogenic and behave as TI-2 antigens. One way to generate an earlier antibody response to such polysaccharides would be to couple a mitogenic entity to them and convert them, in effect, into TI-1 antigens. For example, PC coupled to *B. abortus* stimulates anti-PC antibody formation in neonatal mouse spleen cell cultures several days before PC–KLH or PC–polysaccharides can elicit a response (DEM, unpublished observations).

What is the meaning of the delayed onset of antibody responses to polysaccharide antigens? Two general kinds of explanation have been advanced. The first is that polysaccharides are weak immunogens and that B lymphocytes must undergo considerable maturation to reach the stage when they can be triggered by a polysaccharide. One more specific version of this hypothesis holds that surface immunoglobulin D (sIgD) expression is critical for acquiring responsiveness to polysaccharides, and that most neonatal B cells do not achieve sufficient levels of sIgD expression until some time after birth [37, 46, 55]. Data supporting this hypothesis include the low sIgD expression of *xid* mice [46], and the blocking of TNP–Ficoll but not TNP–*B. abortus* antibody responses by anti-IgD [55]. The alternative explanation for the delayed onset of anti-polysaccharide responses is that a late-appearing B lymphocyte subset is required for such responses. The evidence for this hypothesis is based largely upon studies of the *xid* mutation of CBA/N mice and studies of normal strains using serological reagents generated with *xid* mice [1, 20, 52]. The *xid* mice fail to respond to most polysaccharide antigens, but do generate near-normal antibody responses to most protein antigens [2, reviewed in [46]. One prevalent view of this defect is that *xid* mice lack a late-appearing B-cell subset characterized by high sIgD to sIgM ratio and the expression of the B-cell differentiation antigens Lyb-3, 5, and 7 [37, 50). Data that challenge this interpretation of the *xid* defect have been accumulating recently; these findings will be summarized below.

Characteristics of B cells responding to polysaccharide antigens

Several lines of evidence suggest that the B cells that respond to polysaccharides have unique properties that distinguish them from B cells involved in antibody responses to proteins. In the spleens of rodents, B cells responsive to antigens like TNP–Ficoll reside primarily in the marginal zone [21, 25, 53], whereas protein antigens activate B cells in the periarteriolar lymphoid sheath and follicles [53]. This localization of B cells may be dictated by the presence of specialized marginal zone macrophages or dendritic cells which concentrate and present polysaccharide antigens to B cells [21]. The importance of these specialized cells was demonstrated by a recent study in which selective depletion of marginal zone macrophages abrogated the antibody response to TNP–Ficoll but left intact responses to TNP–KLH and TNP–LPS [13].

The half-life of B cells that respond to polysaccharides *in vivo* is relatively long [45]. Recently we have evaluated the half-life of splenic B cells, using the ratio of sIgM to sIgD on B lymphocytes surviving in recipients as a phenotypic marker of subsets. Figure 1 summarizes experiments in our laboratory that involved the adoptive transfer of cell sorter-purified B lymphocytes into lymphocyte-deficient severe combined immunodeficient (*scid*) recipient mice. The results demonstrate that B cells fall into three categories; a short-lived sIgM > sIgD population, an intermediate-lived sIgD > sIgM population and a long-lived sIgM = sIgD subset. The latter long-

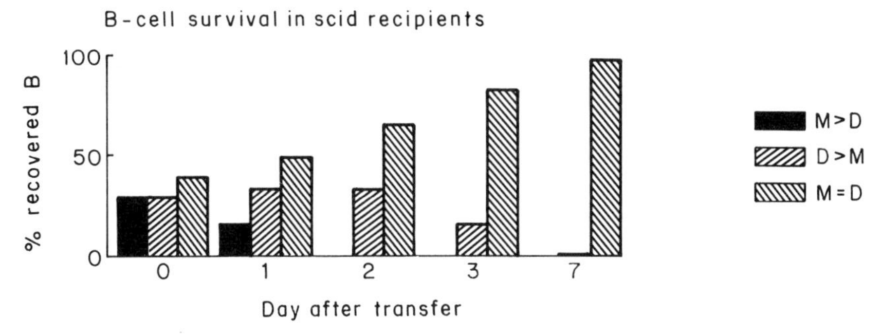

Figure 1. Ten million cell sorter-purified BALB/c splenic B lymphocytes were injected intravenously into C.B-17 *scid* recipients. The number of B cells surviving in the spleen and the sIgM : sIgD ratio was determined by flow cytometry at daily intervals thereafter. The results are presented above as the percentage representation of the three B-cell subpopulations identified by sIgM : sIgD two-colour fluorescence analysis

lived population constitutes the majority of B lymphocytes in peripheral blood and lymph nodes, and about 30% of splenic B cells. Mice immunized 4 weeks after B-cell reconstitution contain only this long-lived subset yet give normal antibody responses to TNP–Ficoll (see Table I below). Lymph node B cells are predominantly long-lived and have been found to reconstitute the TNP–Ficoll response of *xid* mice [45], confirming that much of the antibody response to this prototype TI-2 antigen is derived from long-lived B lymphocytes.

In contrast to these results *in vivo*, the short-lived B-cell population in spleen appears to respond well to TNP–Ficoll as well as TNP–LPS and TNP–*B. abortus* in short-term *in vitro* assays (see Figure 2). This result

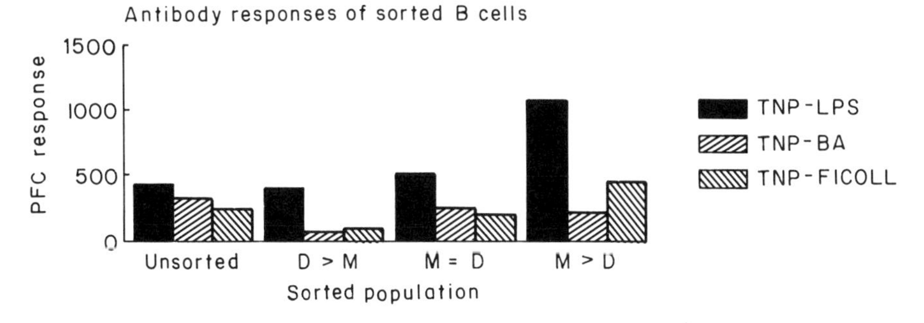

Figure 2. Splenic B lymphocytes were sorted on a flow cytometer into three populations based on the intensity of sIgM and sIgD expression. These sorted B-cell subpopulations were cultured with irradiated, syngeneic spleen filler cells in microculture and stimulated with the TI-1 antigens TNP–LPS and TNP–*B. abortus* (TNP–BA), or with the TI-2 antigen TNP–Ficoll. Anti-TNP antibody formation was determined after 4 days of culture by the plaque-forming cell (PFC) assay

implies that separation of B cells on the basis of sIgD and sIgM expression does not yield functionally distinct subsets, and that many B cells are capable, under the conditions of cell culture, of responding to both TI-1 and TI-2 antigens. The fate of the normally short-lived B cells with sIgM > sIgD could be altered following antigen stimulation, and at least some of this subset could be converted to long-lived cells. Some fraction of B cells activated in the course of a T-dependent antibody response become long-lived memory cells, but it is not clear whether T-independent polysaccharide antigens really stimulate the formation of memory-B cells as opposed to addressing a population of B cells that is already long-lived. Given the high turnover rate of the majority of B lymphocytes [42], it is reassuring to know that protective anti-polysaccharide responses are preserved in a long-lived B-cell population.

In addition to these differences in localization and half-life, B cells responsive to polysaccharide antigens have some unique surface markers in mice. The Lyb-5 and the Lyb-7 alloantigens [1, 52] have been confirmed to be present on B cells responsive to TNP–Ficoll but not on many B cells responsive to TNP–KLH [50]. While the B cells responsive to polysaccharide antigens have been presumed to be high in sIgD and low in sIgM on the basis of the phenotype of neonatal and *xid* B cells, this is not the case, as was demonstrated by the experiment shown in Figure 2. There is thus no correlation between the sIgM : sIgD ratio and the ability of B cells to respond to TI-1 or TI-2 antigens.

Many of the conclusions about B-cell subsets in mice depend upon experiments in neonatal and/or *xid* mice. For instance, the response to PC on either a protein or polysaccharide carrier is absent in neonatal as well as *xid* mice, leading to the conclusion that only the Lyb-5+ subset of B lymphocytes can respond to PC. While this could be the case, it is also possible that neonatal B cells and the defective B cells found in *xid* mice are highly susceptible to tolerance induction by PC-containing antigens and that this is a general property of immature B cells. The failure of PC-containing antigens to trigger *xid* B cells could have explanations that cast little light on the failure of neonatal B cells to respond to PC. Several recent findings detract from the argument that *xid* B cells are a model for immature stages of normal B-cell development (these have been reviewed elsewhere [42]). Briefly, the most potent of these arguments is that the response of *xid* spleen cells to TI-2 antigens can be restored by a variety of lymphokines and immunopotentiating agents such as 8-bromoguanosine, whereas these agents have no effect on TI-2 responses by neonatal B cells [42]. In addition, development of the B-cell lineage in *xid* mice is T-dependent, while the same is not true in conventional mice [51].

A new B-cell subpopulation expressing the Ly-1 differentiation antigen has been identified recently [19, 27]. This subset is prominent in neonates and is elevated in the autoimmune NZB strain [19], but its contribution to anti-polysaccharide responses remains to be determined.

Where does all the above information leave us regarding B-cell subsets and anti-polysaccharide responses? It seems clear that only some B lymphocytes can generate anti-polysaccharide antibody responses, but the precise definition of that subset remains elusive. At best we can say that it appears late in ontogeny, is long-lived, probably expresses the Lyb-3,5, and seven markers, is biased towards IgM and IgG_3 production and does not require T cells for its activation (see below). There is no current evidence to suggest that B cells responsive to polysaccharide antigens fall into a separate lineage, such as the Ly-1+ B-cell lineage, although that remains possible.

T-CELL INDEPENDENCE OF ANTI-POLYSACCHARIDE RESPONSES

The issue of T-cell contribution to anti-polysaccharide responses revolves around two questions: (1) are T cells essential to generating an antibody response, and (2) do T cells regulate the quantity or quality of antibody produced? The classification of polysaccharide antigens as T cell-independent (TI) implies that T cells play no essential role in generating an antibody response to such antigens. Many of the polysaccharide antigens originally were found to be TI by *in vivo* experiments using nu/nu mice or T cell-depleted, bone marrow-reconstituted 'B' mice. That view has been challenged by *in vitro* data showing, for example, that rigorously T-depleted spleen cells fail to respond to TNP–Ficoll [32]. Restoration of T cells allows the antibody response to proceed, but the 'helper effect' of these T cells is quite distinct from the major histocompatibility complex (MHC)-restricted, hapten-carrier-linked T-cell help involved in antibody responses to hapten–-protein conjugates [23]. Thus, T cells seem to be important for the *in vitro* response to a TI-2 antigen, although the nature of the helper effect is poorly defined except to say that it is clearly different from the help involved in classical T-dependent antibody responses. The question of whether or not T cells are essential for optimal *in vivo* responses to polysaccharide antigens would thus seem to be reopened.

In contrast to these *in vitro* results, we have performed experiments recently that strongly suggest that the *in vivo* response to the TI-2 antigen TNP–Ficoll is absolutely independent of T-cell activity. In the course of the *scid* reconstitution experiments described above, we injected cell sorter purified splenic B cells, with or without splenic T cells, into *scid* recipients. Four weeks later the mice were challenged with TNP–Ficoll and the magnitude of the IgM anti-TNP response assayed at 4 days post-immunization. The antibody response was statistically identical in the two groups, and the number of antibody-secreting cells per recovered B cell was similar in the reconstituted *scid* mice and parallel normal controls. No T cells were identified in the *scid* mice that received only B cells initially, whereas recipients of T and B cells had an excess of recovered T cells (60–70%) 4 weeks later. We thus were unable to identify any obligatory contribution of T cells to the response to TNP–Ficoll in these experiments. These experiments are summarized in Table I.

Table I. Antibody responses to TNP–Ficoll of SCID mice reconstituted only with B cells or with T and B cells

Cells used for reconstitution at −4 weeks	PFC response 4 days after 10 μg TNP–Ficoll		
	TNP-specific PFC/spleen	Total IgM PFC/spleen	TNP-specific PFC/10^6 recovered B cells
10^6 B cells	1 398 (1 245–1 571)	18 765 (17 965–19 600)	117 (112–123)
10^6 B cells +3 × 10^6 T cells	1 550 (1 481–1 622)	22 942 (21 813–24 129)	110 (106–114)
None	0	0	0
Normal BALB/c control	30 122 (28 998–31 291)	85 104 (72 059–100 512)	401 (375–431)

This is not to say that T cells cannot be involved in the regulation of anti-polysaccharide responses *in vivo*; substantial evidence suggests that that is the case [5, 9, 33]. The original concept of TI antigens that can elicit effective antibody responses without the participation of T helper cells seems as valid today as when it was first proposed.

What of the role of T cells in regulating anti-polysaccharide responses? We have examined the role of T cells in influencing both the magnitude and the clonal composition of the anti-PC response elicited by R36a *S. pneumoniae* in BALB/c nu/nu mice [40]. As shown in Figure 3, the amount of anti-PC antibody was lower in nu/nu mice than in nu/+ litter-mate controls, but the T15 idiotype dominance of the IgM response was maintained to the same extent in both nu/nu and conventional mice. The antibody response to the PC determinant on a bacterial polysaccharide therefore does not require T-cell help and shows no evidence of regulation of clonal dominance by T cells. The antibody level achieved is higher in the presence of T cells, suggesting a general augmenting activity of T cells in this response. Similar augmenting effects of T cells have been reported in the murine response to type III pneumococcal polysaccharide [5, 9]. Thus it is agreed that T cells can have some positive influences on anti-polysaccharide responses, but the nature of those influences remain poorly defined.

Given that one can show positive non-specific effects of T cells on anti-

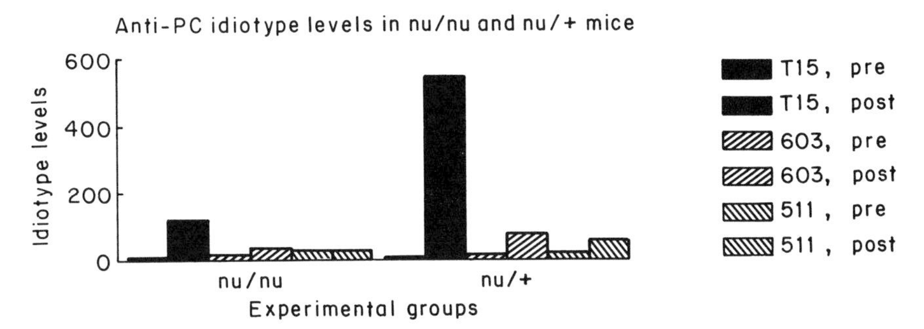

Figure 3. The levels of the three idiotype markets associated with anti-PC antibodies were determined by competitive radioimmunoassay in the serum of BALB/c nu/nu or nu/+ mice before (pre) and after (post) immunization with R36a strain *S. pneumoniae*. The majority of anti-PC antibodies in both nude and normal mice express the T15 idiotype, but the total amount of antibody formed is about fivefold higher in normal *versus* nude mice

polysaccharide responses, it is reasonable to ask whether general activators of T cells, such as adjuvants, are able to augment responses to TI antigens. We have approached this question using supernatants of activated T cells to augment (or suppress) *in vitro* antibody responses to TI-1 and TI-2 antigens. As shown in Table II, we found that supernatants of Concanavalin A-activated rat spleen cells (ConA sup) or mouse mixed lymphocyte cultures (AEF, for allogeneic effect factor) had different effects on each of the antigens tested. The response to TNP–LPS was depressed by both T-cell factors, the response to TNP–*B. abortus* was enhanced by both, and neither factor has a significant effect on the response to the TI-2 antigen TNP–Ficoll. Since most bacterial polysaccharides fall into the TI-2 category, these results are not encouraging for the augmentation of anti-polysaccharide responses by adjuvants or T cell-derived lymphokines, and point to the possibility that such treatments might even diminish the amount of anti-polysaccharide antibody (Table II).

AMPLIFICATION OF NEONATAL ANTI-POLYSACCHARIDE RESPONSES BY ANTIGEN PRIMING

So far, few useful suggestions have been offered for increasing the magnitude of anti-polysaccharide responses other than the procedure of converting a TI-2 antigen into a TI-1 antigen by coupling a small, mitogenic moiety. We [38] and others [47] have demonstrated an effect of neonatal priming with antigen that, if properly applied, holds some potential for augmenting anti-polysaccharide responses. The injection of TNP–Ficoll into mice at the time of birth was found to lead not to antibody formation but to the tenfold

Table II. Effects of T-cell replacing factors on T-independent antibody responses *in vitro*

	Geometric mean IgM anti-TNP PFC/culture (±1 SE)[a]			
Antigen	None	TNP–LPS	TNP–*B. abortus*	TNP–Ficoll
Class	—	TI-1	TI-1	TI-2
T-cell replacing factor				
None	0	663 (585–751)	133 (106–168)	50 (31–79)
ConA sup	10	338 (274–416)	477 (409–556)	45 (28–72)
AEF	13	81 (61–107)	425 (395–458)	73 (46–113)

[a] Cultures consisted of 5 × 10^5 (CBA/N × DBA/2)Fl female spleen cells in a volume of 0.2 ml in RPMI 1640 medium + 5% human serum. Plaque-forming cells (PFC) were assayed using TNP-coupled sheep red blood cells on the fourth day of culture, and the numbers shown represent the geometric mean of five replicate cultures.

expansion of TNP-specific precursors [38], a much greater effect than was seen following immunization of adult animals. Similar results were obtained using inulin either as a bacterial cell wall component or coupled to KLH [47]. It thus appears that there is a stage of B-cell development when polysaccharide antigens trigger cell division but not antibody secretion. Priming at this time would lead to an amplified response to subsequent immunization.

An attempt to extend this neonatal priming strategy to PC-containing antigens led to a better definition of its potential problems. To be effective in amplifying PC-specific precursors, antigens had to be administered between 7 and 10 days of age (unpublished data). Earlier injection of PC led to a suppression of the subsequent anti-PC response, presumably because of B-cell tolerance induction. Any attempt to implement neonatal priming in humans thus would have to take careful consideration of the potential for tolerance induction instead of precursor expansion.

SOMATIC MUTATION OF V GENES DURING ANTI-POLYSACCHARIDE RESPONSES

We have emphasized above that B cells that respond to polysaccharide antigens are probably distinct from those that respond to the same antigenic determinant on a protein carrier. One strategy that has been used [3, 4, 22] to improve the response to poorly immunogenic polysaccharides is to couple them to proteins, which has the dual effect of engaging protein-specific helper

T cells and activating new B cells unresponsive to the polysaccharide alone. This strategy has some important biological consequences that should be understood. One is that antibody production is often switched from IgG_3 (or IgG_2 in humans) to other isotypes that are less effective in affording bacterial protection [10]. Another consequence is the potential loss by somatic mutation of a germline-encoded anti-polysaccharide antibody that has evolved to be optimally protective.

During the course of an antibody response to a T-dependent antigen, there is a clonal evolution which is due both to recruitment of new B-cell clones to the response and somatic mutation of clones activated at the time of initial antigen exposure [7, 28]. Antibody responses to polysaccharide antigens are much more stable and show little clonal evolution [26]. Many of the antibodies generated in mice against common bacterial polysaccharides are encoded by germline V genes [18], and these antibodies are very effective in protection against bacterial infection [11]. The absence of clonal evolution in these responses appears to be due to a very low rate of somatic mutation in the B cells making anti-polysaccharide antibodies. In contrast, during the course of a T-dependent response, the fraction of B cells that retain expression of the original germline antibody sequence rapidly diminishes [7, 28]. This is true, for instance, for the expression of the T15 clone in the antibody response to PC–KLH; this clone is dominant in the primary response, but is almost absent from the secondary anti-PC–KLH response [12, 17, 54]. Since T15 anti-PC IgG_3 antibody is the most protective against bacterial infection, the consequence of repeated immunization with PC–KLH is actually to decrease the concentration of protective antibody.

The cost to the overall immune response of the fine tuning imposed by T cells is quite high. The rate of V region somatic mutation in the T cell-dependent antibody response to influenza haemagglutinin has been estimated to be one mutation per 1000 base pairs per cell generation [29]. This high rate means that after several rounds of B-cell division, fewer than 10% of the original clonal progeny will survive to produce detectable antibody, and very few B cells will produce unmutated germline-encoded antibody. Clearly, the adaptability of the antibody response is achieved at the expense of stability. While the value of being able to respond to new influenza haemagglutinin variants is readily apparent, polysaccharide antigens are stable and it is equally important that B lymphocytes do not 'forget' how to generate effective antibody responses to them. This may well be why T-dependent and T-independent antibody responses have evolved, and it should be made as clear as possible that converting a T-independent polysaccharide antigen to a T-dependent conjugate vaccine is a strategy with some perils. In the clinical setting, it may be imperative to generate some anti-polysacharide response (regardless of isotype or efficiency). However, immunization with polysaccharide–protein conjugates in situations where there is some pre-existing anti-polysaccharide response may interfere with the expansion and preservation of long-lived clones of B cells producing effective anti-bacterial antibody. The secondary antibody response to PC–KLH illustrates another potential hazard of conjugate vaccines. Most of the antibody formed in this response has higher affinity for the diphenyl–PC (DPPC) determinant created by conjugating PC to KLH and lower affinity for PC [12, 44]. The new determinant generated by the conjugation procedure apparently selects B cells expressing somatically mutated antibodies at the expense of PC-binding antibodies. These antibodies with higher affinity for DPPC and lower affinity for PC should bind PC-containing bacterial polysaccharides less well, and thus would be less protective against bacterial infection. There is also evidence to suggest that polysaccharide–protein conjugate immunization leads to a short-term response that does not prime for subsequent responses to the polysaccharide alone [22]. Conjugate polysaccharide vaccines for neonates thus may not be a panacea for bacterial infections, and could lead to a long-lasting interference with normal B-cell responses to polysaccharides.

SUMMARY

The antibody response of mice to many polysaccharide antigens seems to involve the T cell-independent activation of a subset of B lymphocytes to produce antibody of limited heterogeneity and isotype distribution. The majority of B cells responding to a model TI-2 polysaccharide antigen such as TNP–Ficoll are long-lived and comprise a major B-cell fraction in the peripheral blood and lymph nodes and a minor fraction of splenic B cells. T lymphocytes have no discernible effect on the *in vivo* antibody response to TNP–Ficoll, but T cells do appear to increase the magnitude of the anti-PC response elicited by R36a *S. pneumoniae*. Products of activated T cells had quite variable effects on different T-independent antibody responses *in vitro*, with the TNP–Ficoll response showing no increase from control values. A consistent role for T lymphocytes or their products in the augmentation of anti-polysaccharide responses is difficult to discern from our data. The strategy of augmenting anti-polysaccharide responses by increasing non-specific T-cell helper effects thus seems to hold little promise.

The alternative strategy of converting polysaccharide antigens to a T-dependent form by coupling them to protein carriers is known to work, but the strategy has a significant cost. T-dependent antigens, such as PC–KLH, are known to elicit high rate somatic mutation of antibody V region genes among responding B cells. The consequence of this mutation may be the loss of a germline-encoded antibody that is effective for bacterial protection. The strategy of generating anti-polysaccharide responses by using polysaccharide : protein conjugate vaccines thus has the risk of diverting B cells from the production of protective antibody to the synthesis of new or somatic variant antibodies which are less protective.

The best strategy for enhancing anti-polysaccharide antibody responses may be to alter polysaccharide antigens to convert them from TI-2 to TI-1, TI-1 antigens being defined as those T-independent antigens which contain a mitogenic component that allows them to activate the immature B-cell subset not normally stimulated by most polysaccharides.

ACKNOWLEDGEMENTS

Much of the work reported here has been supported by NIH grants AI-22792 and AI-22871. We thank Peter Lopez and Charles Sylvester for assistance with the cell sorter experiments, Marian Mastrangelo, Susan Shinton and Eileen Walsh for technical assistance and Dr Roy Riblet for his helpful comments on the manuscript. We also appreciate the secretarial assistance of Debby Adler. This is manuscript No. 106 from the Medical Biology Institute, La Jolla, CA.

REFERENCES

1. Ahmed, A., Scher, I., Sharrow, S. O., Smith, A. H., Paul, W. E., Sachs, D. H., and Sell, K. W. B-lymphocyte heterogeneity: Development and characterization of an allo-antiserum which distinguishes B-lymphocyte differentiation alloantigens. *J. Exp. Med.*, **145**, 101–10 (1977).
2. Amsbaugh, D. F., Hansen, C. T., Prescott, B., Stashak, P. N., Barthold, D. R., and Baker, P. J. Genetic control of the antibody response to type III pneumococcal polysaccharide in mice. I. Evidence that an X-linked gene plays a decisive role in determining responsiveness. *J. Exp. Med.*, **136**, 931–9 (1972).
3. Anderson, P., Pichichero, M. W., and Insel, R. A. Immunogens consisting of oligosaccarides from the capsule of *Haemophilus influenzae* type b coupled to diphtheria toxoid or CRM197. *J. Clin. Invest.*, **76**, 52–9 (1985).
4. Anderson, P., Pichichero, M. E., Insel, R. A. Immunization of 2-month old infants with protein-coupled oligosaccharides derived from the capsule of *Haemophilus influenzae* type b. *J. Pediatr.*, **107**, 346–51 (1985).
5. Baker, P. J., Stashak, P. W., Amsbaugh, D. F., and Prescott, B. Characterization of the antibody response to type III pneumococcal polysaccharide at the cellular level. I. Dose response studies and the effect of prior immunization on the magnitude of the antibody response. *Immunology*, **20**, 469–79 (1971).
6. Barrett, D. J., and Ayoub, E. M. IgG2 subclass restriction of antibody to pneumococcal polysaccharides. *Clin. Exp. Immunol.*, **63**, 127–34 (1986).
7. Berek, C., Griffiths, G. M., and Milstein, C. Molecular events during maturation of the immune response to oxazolone. *Nature*, **316**, 412–18 (1985).
8. Bona, C., Lieberman, R., Chien, C. C., Mond, J., House, S., Green, L., and Paul, W. E. Immune response to levan. I. Kinetics and ontogeny of anti-levan

and anti-inulin antibody response and of expression of cross-reactive idiotype. *J. Immunol.*, **120**, 1436–42 (1978).
9. Braley-Mullen, H. Secondary IgG responses to type III pneumococcal polysaccharide. II. Different cellular requirements for induction and elicitation. *J. Immunol.*, **116**, 904–12 (1976).
10. Briles, D. E., Claflin, J. L., Schroer, K., and Forman, C. Mouse IgG3 antibodies are highly protective against infection with *Streptococcus pneumoniae. Nature*, **294**, 88–90 (1981).
11. Briles, D. E., Forman, C., Hudak, S., and Claflin, J. L. Anti-phosphorylcholine antibodies of the T15 idiotype are optimally protective against *Streptococcus pneumoniae. J. Exp. Med.*, **156**, 1177–85 (1982).
12. Chang, S. P., Brown, M., and Rittenberg, M. B. Immunologic memory to phosphorylcholine. II. PC-KLH induces two antibody populations that dominate different isotypes. *J. Immunol.*, **128**, 702–6 (1982).
13. Claassen, E., Kors, N., and vanRooijen, N. Influence of carriers on the development and localization of anti-2,4,6-trinitrophenyl (TNP) antibody-forming cells in the murine spleen. II. Suppressed antibody response to TNP–Ficoll after elimination of marginal zone cells. *Eur. J. Immunol.*, **16**, 492–7 (1986).
14. Claflin, J. L. Uniformity in the clonal repertoire of the immune response to phosphorylcholine in mice. *Eur. J. Immunol.*, **6**, 669–74 (1976).
15. Cohen, P. L., Scher, I., and Mosier, D. E. *In vitro* studies of the genetically determined unresponsiveness to thymus-independent antigens in CBA/N mice. *J. Immunol.*, **116**, 301–4 (1976).
16. Cosenza, H., and Kohler, H. Specific inhibition of plaque formation to phosphorylcholine by antibody against antibody. *Science*, **176**, 1027–30 (1972).
17. Feeney, A. J., and Mosier, D. E. Helper T lymphocytes from *xid* and normal mice support anti-phosphocholine antibody responses with equivalent T15, 511 and 603 idiotypic composition. *J. Immunol.*, **133**, 2868–73 (1984).
18. Gearhart, P. J., Johnson, N. D., Douglas, R., and Hood, L. IgG antibodies to phosphorylcholine exhibit more diversity than their IgM counterparts. *Nature*, **291**, 29–34 (1981).
19. Hayakawa, K., Hardy, R. R., Honda, M., Herzenberg, L. A., Steinberg, A. D., and Herzenberg, L. A. Ly-1 B cells: functionally distinct lymphocytes that secrete IgM autoantibodies. *Proc. Natl. Acad. Sci. USA*, **81**, 2494–8 (1984).
20. Huber, B. T., Gershon, R. K., and Cantor, H. Identification of a B-cell surface structure involved in antigen-dependent triggering: absence of this structure on B cells from CBA/N mutant mice. *J. Exp. Med.*, **145**, 10–20 (1977).
21. Humphrey, J. H., and Grennan, D. Different macrophage populations distinguished by means of fluorescent polysaccharides. Recognition and properties of marginal-zone macrophages. *Eur. J. Immunol.*, **3**, 221–8 (1981).
22. Insel, R. A., and Anderson, P. W. Response to oligosaccharide-protein conjugate vaccine against *Hemophilus influenzae* b in two patients with IgG2 deficiency unresponsive to capsular polysaccharide vaccine. *N. Engl. J. Med.*, **315**, 499–503 (1986).
23. Katz, D. H., Hamaoka, T., and Benacerraf, B. Cell interactions between histoincompatible T and B lymphocytes. II. Failure of physiologic cooperative interactions between T and B lymphocytes from allogeneic donor strains in humoral response to hapten-protein conjugates. *J. Exp. Med.*, **137**, 1405–18 (1973).
24. Klinman, N. R., and Press, J. L. The characterization of the B-cell repertoire specific for the 2,4-dinitrophenyl and 2,4,6-trinitrophenyl determinants in neonatal BALB/c mice. *J. Exp. Med.*, **141**, 1133–46 (1975).

25. MacLennan, I. C. M., Gray, D., Kumararatne, D. S., and Bazin, H. The lymphocytes of splenic marginal zones: a distinct B cell lineage. *Immunol. Today*, **3**, 305–7 (1982).
26. Maizels, N., and Bothwell, A. The T-cell-independent immune response to the hapten NP uses a large repertoire of heavy chain genes. *Cell*, **43**, 715–20 (1985).
27. Manohar, V., Brown, E., Leiserson, W. M., and Chused, T. M. Expression of Lyt-1 by a subset of B lymphocytes. *J. Immunol.*, **129**, 532–8 (1982).
28. Manser, T., Wysocki, L. J., Gridley, T., Near, R. I., and Gefter, M. L. The molecular evolution of the immune response. *Immunol. Today*, **6**, 94–101 (1985).
29. McKean, D., Huppi, K., Bell, M., Staudt, L., Gerhard, W., and Weigert, M. Generation of antibody diversity in the immune response of BALB/c mice to influenza virus hemagglutinin. *Proc. Natl. Acad. Sci. USA*, **81**, 3180–4 (1984).
30. Mond, J. J., Lieberman, R., Inman, J. K., Mosier, D. E., Paul, W. E. Inability of mice with a defect in B cell maturation to respond to phosphorylcholine. *J. Exp. Med.*, **146**, 1138–42 (1977).
31. Mond, J. J., Scher, I., Mosier, D. E., Blaese, M., and Paul, W. E. T-independent responses in B cell defective CBA/N mice to *Brucella abortus* and to TNP-conjugates of *Brucella abortus. Eur. J. Immunol.*, **8**, 459–63 (1978).
32. Mond, J. J., Mongini, P. K., Sieckmann, D., and Paul, W. E. Role of T lymphocytes in responses to TNP–AECM Ficoll. *J. Immunol.*, **125**, 1066–70 (1980).
33. Mongini, P. K. A., Stein, K. E., and Paul, W. E. T cell regulation of IgG subclass antibody production in response to T-independent antigens. *J. Exp. Med.*, **153**, 1–10 (1981).
34. Mosier, D. E., Scher, I., and Paul, W. E. *In vitro* responses of CBA/N mice: spleen cells of mice with an X-linked defect that precludes immune responses to several thymus-independent antigens can respond to TNP-lipopolysaccharide. *J. Immunol.*, **117**, 1363 (1976).
35. Mosier, D. E., Mond, J. J., and Goldings, E. A. The ontogeny of thymic-independent antibody responses *in vitro* in normal mice and mice with an X-linked B cell defect. *J. Immunol.*, 119, 1874–8 (1977).
36. Mosier, D. E., Zaldivar, N., Goldings, E., Mond, J., Scher, I., and Paul, W. E. Ontogeny of the response to T-independent antigens in the neonatal mouse. *J. Infect. Diseases*, **136**, 514 (1977).
37. Mosier, D. E., Zitron, I. M., Mond, J. J., Ahmed, A., Scher, I., and Paul, W. E. Surface immunoglobulin D as a functional receptor for a subclass of B lymphocytes. *Immunol. Rev.*, **37**, 89–104 (1977).
38. Mosier, D. E. Induction of B cell priming by neonatal injection of mice with thymic-independent (type 2) antigens. *J. Immunol.*, **121**, 1453–9 (1978).
39. Mosier, D. E., and Subbarao, B. Thymus-independent antigens – complexity of B lymphocyte activation revealed. *Immunol. Today*, **3**, 217–22 (1982).
40. Mosier, D. E., and Feeney, A. J. Idiotype regulation in the antibody response to phosphocholine. Antigen selection of B-lymphocyte subsets with differential idiotype expression? In *The Biology of Idiotypes*, (ed. M. Green and A. Nisonoff), Plenum Press, New York, 1984, pp. 403–15.
41. Mosier, D. E. Are *xid* B lymphocytes representative of any normal B cell population? *J. Mol. Cell. Immunol.*, **2**, 70 (1985).
42. Osmond, D. G., and Nossal, G. J. V. Differentiation of lymphocytes in mouse bone marrow. II. Kinetics of maturation and renewal of anti-globulin-binding cells by double labelling. *Cell Immunol.*, **13**, 132–45 (1974).
43. Perlmutter, R. M., Nahm, M., Stein, K. E., Slack, J., Zitron, I. Paul, W. E.,

and Davie, J. M. Immunoglobulin subclass-specific immunodeficiency in mice with an X-linked B lymphocyte defect. *J. Exp. Med.*, **149**, 993–8 (1979).
44. Rodwell, J. D., Gearhart, P. J., and Karush, F. Restriction in IgM expression. IV. Affinity analysis of monoclonal anti-phosphorylcholine antibodies. *J. Immunol.*, **130**, 313–16 (1983).
45. Ron, Y., and Sprent, J. Prolonged survival *in vivo* of unprimed B cells responsive to a T-independent antigen. *J. Exp. Med.*, **161**, 1581–6 (1985).
46. Scher, I. The CBA/N mouse strain: an experimental model illustrating the influence of the X-chromosome on immunity. *Adv. Immunol.*, **33**, 1–35 (1982).
47. Shahin, R. D., and Cebra, J. J. Rise in inulin-sensitive B cells during ontogeny can be prematurely stimulated by thymus-dependent and thymus-independent antigens. *Infection and Immunity*, **32**, 211–15 (1981).
48. Sher, A., and Cohn, M. Inheritance of an idiotype associated with the immune response of inbred mice to phosphorylcholine. *Eur. J. Immunol.*, **2**, 319–24 (1972).
49. Sigal, N. H., Pickard, A. R., Metcalf, E. S., Gearhart, P. J., and Klinman, N. R. Expression of phosphorylcholine-specific B cells during murine development. *J. Exp. Med.*, **146**, 933–48 (1977).
50. Singer, A., Morrissey, P. H., Hathcock, K. S., Ahmed, A., Scher, I., and Hodes, R. J. Role of the major histocompatibility complex in T cell activation of B cell subpopulations. Lyb5$^+$ and Lyb5$^-$ B cell subpopulations differ in their requirements for major histocompatibility complex-restricted T cell recognition. *J. Exp. Med.*, **154**, 501–16 (1981).
51. Sprent, J., and Bruce, J. Physiology of B cells in mice with X-linked immunodeficiency (*xid*). II. Influence of the thymus and mature T cells on B cell differentiation. *J. Exp. Med.*, **160**, 335–40 (1984).
52. Subbarao, B., Ahmed, A., Paul, W. E., Scher, I., Lieberman, R., and Mosier, D. E. Lyb 7, a B cell alloantigen controlled by genes linked to the IgC_H locus. *J. Immunol.*, **122**, 2279–85 (1979).
53. van Rooijen, N., Claassen, E., and Eikelenboom, P. 'Is there a single differentiation pathway for all antibody-forming cells in the spleen?' *Immunol. Today*, **7**, 193–6 (1986).
54. Wicker, L. S., Guelde, G., Scher, I., and Kenny, J. J. The asymmetry in idiotype-isotype expression in the response to phosphocholine is due to divergence in the expressed repertoires of Lyb-5$^+$ and Lyb-5$^-$ B cells. *J. Immunol.*, **131**, 2468–76 (1983).
55. Zitron, I. M., Mosier, D. E., and Paul, W. E. The role of surface IgD in the response to thymic-independent antigens. *J. Exp. Med.*, **146**, 1707–18 (1977).

DISCUSSION – Chaired by Professor G. L. Ada

ROBBINS: Dr Mosier, then you would suggest that perhaps lipids could be covalently bound to an antigen, what would it recognize, a primitive cell or something that would be stimulant for a primitive cell? What would you suggest to start off to look at that possibility in the mouse?
MOSIER: Well, the most obvious candidate would be lipid A or lipid X, since both of those molecules are known to activate relatively immature B cells. The absolute concentration of those molecules would be important because

at high concentrations they polyclonally activate many B cells. They should be used at low conjugation ratios and low concentrations of polysaccharides so that they are focused only on the appropriate B cells.

MÄKELÄ: What is the relationship of the long-lived B cells *versus* short-lived B cells and Bl B cells *versus* B2 B cells?

MOSIER: I didn't answer that question because it is not altogether clear. It appears that most of the long-lived B cells belong to the B2 subpopulation. There is a slight confounding effect and that is that recently activated B cells tend to decrease their expression of surface IgD and so end up this high sIgM, low sIgD population. We don't really know the fate of those recently activated B cells.

MÄKELÄ: Can I also ask whether there is any evidence that human beings have the equivalent of B1 and B2?

MOSIER: Well, we tried very hard to answer that question by extending our mouse experiments to humans and we don't have any convincing evidence that there is a subset of B cells that respond to pneumonococcal polysaccharides. We were successful in inducing an *in vitro* response to pneumococcal polysaccharides in human peripheral blood lymphocytes, and then we asked if there were any of the available subset markers for human B cells that identified the B cells, giving rise to this response. The answer was simply negative. None of the markers, including FMC7 monoclonal antibody, Bl and Bl, or the mouse erythrocyte receptor, appeared to define a subpopulation of human B cells that responded to polysaccharide antigens. So the concept of human B-cell subsets remains a viable hypothesis I think, but there is no direct evidence supporting the possibility.

SÖDERSTRÖM: If you coupled the polysaccharides to thymus independent type 1 antigens, what would be the reason not to expect that such conjugates would induce very short-lived clones?

MOSIER: The argument for saying that they would produce more long-lived responses is simply that the response to TNP–LPS itself is of long duration, not of short duration.

ADA: How do you distinguish between long-lived B cells that are producing your antibody and short-lived ones and continual recruitment of B cells?

MOSIER: The arguments for distinguishing these is that we see no evidence of phenotypic conversion. If we transfer, for instance, lymph-node B cells, which seem to be a very stable population with very low cycling time, we see no evidence of recruitment of new B cells to that pool in the *scid* mouse. There must, of course, be some mechanism by which some short-lived B cells get to be longer-lived, since the consequence of every B cell being short-lived would, of course, be that there are no long-lived B cells, and that seems unacceptable.

ROBBINS: Regarding Dr Mäkelä's findings that the conjugate and the polysaccharide just differ qualitatively and not quantitatively in the type of antibody they elicit. How would you map that out with your view of the cellular basis for this?

MOSIER: First of all, I am somewhat surprised that Dr Mäkelä sees so much IgG_1 in the response, but the differences between the pure polysaccharide and the conjugate are not all that outstanding. I would suggest that, when you use a large molecular weight polysaccharide on a carrier protein, what you are doing is engaging some non-specific help which is relatively inefficient at driving class switching or somatic mutation. I spoke briefly of the B2 type of cell being susceptible to non-specific helper effects *in vitro*. Such sensitivity to bystander help has never been demonstrated convincingly *in vivo*, but it is possible that when you use something like a tetanus toxoid coupled to high molecular weight polysaccharide antigen, what you are doing is simply focusing T cells in the vicinity of responding B cell and there is a non-specific, factor-mediated T-cell help which is not very efficient at driving class-switching and somatic mutation but does amplify the clonal burst size of the responding B cells.

MORENO: When you mentioned the possibility of transforming type 2 TI antigens to type 1, maybe an alternative to the one you suggested is the use of the so-called Braun's lipoprotein, that is also a B-cell activator and could function in a similar way (V. Braun and V. Bosch, *Proc. Natl. Acad. Sci., USA*, **69**, 970–4 (1972)).

MODABBER: I was wondering whether long-term B cells require antigen to sustain their antibody formation? If not, then that might be an advantage in favour of carbohydrates.

MOSIER: I really can't answer that question. We have done tracer studies with TNP–Ficoll and it essentially persists for the life of the animal. So, in essence, there is no way of eliminating the possibility of residual antigen stimulation in these kinds of experiments.

ADA: Is there a role for anti-idiotypes in the long-lived production of antibodies?

MOSIER: No, we feel fairly strongly that in these pure B-cell mice, anti-idiotype is not regulating the response because every anti-idiotype I know is T-dependent for its production.

SÖDERSTRÖM: Jerne has argued that, in addition to the very long-lived T and B cells, there are also long-lived immunoglobulins. Was there any evidence that the immunoglobulins produced by the different cells differed in half-life?

MOSIER: No, not really. We only analysed the isotype distribution over the course of response and this is a response that is IgM predominant and has a fairly good representation of IgG_3 antibodies. The relative proportion of those isotypes was fairly constant over the period of time. Since, *in vivo*, IgM has a shorter half-life than IgG_3, I think that these results suggest the stable production of both classes of antibody by long-lived B cells.

MÄKELÄ: It was thought at one time that the *xid* type B cell is less mature than the l cell and you used the word 'immature' B cell at the beginning of your talk. Are you now fairly convinced that there is not a difference in maturity?

MOSIER: The only evidence for the importance of maturation is the sequence of appearance in ontogeny. In the mature mouse, it is not clear that the maturity of the B cells has anything to do with these two subsets. I think the *xid* model has been somewhat misleading because, the more we study those B cells, the more we find they resemble no naturally occurring B cell in quite a number of respects. Their differentiation is very T-cell dependent, yet normal B-cell differentiation in B-cell reconstituted *scid* mice is totally independent of T cells. There are many factors which will activate normal neonatal B cells which fail to act on *xid* B cells and I think that the current view of *xid* mutation is that these B cells fail to express the whole series of surface glycoproteins which renders them functionally incompetent. They are not a clear model for an immature B cell.

ROBBINS: Dr Mosier, you know we have always tried very hard to extrapolate information as far as we could from mice to humans. Let me just tell you our experience, our long list of failures, in trying to make our polysaccharides more suitable for infants. Just to illustrate one failure of our and other laboratories: we would mix the polysaccharides with other macromolecules that had opposite charge – lysozyme, methylated bovine albumin, outer membrane proteins – and when these complexes, that were not covalently formed, were injected intraperitoneally or intravenously into mice, they elicit high levels of polysaccharide antibodies, in contrast to the polysaccharide alone (which was either poorly or non-immunogenic). But when the non-covalent 'complexes' were injected subcutaneously, they failed to induce polysaccharide antibody. Many of the mouse experiments used the intraperitoneal or intravenous route of immunization and it may circumvent one immune process which can't be circumvented in humans and may give an immune response that might not be exactly comparable to what you have to deal with in the human situation.

ADA: A lesson to be learned.

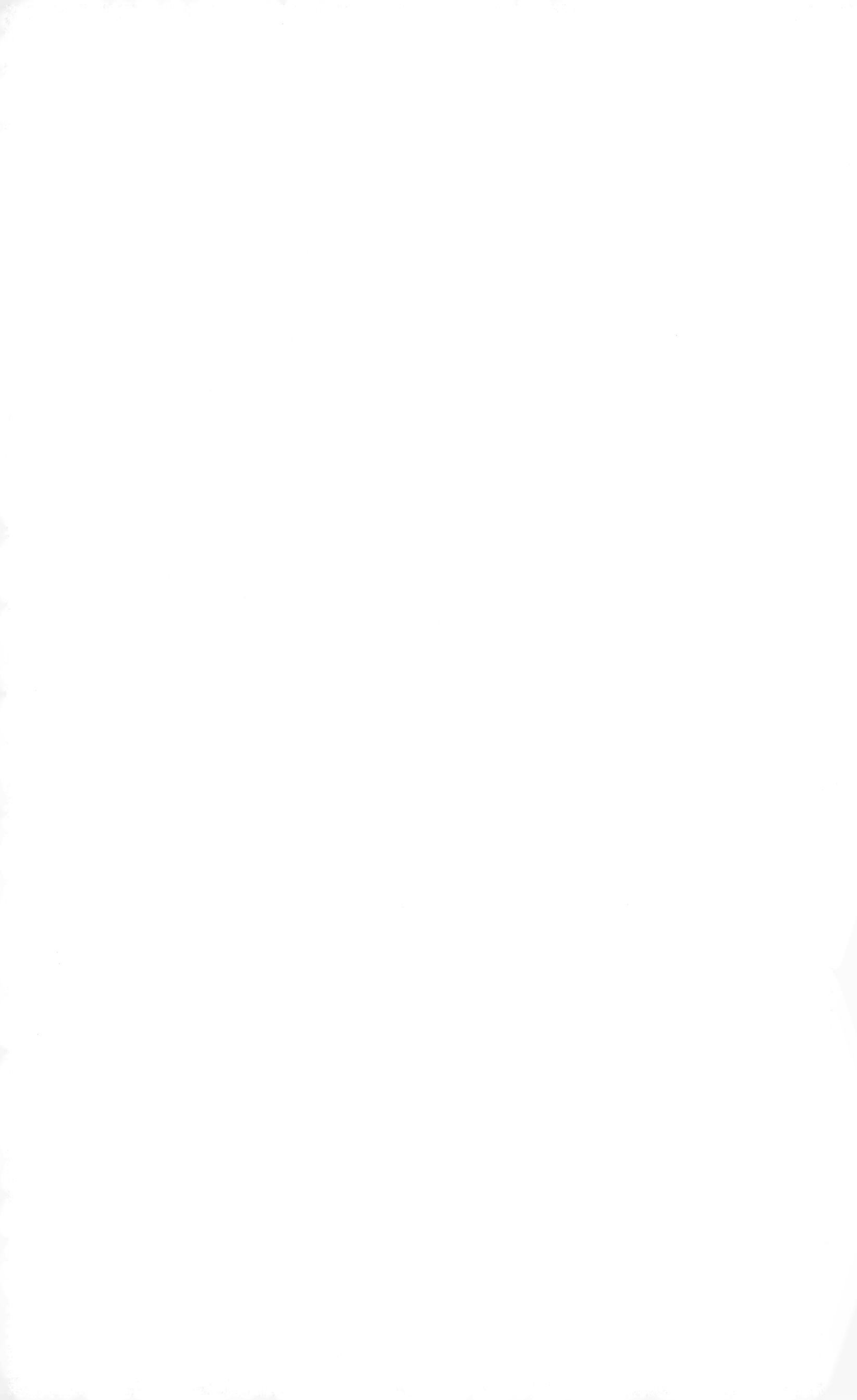

Towards Better Carbohydrate Vaccines
Edited by R. Bell and G. Torrigiani

Published by John Wiley & Sons Ltd

19

Carbohydrates as immunogens and tolerogens. Antibody *versus* cell-mediated immune responses

CARLOS MORENO
Medical Research Council Tuberculosis and Related Infections Unit, Hammersmith Hospital, London W12 0HS, UK

It became apparent to me after accepting the invitation to participate in this symposium – an invitation I am truly grateful for – that one should opt out of the rather comfortable, conventional presentation full of data already published that would illustrate our own contribution to the field of tolerance and immunity to bacterial polysaccharides, tossed here and there with pertinent slides. But, we have been convoked here – so I gather – to act as something like Sibyls and read the future. A conventional, down-to-earth lecture, full of facts and little else will not do. Where do we go from here? Which new avenues can be sensibly opened to lead research in the field of immunity and vaccination with carbohydrate antigens? To tackle this kind of problem, many people would resort to a different, multidisciplinary approach, from where a new, fresh vision could be hoped to emerge.

At this point and on this province I must quote Stafford Beer [32] because he has seen the problem with a lucidity that I will never be able to master:

> The contemporary University is an iron maiden in whose secure embrace scholarship is trapped. The number of papers increases exponentially, knowledge grows by infinitesimals but understanding of the world actually recedes.

> There has been some recognition of this, and inter-disciplinary studies are now common place in every University. . . . Unfortunately, interdisciplinary studies often consist of a group of disciplinarians holding hands in a ring of mutual comfort. The ostensible topic has slipped down the hole in the middle.

Consequently, I decided to attempt a different approach. No data will be presented on this occasion, but rather what I could extract from them in the context of this discussion. Unfortunately, the discussion has been parcelled from the very beginning by asking me and others to speak about something rather restricted. I insist upon the word 'restricted' because it is very different from the word 'specific' and even more so from the word 'precise'. Alas, one can speak about generalities and be very precise, whereas I find it difficult to give overall views while forced to look at things through a very narrow (restricted) window.

The issues I intend to approach are germane to the way by which the immune system (a) handles a polysaccharide when it is injected, (b) the outcome of such interaction and (c) some possible ways to manipulate and control the interactions in such a fashion that the dream of every vaccinator, i.e. to achieve protective immunity, can be fulfilled in the most effective way without unwanted side effects.

If there were a mathematical equation for effective vaccination it should contain at least six variables that, for discussion purposes, I have paired in three groups, although the two factors in each pair should not be considered necessarily as polar or mutually exclusive.

(I) Immunity and tolerance.
(II) Thymus dependence (TD) and thymus independence (TI).
(III) Non-specific stimulation and immunosuppression.

I. IMMUNITY AND TOLERANCE

The situation for the first pair of factors may be illustrated with many examples from the literature (see [37] [43] and [45] for reviews on the subject). Regardless of the route, dose or animal model employed, experimental evidence so far accumulated indicates that immunity to polysaccharide determinants takes the form of B-cell responses. In my view, it would be quite unsafe to consider the meagre data available in the literature [12, 26] as evidence for cellular immunity (T-cell responses); maybe this type of response to carbohydrates does exist, but I have no way to judge that it does. Purified bacterial polysaccharides, on the other hand, are perfectly capable of eliciting humoral responses, i.e. circulating antibodies, and there is a growing body of evidence indicating that at least some polysaccharides are capable of eliciting B-cell memory [23, 38]. However, demonstrable B-cell memory does not seem to play a significant role in schemes of secondary immunization in which no rise of titre is achieved after a primary immunization [7]. It is possible that, in many cases, partial tolerance overshadows memory.

More important than the quantitative aspect of the secondary immunization, i.e. the amount of antibody in circulation, are the qualitative changes resulting from this primary interaction. For instance, in migration of antigen specific B cells from the marginal zones of the spleen after a single dose of purified polysaccharide [24]. Other related phenomena have been examined in detail using animal models [4, 31] and some of its features should serve as a basis for future vaccine development.

Returning to the problem of tolerance *versus* immunity, I will make four general statements:

1. For supraoptimal doses of polysaccharide antigen, immunity anti-parallels tolerance and both are related to the dose of antigen injected. Specific tolerance is in most cases a B-cell phenomenon. Although immunogenicity is directly related to the molecular weight of the antigen [22, 27] tolerogenicity is not necessarily so [34, 35].
2. In mature immune systems, TI tolerogenesis is not accompanied by clonal deletion; rather a state of anergy [42, 48] is achieved from which antibody-producing cells can be rescued only if antigen is removed from the system [36, 42]. Since many polysaccharides persist for a very long time, tolerance can last for years. There is evidence however, that clonal elimination does take place during ontogenesis [41].
3. The presence of TD antigen-specific suppressor activity, although it appears as demonstrable in some specific cases of which pneumococcal type III is probably the best characterized [2, 3, 8], it does not constitute a general phenomenon applicable to most polysaccharides.

Another example cited rather often nowadays is the T-suppressor system described to be specific for the phenolic glycolipid I of *Mycobacterium leprae* [33]. Once again, a direct demonstration of antigen specificity, i.e. that the putative suppressor cells found in lepromatous patients is recognizing specifically the antigen *via* T-cell receptors, is sadly missing.

4. Secondary immunization with purified polysaccharides usually leads to no increase in antibody titre. The outcome of these further immunizations could be taken as a clear indication that they ought to be avoided. However, exceptions to this rule, ostensibly meningococcal Group A polysaccharide [19], are important enough to be cited because in this particular case it has prompted the introduction of a two-injection schedule for vaccination of children. Unfortunately, we have no experimental data to explain the phenomenon in a completely satisfactory way, but will return to this point later.

I would prefer also to regard B-cell tolerance as specific, as far as the signals triggering it are concerned, although there is also a contribution from non-specific (non-epitopic) elements in the induction and maintenance of it [44]. Claims that the signals for triggering tolerance are non-specific [15] I would discard, both on theoretical and experimental grounds. However, in the context of this discussion and having vaccination in mind, we need not worry particularly about profound B-cell tolerance; usually achieved with very high doses of polysaccharide, but with a partial state of tolerance resulting in suboptimal immunization. The potential differences in tolerogenicity of polysaccharides after manipulation such as splenectomy should also be our concern [1, 20].

If the incapacity of the immune system to respond to a secondary injection of a TI polysaccharidic antigen is a direct consequence of its persistence in the organism, then it follows that degradation of those polysaccharides *in vitro* would restore the immune responsiveness. This can be done experimentally by injecting the tolerant animals with hydrolytic enzymes. Indeed, this is the case for TI and TD responses to the $\alpha(1 \rightarrow 6)$ specific determinants of dextran [15, 36] as was demonstrated many years ago for SIII pneumococcal polysaccharide [10]. Upon reflection this might also be the case for meningococcal Group A immunization in humans where, as I mentioned before, two doses of purified polysaccharide are recommended instead of one. This polysaccharide degrades rather quickly *in vitro* and probably also *in vivo*. An extreme case is B polysaccharide of *Neisseria menigitidis* that, in a purified form, is neither immunogenic nor tolerogenic [38], its antigenic determinants being very labile both *in vivo* and *in vitro*. Here the epitope being recognized by all the antibodies so far examined seems to be discontinuous and conformational, with its integrity entirely dependent on the presence of long stretches of $\alpha(2 \rightarrow 8)$-linked *N*-acetyl neuraminic (NANA) acid whose secondary structure can be easily disturbed by mild acidification, leading to internal sterification, or enzymatic degradation with neuraminidases [30].

If I extend a little on the properties of this polysaccharide it is because I think it constitutes a beautiful analogy to self-antigens, like nucleic acids, with which a cross-reactivity has been reported [28], and collagen, that have properties akin to those defining TI antigens and also because the linear epitope represented by $\alpha(2 \rightarrow 8)$-linked NANA is also present in sialogangliosides.

In sighting vaccination, there is a question pending in relation to immunity (and tolerance) to polysaccharides: would we want immune memory or high levels of antibody circulating for a long time? It seems that with purified polysaccharides it will be unlikely that we can optimize for both, or can we?

Tolerance and immunity as concepts define the state of the immune system in reference to an antigen or a group of antigens. Thus, in itself, tolerance is defined regardless of the mechanism by which such a state was achieved. Only in this sense do I find the concept useful. However, understanding the mechanisms by which such a state of tolerance is achieved is paramount, and when we look at the list of polysaccharides used for vaccination I must own that true understanding of both processes is rather poor. So busy have we been working for the answers that we have failed to see the question, and our understanding of immune responses *in vivo* has been summarized already: few principles and much ignorance [25].

Some of the difficulties lie deep into the way the subject has been approached. Since we try to understand tolerance in a restricted, narrow view as a problem on its own, perhaps the answer to many problems of tolerance induction will be solved when a more basic problem, i.e. antigen recognition, is finally cracked.

II. THYMUS-DEPENDENT AND THYMUS-INDEPENDENT ANTIGENS

The terms of reference for the second aspect I want to touch upon, i.e. the problem of TD, has necessarily to be based upon the definition of TI antigens.

Thymus independence can be seen as the absence of an absolute requirement for T cells, whether antigen specific or non-specific, to mount a B-cell response. It can be a useful definition but, as always with any definition, one can make nonsense of it by applying the concept to situations in which it is not valid, like the maturation of the immune system in athymic mice, for instance, where the absence of T cell-derived factors does affect the maturation of B cells. According to the restrictive notion of TI just given, it has been found [49] that antigens with repetitive epitopes of similar or identical specificity, are usually (but not always) non-degradable [21], or poorly degradable *in vivo*, this being an essential requisite to trigger B cells into TI antibody production. But this is not always so. Some of the determinants, for instance those at the non-reducing end of linear carbohydrates, are to be found only once per molecule. Moreover, the resistance of polysaccharides to degradation varies enormously. Meningococcal Group B polysaccharide is degraded and removed from spleen or liver far more quickly than linear dextran of similar molecular weight (Moreno *et al.*, unpublished results) although under some conditions behaves like a truly TI antigen [39].

The capacity of T cells of *any* description to recognize carbohydrate determinants has never been proved in a satisfactory way and it is perfectly possible that they do not recognize them. This could be due to the chemical characteristics of carbohydrates that do not permit interaction with Ia molecules in a form recognizable by the T-cell receptor; alternative explanations, however, are conceivable. It is a pity that this problem has not been the subject of more fruitful experimental research and brings up the question of how carbohydrates would be modified for such interactions to take place. It points out the difficulties, however, with T-suppressor cells conceived to explain the control of B-cell responses to some polysaccharides and it is more than likely that, if those suppressor cells do exist, they regulate the response indirectly *via* idiotype and anti-idiotypes, as has been established for the DNP–Ficoll response in the mouse [16, 17, 46] and also for levan [6]. Nevertheless, it must be pointed out that I have some problems with the generation of idiotypic antibodies that, by definition, are the result TD responses. How is it triggered when the original stimulus is TI? How is the T-helper activity generated and which is its specificity? The most likely candidate is the idiotypic determinant itself, but this imposes severe restrictions on the triggering mechanism generating the response that, to my knowledge, has not been elucidated. The helper-T cell activity must come, in most cases, from proteins or peptides complexed non-covalently or covalently. It is possible that the specific anti-carbohydrate antibody acts as carrier, but still leaves the problem of identification of the specificity for the T-helper cells to be sorted out.

Returning to the problem of cell triggering, it is useful to ask whether the question of the one *versus* two signals for B-cell activation [9] is still pertinent. The first signal is the one delivered *via* the membrane-bound immunoglobulin receptor. In most cases this is completely insufficient to trigger antibody production and leads to cell anergy. If additional stimuli, both positive and/or negative are provided, either of specific nature (T-cell help) or lymphokines, it would lead to one more of five events: (a) cell proliferation; (b) cell differentiation; (c) antibody secretion (d) B-cell memory and (e) gene rearrangement, followed by a switch to other immunoglobulin classes. The question is therefore the more-than-one signal problem. In the case of TI (carbohydrate) antigens, if we accept (and it is provisional) the fact that these antigens cannot be presented in the context of Ia, the specific T-cell signals have to be delivered *via* idiotypic receptors and one envisages fragments of the idiotype-bearing immunoglobulins being trapped by the B cells as Ag–Ab complexes and re-expressed on their surface complex in true context of Ia molecules [29]. Alternatively, one could see the system relying heavily on the professional antigen-presenting cell, provided it is physically close enough to the B cell. Since I prefer to stress the relative importance of this second mechanism in the regulation of the response to carbohydrates, it follows that the micro anatomy of the immune system and its cellular interactions is paramount in understanding the events that ensue.

Many scientists have turned to tetanus and diphtheria toxoids as good 'acceptable' carriers to bestow carbohydrate antigens with T-helper activity. Although I have nothing against attempts of that kind, I find it surprising that for such a long time it has been decided to leave aside the objection that helper activity of such specificity would be of little significance when mounting an antibody response to the infecting organism itself. One must also bear in mind that TD responses are usually higher than TI ones, but we really do not know whether very high levels of antibody in circulation are really critical for protection when the B- and T-cell memory are really strong. It might very well be that very low levels of circulating antibody will protect well if the T-helper memory is of the right specificity. Nevertheless, it would appear more logical to increase the effort at production and study of TD forms of carbohydrate vaccines where the carrier proteins are more closely related to the infective organism in question. Moreover, the use of toxoids as carriers would force a continued reanalysis of their effect, not only in terms of the immune response to the carbohydrates but also to the toxoids themselves as vaccines.

The events that follow interaction of a B-cell receptor with a carbohydrate antigen, when this is still part of the bacterial envelope, are completely different from those that follow interaction with a purified one, even if in both cases we are examining only the TI component of the response. The stimulation *via* epitopes is accompanied by several other stimuli that could act as polyclonal cell activators, such as lipopolysaccharide or lipoprotein from gram negatives, and these substances can affect the immune and tolerant status [11]. This, in my opinion constitutes the basis for the distinction between TI-1 and TI-2 antigens [40]. Some of these components can deliver negative, rather than stimulatory signals. The outcome is not the result of one *versus* two signals but the overall balance of many. Immunity as the outcome of this interaction can have, and usually has, a protective value against bacterial infections that differs enormously from that generated with the purified polysaccharide where, until now, only antibody titres in circulation matter to the vaccinator. A reassesment of this view is very much needed.

III. IMMUNOSTIMULATION AND IMMUNOSUPPRESSION

Many polysaccharides, some dextrans and levans included, are very good mitogens [35] even though this property seems to manifest itself only in the presence of macrophages [13]. This, or a closely related property, is probably linked, for instance, to the adjuvant properties of tapioca and the increase in the antigen-specific T-cell proliferation *in vitro* that we have observed in our laboratory (J. Lamb *et al.*, unpublished observations), that also depends on antigen processing and presentation by macrophages. Some polysaccharides exhibit a clear anti-tumour activity *in vivo*, when the tumour under study is particularly susceptible to activated macrophages [5].

Although common, immunopotentiation by polysaccharides is not universal. Moreover, there are polysaccharides that show clear immunosuppressive activity, as has been demonstrated for mycobacterial arabinomannans [14] that inhibit T-cell mediated immunity, apparently by interfering with antigen processing and presentation. So, although purified polysaccharides are incapable of generating T-cell responses, they do affect T-cell responsiveness in a non-specific manner, but this property(ies) has to be defined for each carbohydrate in particular. The same is valid for polyclonal B-cell stimulation. It is tempting to suggest that carbohydrate vaccines of the future could be designed considering these two properties as if they could be manipulated, increasing or minimizing them according to the specific vaccine requirements.

As our knowledge of B-lymphocyte surface markers increases [18] we are in a position to study their role in B-cell differentiation. Also, the experimental evidence available indicating the pivotal function of surface IgD in immunity [4] and tolerance [47] could make it possible to use these principles in designing more effective vaccines than those based on purified polysaccharides which must, eventually, yield the way to more practical and manageable ones. Let us hope.

REFERENCES

1. Amlot, P. L., Grennan, D., and Humphrey, J. H. Splenic dependence of the antibody response to thymus-independent antigens. *Eur. J. Immunol.*, **15**, 508–12 (1985).
2. Baker, P. J., Stashak, P. W., Amsbaugh, D. F., and Prescott, B. Regulation of the antibody response to type III pneumococcal polysaccharide. IV. Role of suppressor T cells in the development of low dose paralysis. *Immunol.*, **112**, 2020–7 (1974).
3. Baker, P. J., and Prescott, B. Regulation of the antibody response to pneumococcal polysaccharides by thymus-derived (T) cells: mode of action of suppressor and amplifier T cells. In *Immunology of Bacterial Polysaccharides* (ed. J. A. Rudbach and P. J. Baker), Elsevier (North-Holland), New York, Amsterdam, Oxford, 1979, pp. 67–104.
4. Bazin, H., Gray, D., Platteau, B., and MacLennan, I. C. M. Distinct δ-positive and δ-negative B lymphocyte lineages in the rat. *Ann. N.Y. Acad. Sci.*, 1982; part IV: 157–174.
5. Bomford, R., and Moreno, C. Mechanism of the anti-tumour effect of glucans and fructosans: a comparison with *C. parvum*. *Br. J. Cancer*, **36**, 41–8 (191977).
6. Bona, C., Lieberman, R., House, S., Green, I., and Paul, W. E. Immune response to levan. II. T independence of suppression of cross-reactive idiotypes by anti-idiotype antibodies. *Immunol.*, **122**, 1614–19 (1979).
7. Braley-Mullen, H. Antigen requirements for induction of B-memory cells. Studies with dinitrophenyl coupled T-dependent and T-independent carriers. *J. Exp. Med.*, **147**, 1824–31 (1978).
8. Braley-Mullen, H. Selective suppression of primary IgM responses by induction of low dose paralysis to type III pneumococcal polysaccharide. *Cell Immunol.*, **37**, 77–85 (1978).
9. Bretscher, P. A., and Cohn, M. A theory of self-nonself discrimination: paralysis and induction involve the recognition of one and two determinants on an antigen, respectively. *Science*, **169**, 1042–9 (1970).

10. Brooke, M. S. Breaking of immunological paralysis by injection of a specific depolymerase. *Nature*, **204**, 1319–20 (1964).
11. Brooke, M. S. Conversion of immunological paralysis to immunity by endotoxin. *Nature (London)*, **206**, 635–6 (1965).
12. Crowle, A. J., and Hu, C. C. Delayed hypersensitivity in mice to dextran. *Int. Arch. All. and Appl. Immunol.*, **31**, 123–44 (1967).
13. Desaymard, C., and Ivanyi, L. Comparison of *in vitro* immunogenicity, tolerogenicity and mitogenicity of dinitrophenyl-levan conjugates with varying epitope densities. *Immunology*, **30**, 647–53 (1976).
14. Ellner, J. J., and Daniel, T. M. Immunosuppression by mycobacterial arabinomannan. *Clin. exp. Immunol.*, **35**, 250–7 (1979).
15. Fernandez, C., and Moller, G. Irreversible immunological tolerance to thymus-independent antigens is restricted to the clone of B cells having both Ig and PBA receptors for the tolerogen. *Scand J. Immunol.*, **7**, 137–44 (1978).
16. Goidl, E. A., Thorbecke, G. J., Weksler, M. E., and Siskind, G. W. Production of auto-anti-idiotypic antibody during the normal immune response: changes in the auto-anti-idiotypic antibody response and the idiotype repertoire associated with aging. *Proc. Natl. Acad. Sci. USA*, **77**, 6788–92 (1980).
17. Goidl, E. A., Schrater, A. F., Thorbecke, G. J., and Siskind, G. W. Production of auto-anti-idiotypic antibody during the normal immune response. IV. Studies of the primary and secondary responses to thymus-independent and thymus-independent antigens. *Eur. J. Immunol.*, **10**, 810–14 (1980).
18. Golay, J. T. Functional B-lymphocyte surface antigens. *Immunology*, **59**, 1–5 (1986).
19. Gold, R., Lepow, M. L., Goldschneider, I., Draper, T. L., and Gotschlich, E. C. Clinical evaluation of group A and group C meningococcal polysaccharide vaccines in infants. *J. Clin. Invest.*, **56**, 1536–47 (1975).
20. Gray, D., Chassoux, D., MacLennan, I. C. M., and Bazin, H. Selective depression of thymus-independent anti-DNP antibody responses induced by adult but not by neonatal splenectomy. *Clin. exp. immunol.*, **60**, 78–86 (1985).
21. Hardy, B., and Mozes, E. Expression of T cell suppressor activity in the immune response of newborn mice to a T-independent synthetic polypeptide. *Immunology*, **35**, 757–62 (1978).
22. Howard, J. G., Vicari, G., and Courtenay, B. M. Influence of molecular structure on the tolerogenicity of bacterial dextrans. I. The α 1-6 linked epitope of Dextran B512. *Immunology*, **29**, 585–97 (1975).
23. Hosokawa, T. Studies on B-cell memory. II. T-cell independent antigen can induce B-cell memory. *Immunology*, **38**, 291–9 (1979).
24. Humphrey, J. H. The fate of antigens. In *Clinical Aspects of Immunology*, 4th edn (ed. P. J. Lachmann and D. K. Peters), Blackwell Scientific Publications, Oxford, 1982, pp. 161–86.
25. Humphrey, J. H. Regulation of *in vivo* immune responses: few principles and much ignorance. Synthetic peptides as antigens. *Ciba Foundation Symposium* (Pitman, London), **119**, 6–24 (1986).
26. Jackson, S., Folks, T. M., Wetterskog, D. L., and Kindt, T. J. A rabbit helper T cell clone reactive against group-specific streptococcal carbohydrate. *J. Immunol.*, **133**, 1553–7 (1984).
27. Kabat, E. A., and Bezer, A. E. The effect of variation in molecular weight on the antigenicity of dextran in man. *Arch. Biochem. Biophys.*, **78**, 308–18 (1958).
28. Kabat, E. A., Nickerson, K. G., Liao, J., Grossbard, L., Lott, F. I. I., Osserman, F., Glickman, E., Chess, L., Robbins, J. B., Schneerson, R., and Yang, Y. A

human monoclonal macroglobulin with specificity for α(2 → 8)-linked poly-*N*-acetyl neuraminic acid, the capsular polysaccharide og roup B meningococci and *Escherichia coli* K1, which crossreacts with polynucleotides and with denatured DNA. *J. Exp. Med.*, **164**, 642–54 (1986).

29. Lanzavecchia, A. Antigen-specific interaction between T and B cells. *Nature*, **314**, 537–9 (1985).
30. Lifely, M. R., Moreno, C., and Lindon, J. C. An integrated molecular and immunological approach towards a meningococcal group B vaccine. *Vaccine*, **5**, 11–26 (1987).
31. MacLennan, I. C. M., and Gray, D. Antigen-driven selection of virgin and memory B cells. *Immunol. Rev.*, **91**, 61–85 (1986).
32. Maturana, H. R., and Varela, F. J. *Autopoiesis and Cognition. The Realization of the Living*, Boston Studies in the Philosophy of Science (ed. R. S. Cohen and M. W. Wartofsky), D. Reidel Co., Dordrecht, the Netherlands, 1980, Vol. 42, pp. 63–72.
33. Mehra, V., Brennan, P. J., Rada, E., Convit, J., and Bloom, B. R. Lymphocyte suppression in leprosy induced by unique *M. leprae* glycolipid. *Nature*, **308**, 194–6 (1984).
34. Moreno, C., Courtenay, B. M., and Howard, J. G. Molecular size and structure in relation to the tolerogenicity of small fructosans (levans). *Immunochemistry*, **13**, 429–35 (1976).
35. Moreno, C., Hale, C., and Ivanyi, L. The mitogenic, immunogenic and tolerogenic properties of dextrans and levans. Lack of correlation according to differences of molecular structure and size. *Immunology*, **33**, 261–7 (1977).
36. Moreno, C., Hale, C., Hewett, R., and Esdaile, J. Induction and persistence of B-cell tolerance to the thymus-dependent component of the α(1 → 6) glucosyl determinant of dextran. Recovery induced by treatment with dextranase *in vivo*. *Immunology*, **44**, 517–27 (1981).
37. Moreno, C. Tolerance. In *Clinical Aspects of Immunology*, 4th edn (ed. P. J. Lachmann and D. K. Peters), Blackwell, Oxford, 1982, pp. 199–242.
38. Moreno, C., Lifely, M. R., and Esdaile, J. Immunity and protection of mice against *Neisseria meningitidis* group B by vaccination using polysaccharide complexed with outer membrane protein: a comparison with purified B polysaccharide. *Infec. Immunity*, **47**, 527–33 (1985).
39. Moreno, C. Esdaile, J., and Lifely, M. R. Thymic-dependence and immune memory in mice vaccinated with meningococcal polysaccharide group B complexed to outer membrane protein. *Immunology*, **57**, 425–30 (1986).
40. Mosier, D. E., and Subbarao, B. Thymus-independent antigens: complexity of B-lymphocyte activation revealed. *Immunology Today*, **3**, 217–22 (1982).
41. Nossal, G. J. V., Pike, B. L., Teale, J. M., Layton, E., Kay, T. W., and Battye, F. L. Cell fractionation methods and the target cells for clonal abortion of B lymphocytes. *Immunol. Rev.*, **43**, 185–216 (1979).
42. Nossal, G. J. V., and Pike, B. L. Clonal anergy: persistence in tolerant mice of antigen-binding B lymphocytes incapable of responding to antigen or mitogen. *Proc. Natl. Acad. Sci. USA*, **77**, 1602–6 (1980).
43. Nossal, G. J. V. Cellular mechanisms of immunologic tolerance. *Ann. Rev. Immunol.*, **1**, 33–62 (1983).
44. Paul, W. E., Karpf, M., and Mosier, D. E. Activation of and tolerance induction in DNP-specific B cells: analysis with three distinct DNP-carrier conjugates. In *Immunological Tolerance. Mechanisms and Potential Therapeutic Applications*

(ed. D. H. Katz and B. Benacerraf), Academic Press, New York, 1974, pp. 141–58.
45. Richter, A. W. The immune response to polysaccharides. In *Developments in Immunology, Clinical Immunology and Allergology* (ed. C. Steffen and H. Ludwig), Elsevier/North-Holland Biomedical Press, Amsterdam, 1980, Vol. 14, pp. 235–46.
46. Schrater, A. F., Goidl, E. A., Thorbecke, G. J., and Siskind, G. W. Production of auto-anti-idiotypic antibody during the normal immune response to TNP–F-icoll. III. Absence in nu/nu mice: evidence for T-cell dependence of the anti-idiotypic-antibody response. *J. Exp. Med.*, **150**, 808–17 (1979).
47. Scott, D. W., Layton, J. E., and Nossal, G. J. V. Role of IgD in the immune response and tolerance. I. Anti-δ pretreatment facilitates tolerance induction in adult B cells *in vitro*. *J. Exp. Med.*, **146**, 1473–83 (1977).
48. Scott, D. W., Venkataraman, M., and Jandinski, J. J. Multiple pathways of B lymphocyte tolerance. *Immunol. Rev.*, **43**, 241–80 (1979).
49. Sela, M., Mozes, E., and Shearer, G. M. Thymus-independence of slowly metabolised immunogens. *Proc. Nat. Acad. Sci. USA*, **69**, 2696 (1972).

DISCUSSION – Chaired by Professor G. L. Ada

MOSIER: I would like to address two points you made. The first has to do with generation of B-cell memory to polysaccharide antigens. In my experience this can happen, but it certainly seems to be an exception rather than the rule. One interesting situation in which one can see large-scale expansion of antibody-specific precursors is when one neonatally primes mice with antigens like TNP–Ficoll, and that priming is somewhat unusual because it seems to result from activating B cells at a stage where they can proliferate following antigenic stimulation, but do not differentiate to antibody-secreting cells. That is a very transient stage of B-cell development, and one can only achieve this kind of priming for a limited period of life, during the neonatal period. I have never seen any instance of this kind of priming in adult animals.

The second comment I want to make has to do with the role of anti-idiotype production in regulating anti-polysaccharide responses. To my way of thinking, this field is littered with bad data, and I would just like to cite two examples of our own work, where we do not find any evidence for anti-idiotype regulation. This is a response to TNP–Ficoll and a response phosphorylcholine as a component of R36A *Streptococcus pneumoniae* in nude mice. We find absolutely no difference in the course of the antibody response between nudes and litter mates with T cells, even though anti-idiotype antibodies can only be formed in the latter instance.

ADA: Do you get the fluctuation? That is often taken as some sort of evidence.

MOSIER: We do get fluctuation, and I think that is an intrinsic part of the B-cell response. It has nothing at all to do with the anti-idiotype regulation. In the anti-phosphorylcholine system, we have a very sensitive measure for the existence of anti-idiotypes, since it is only the anti-T15 idiotype that is regulatory. Anti-TIS antibodies do not exist in nude mice, and they do exist in normal mice. Yet one sees no difference in the course of the response. I think this question of idiotype regulation of T-independent responses is totally up in the air. I do not see any convincing evidence that it happens *in vivo*.

HANDMAN: I may have missed the point of the conjugate, I cannot see the problem of injecting conjugates of proteins and carbohydrates. I can understand that you may add epitopes, but I cannot see in what way you change the carbohydrate epitopes and also I cannot see the problem with future immune responses to the protein carrier. If anything, I can imagine that it would act as a booster.

MORENO: The epitopes will not change. All I am saying is that, if we want to use the potential of the immune system to use memory as a protective element, then these carriers are out. We cannot use them because they are completely unrelated to the agent causing the disease. We have good examples with meningococcal Group B polysaccharides, in which the carrier is the protein from the outer membrane of these polysaccharides in which, not only we promote immunity and protection across type. If we immunize with type 6, we get protection against type 2 and a secondary response for the anti-Group B antibodies. This is, therefore, an example where we can take advantage of memory to the carriers but, even more so, because, if we leave those mice until the anti-B response declines and is undetectable, we can still demonstrate protection when those mice are challenged with live meningococcal organisms. It is not the ideal protection system, I agree, but it is a demonstration that the potential to evoke a secondary response that is protective is there, even though we are not using the same organism for challenge as the one used for the original immunization scheme.

The second point I raised refers to monitoring the immune response of the population against diphtheria or tetanus toxoids when one is continuously boosting them with the same carrier. In some cases one could over-immunize and provoke a depression of the immune response. Unless you have a complete demonstration that it is safe to use and reuse the same carrier, or that very high titres are safe, you cannot use the same carrier again. So there are problems: you need to know the immune state of that population. It is possible to monitor it in a few individuals but not in a population. That was the point I wanted to make.

MÄKELÄ: You mentioned that the meningococcal B polysaccharide disappears in hours. Did you mean that it disappears from the circulation of the injected individual, or that it disintregated completely?

MORENO: The experiments were done (they have not been published) injecting radioactive polysaccharide and following the radioactivity in the spleen and liver. We measured and compared the rate of decreasing radioactivity in the spleen and liver with the rate of removal of dextran of comparable molecular weight, whereas dextran remained for weeks in the spleen and liver, B polysaccharide disappeared, as far as radioactivity is concerned, in 24 to 48 hours.
MÄKELÄ: How was it made radioactive?
MORENO: By iodination.
MÄKELÄ: Could it be that the iodine was digested away?
MORENO: It is possible.
SÖDERSTRÖM: Regarding the comments of Dr Mosier, we have also tried to prime adult mice with anti-idiotypic antibodies in the *Escherichia coli* K13 system. The results are disappointingly negative.
MOSIER: I think that the timing of when B cells first see antigen can be critical for whether they are tolerized or primed. I set as an example a neonatal priming with TNP–Ficoll. If one tries the same kind of priming with a phosphorylcholine conjugate Ficoll, one induces tolerance rather than immunity by neonatal injection. It is only when if one waits until the mice are 2 weeks old and then prime with PC that you can see any kind of priming effect there. So one would infer from that kind of experiment that exposure of developing B cells to relatively high doses of naturally occurring polysaccharides could have a tolerogenic effect in the neonatal period. In that case one would only see a response much later, as is the case of levan, when a small pool of mature B cells emerges.
ROBBINS: It would take a long time to review the clinical experience with polysaccharides, but there are some patterns of immune response that differ among them. For instance, with meningococcus Group A, a single injection before 24 months allows the second injection given in that time to induce a higher response than a primary. The opposite occurs with Group C. Group C injected within 24 months seems to depress the reaction to a second injection, but that disappears after 2 years and is not seen in later life. With *Haemophilus influenzae* type b, a single injection under 2 years of age, followed by an injection at intervals thereafter, has no effect. The second injection induces a primary response. That seems to be the case with all the pneumococcal polysaccharides. This, of course, could be a dosage effect. Tolerance in its traditional sense has not been seen in humans, except for the one experience with meningococcus Group C and there, since the word 'tolerance' is poorly defined anyhow, you could say that reinjection produces a lesser response than a primary, and if there would be partial tolerance, that would be one, but it disappears.
MORENO: Yes, precisely. My intention was to stress that we do not know the explanation for those differences and they ought to be explored and clarified

in terms of finding not only the practicalities of what is best, but why is it occurring? The knowledge there is completely insufficient. Coming back to the problem raised by Dr Mosier. Yes, I agree completely, with the fact that this B-cell memory is poor, probably occasional and not easy to demonstrate. It is my point that probably it could be improved and optimized, in some instances, and to take advantage of it. I see a potential there. As far as anti-idiotypes are concerned, I do not see any disagreement with the fact that these types of responses are occasional. There are not very many systems that seem to be regulated by anti-idiotypes and I do not think I can add anything further to it. But, if any advantage is to be taken of that, further clarification is required of how, if these phenomena exist, and in which systems they exist. Further study is required before anything can be taken as a potential for development.

HANDMAN: You brought up a problem that concerns me very much. The problem of the purity of polysaccharide antigens, and the problem as I see it, coming from the background of protein chemistry, is how does one determine purity in a population of molecules that is heterogeneous and poly-dispersed by its nature? I get asked this question all the time. Is your antigen pure?

MORENO: I think that the question asked in the air like that is of very little use. Actually what you are asking is to characterize. If you say, 'We have found that the percentage of protein in our preparation is 1, or 2%', you are saying something. If you say, 'What we find is lipopolysaccharide below 0.5%', you are saying something. If you do not commit yourself and say, 'We purify the polysaccharide by the methods of so and so' and you are happy with that, then this is where the problem emerges. Now, in many studies using polysaccharides for defining the specificity of the immune response, this element of definition of minimal concentration of impurities is missing, because they did not even bother to measure them, or they got it from somebody, as if the problem of defining the purity remains with the person who sent the stuff. Therefore, particularly with T cells, it is very difficult to define the specificity because they rely on T-cell proliferation. Therefore, it is not an antibody as a tool to define a specificity and, therefore, it requires extra care. So in that sense, I stress, it is a problem. The question is 'how pure is your thing' or 'how pure is pure' in general terms, is of very little use? Do I make myself clear.

ADA: I think in your case Dr Handman, Dr Moreno would say that you should show that your preparation contains less than a given % of protein. You cannot do very much more than that.

KABAT: With respect to polysaccharides which are intrinsically heterogeneous, I do not think that, because a substance is heterogeneous, it is not necessarily pure with respect to the antigenic groups which it contains – or something like this. I think that what is usually asked, from the days when they thought that allergic reactions to dextran were being caused because there was contamination with proteins, is whether the impurities were related to the presence of extraneous non-dextran substances. I think that that holds with polysaccharides as well. Now, of course, you could have your dextran contaminated with some other polysaccharide and that too would be an impurity. But just heterogeneity, with the same basic structural composition of repeating unit, I do not think falls under the commonly accepted definition of purity or impurity.

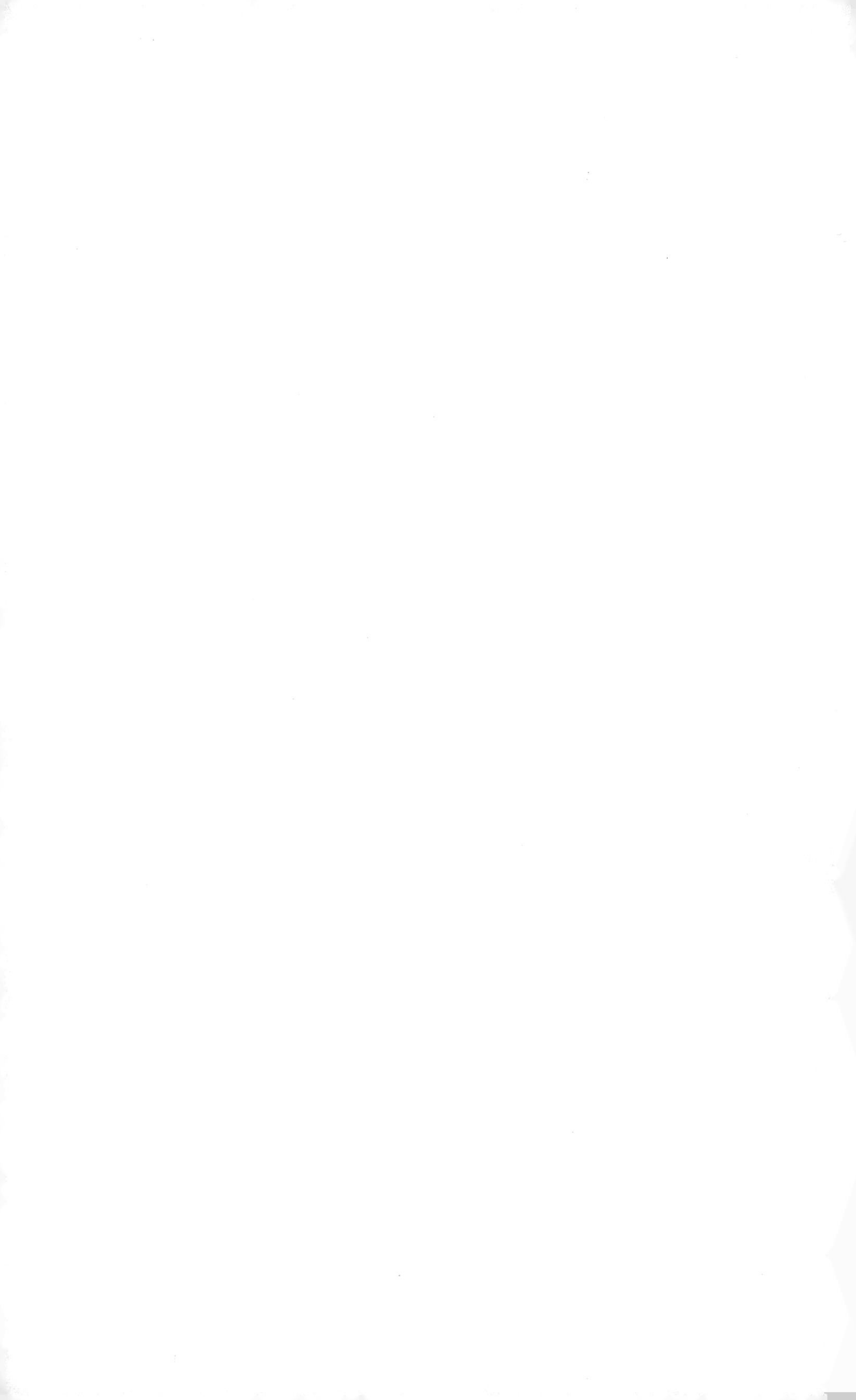

Towards Better Carbohydrate Vaccines
Edited by R. Bell and G. Torrigiani

Published by John Wiley & Sons Ltd

20

Artificial glycoproteins of predetermined multivalent antigenicity as a new generation of candidate vaccines to prevent infections from encapsulated bacteria: analysis of antigenicity *versus* immunogenicity

Massimo Porro*
Sclavo SpA, Siena 53100, Italy

ABSTRACT

Several artificial glycoproteins have been synthesized using different proteins, such as the non-toxic mutant protein CRM197, related to diphtheria toxin, and tetanus toxoid (TT) as carriers supporting covalently bound oligosaccharide haptens derived from the native capsular polysaccharides of *Streptococcus pneumoniae* type 6A, *Neisseria meningitidis* group B and C and *Haemophilus influenzae* type b.

The antigens were synthesized by the same procedure and were analysed by physico-chemical characteristics in order to control the reproducibility of the model employed in the synthesis procedure. Molecular mapping of the antigens by monoclonal and polyclonal antibodies defined the immunochemical characteristics in order to determine the required specific antigenicity. Finally, the immunogenicity of these antigens was evaluated in animal models as quantity of specifically induced antibodies and was compared to their immunochemical characteristics with the purpose of relating antigenicity and immunogenicity.

* Present address: PRAXIS BIOLOGICS, INC., Rochester, New York 14623, USA.

INTRODUCTION

The protection of infants from diseases related to encapsulated bacterial infection by *Haemophilus influenzae*, *Neisseria meningitidis* and *Streptococcus pneumoniae*, that is, otitis media and cerebrospinal meningitis, is still an unsolved problem despite the introduction in the past decade of highly purified capsular polysaccharide vaccines [6, 14, 15, 22, 23, 39, 40, 45].

These polysaccharide-based vaccines have been shown to be safe and immunogenic in children older than 2 years as well as in adults but, for reasons not yet well understood, they are inefficient in the infant population.

Polysaccharides have been classified as thymic-independent (TI-2) antigens in animals, that is, helper-T cells do increase the antibody response against the carbohydrate antigen but are not required to activate the immunological response [42]. A similar classification has also been recently introduced to define the immunological properties of these antigens in humans [52]. In addition, highly purified polysaccharides do not elicit a memory antibody response after reinjection, either in animals or in humans, and only a limited number of B-cell clones are activated, resulting in the secretion of isotype antibody with restricted structural heterogenicity [27, 32, 36].

A strategy to overcome the problems associated with the use of polysaccharide antigens as vaccines involves the use of thymic-dependent antigens (e.g. proteins) as carriers for oligosaccharides or polysaccharides, in order to stimulate carrier-specific T-helper cells playing a role in the induction of anticarbohydrate antibody synthesis [44]. This strategy goes back to the pioneering and elegant studies of immunochemistry, using synthetic haptens, performed by Avery and Goebel [7, 20].

In the past few years, several models of artificial glycoproteins (glycoconjugates) have been described and proposed as potential vaccines for encapsulated bacteria [2, 9, 31, 48, 49, 50, 54]. All these antigens have been proved immunogenic in animal models so far as acquired thymic dependency of the carried polysaccharides or oligosaccharide haptens is concerned, indirectly evidenced by the induction of boostable IgG isotype antibodies. Preliminary results obtained in clinical trials after injection of some of these models in adults [3, 55] and in infants [4] generally support the observations reported in animal models, although in some cases the failure of induction of significant levels of polysaccharide-specific antibody in infants less than 6 months of age has been documented [24]. An analysis of the clonotype and isotype antibodies induced in infants immunized with a model of oligosaccharide–protein conjugate antigen also showed a restriction in their structural heterogeneity [28], paralleling the findings mentioned previously on immunization with highly purified polysaccharide antigens. In this case, however, the antigen clearly resembled the characteristics of a thymic-dependent antigen.

Altogether these results appear very encouraging in the perspective of new vaccines against epidemiologically significant encapsulated bacteria.

However, several basic problems involved in understanding the immunological activity at cellular level of these synthetic molecules, as well as their physico-chemical and antigenic composition, remain to be elucidated. In particular, the following questions need further study:

1. The molecular basis by which a T helper-independent carbohydrate antigen acquires the typical property of a T helper-dependent protein in the induction of the immunological memory specific for the carried carbohydrate antigen or hapten.
2. The immunological role of hybrid determinants (if any) present in the linking region between the carbohydrate and the carrier protein.
3. The importance of a determined stechiometry in terms of carbohydrate/protein ratio (w/w).
4. The minimal structure for a given carbohydrate hapten able to induce a specific immunological response after the conjugation with the carrier protein.
5. The importance for a given oligosaccharide epitope to be exposed on the surface of the carrier protein.
6. How the immunochemical and immunological properties of a given carrier protein change after the conjugation with the carbohydrate moiety.
7. The kind of laboratory controls sufficient for accurate standardization of these synthetic antigens from the physico-chemical, immunochemical and immunological points of view.
8. The kind of correlation that exists (if any) between immunogenicity in animal models and human infants in order to control the biological activity of these hybrid molecules.

In this chapter, some of these problems will be analysed on the basis of antigenicity *versus* immunogenicity either for the carried carbohydrate hapten(s) or the carrier protein(s) used in the preparation of chemically defined artificial glycoproteins synthesized according to the model previously described [48, 50]. The creation of this model involved the following strategy:

(A) Preparation of oligosaccharide haptens from their homologous, highly purified capsular polysaccharides.
(B) Physico-chemical and immunochemical characteristics of the haptens.
(C) Synthesis and characterization of the artificial glycoprotein, using monovalent-activated oligosaccharides in order to achieve their exposure on the surface of the carrier protein and to avoid undefined cross-linked products.
(D) Molecular mapping by monoclonal and polyclonal antibodies of the epitopes present in the artificial glycoprotein.
(E) Immunogenicity in animal models of the artificial glycoprotein containing predetermined epitopes.

MATERIALS AND METHODS

The following artificial glycoproteins were analysed for their characteristics in this work.

CRM197–Oligo 6A

This antigen was synthesized using the non-toxic mutant protein CRM197 (cross-reacting material), serologically related to diphtheria toxin [43, 46, 57], and an oligosaccharide hapten derived from the high molecular weight capsular polysaccharide of *S. pneumoniae* type 6A (serologically cross reacting with type 6B [35, 51]). The antigen, as well as all the techniques involved in its preparation and characterization, has been previously reported [48]. The goal of using this bivalent antigen was the induction of antibodies specific for the capsule of *S. pneumoniae* type 6A and 6B (Group 6) as well as neutralizing the toxicity of diphtheria toxin *in vivo*.

CRM197–Oligo 6A – Oligo MenC

This antigen was synthesized using the non-toxic mutant protein CRM197 and two oligosaccharide haptens, respectively derived from the high molecular weight capsular polysaccharides of *S. pneumoniae* type 6A and *N. meningitidis* Group C. The antigen and the techniques involved in its preparation and characterization have been reported recently [50]. The goal of using this multivalent antigen was the induction of antibodies specific for the capsule of *S. pneumoniae* type 6A and 6B (Group 6), *N. meningitidis* Group C and neutralizing the toxicity of diphtheria toxin *in vivo*.

CRM197 – Oligo Hib

This antigen has been synthesized using the non-toxic mutant protein CRM19/ and an oligosaccharide hapten derived form the high molecular weight capsular polysaccharide of *H. influenzae* type b [13]. The synthesis procedure was similar to those previously reported and involved the following.

Preparation of the oligosaccharide hapten The capsular polysaccharide of *H. influenzae* was purified, basically according to the procedure reported for meningococcal polysaccharides present in the human vaccine [61]. The derived oligosaccharide hapten was obtained from the acid hydrolysis (10 mM CH_3COOH, pH 3.4) of a solution of capsular polysaccharide (10 mg/ml), by heating at 100 °C × 1–2 hours. The oligosaccharide hapten eluted from Sephadex G-50 gel chromatography as a bell-shaped curve with K_d =

0.48. Molar ratio among ribose : phosphorus : reducing groups was 6 : 6 : 1, as estimated by the chemical assays reported [48]. These results identified the hapten as an oligosaccharide consisting of approximately six basic repeating units with an average molecular weight of 2400.

Chemical activation of the oligosaccharide hapten The oligosaccharide hapten was activated by the introduction of a primary amino group at the end-reducing ribose residue of its structure, basically using the conditions reported [48] except for a shorter reaction time (3 days). After chemical activation, the oligosaccharide was purified on Sephadex G-15 column and a 'shift' of the Kd value to 0.56 on Sephadex G-50 was observed. Stechiometry in terms of molar ratio ribose : phosphoros : amino group, was 4 : 4 : 1. The oligosaccharide was freeze-dried and then resolubilized in dimethyl sulphoxide: H_2O (95 : 5 v/v) at the concentration of 10 mg/ml. The oligosaccharide was then dropped in a solution of disuccinimidyl ester of adipic acid in dimethyl sulphoxide, as previously reported [48].

Conjugation of the activated oligomer to CRM197 The organic solution containing the monoester-activated oligosaccharide hapten was reacted overnight at room temperature with an aqueous solution of CRM197 (2 mg/ml) in such a way that a solvent composed of dimethylsulphoxide: H_2O = 20 : 80, was obtained. The glycoprotein was recovered by Sephadex G-100 gel chromatography equilibrated in 0.2 M NaCl pH = 7.0, as published [48].

Physico-chemical characterization of the glycoprotein

SDS–PAGE analysis and chemical characterization in terms of substitution degree (SD) for the oligosaccharide hapten, was performed as reported for the other glycoproteins previously synthesized [48, 50]. The antigen consisted of a molecule of apparent average molecular weight (MW) = 7.3×10^4 with a carbohydrate protein ratio = 0.17 (w/w) and SD = 6 considering for the activated linear oligosaccharide hapten an average MW = 1800 (K_d = 0.56 on Sephadex G-50) corresponding to about four repeating units of the polysaccharide structure [13].

Immunochemical analysis of the glycoprotein

Molecular mapping of the epitopes still present in the carrier protein CRM197 after the synthesis procedure was performed by ELISA as published [50], using a monoclonal antibody collection recently developed [65]. The presence of antigenically active oligosaccharides on the surface of the carrier protein was tested by specific polyclonal antibodies (DIFCO Laboratories) using differential immunoelectrophoresis with the conditions similar to those reported [48].

Tetanus toxoid – Oligo MenB

This antigen was synthesized using TT and an oligosaccharide hapten derived from the high molecular weight capsular polysaccharide of *N. meningitidis* Group B. The synthesis procedure was the same as previously reported for the preparation of the other glycoproteins [48, 50] and involved the following.

Preparation of the oligosaccharide hapten

The Group B oligosaccharide hapten was obtained by acid hydrolysis of the homologous capsular polysaccharide, purified according to Gotschlich [22], in 10^{-2} M acetic acid solution for 10 hours at 50 °C, in sealed vials. The oligosaccharide hapten eluted from Sephadex G-50 gel chromatography as a bell-shaped curve with a K_d = 0.50. This value was assumed as corresponding to an average MW = 1800 based on the observations previously reported for a linear oligosaccharide hapten characterized by ^{13}C-NMR spectroscopy and showing a comparable Kd value on gel chromatography [48]. According to the structure of the Group B capsular polysaccharide, (2,8-α-D-*N*-acetylneuraminic acid), [10], this average MW would correspond to six *N*-acetylneuraminic acid $(NANA)_6$ residues.

Chemical activation of the oligosaccharide hapten

The method and the conditions used for the chemical activation of the oligosaccharide hapten were similar to those reported [48] and mentioned above.

Conjugation of the activated oligosaccharide to tetanus toxoid

The monosuccinimidyl ester-activated oligosaccharide was conjugated to TT (purity level = 2600 limit flocculation unit (L_f) for mg of protein nitrogen [62]) using the same schedule of reaction described previously [48] but with two different stechiometry of reaction in order to synthesize two artificial glycoproteins characterized by two different SD, respectively with 4 and 10 moles of oligosaccharide haptens per mole of TT carrier protein. These two artificial glycoproteins, referred to in the text as TT–$(NANA)_6$(SD4) and TT–$(NANA)_6$(SD10), were synthesized to study the role played by the chemical glycosylation on the immunological characteristics of the carrier protein.

Physico-chemical characterization of the two glycoproteins

The apparent average MW, as detected by SDS–PAGE [37], was 1.9×10^5 in the case of SD = 4 and 2.1×10^5 in the case of SD10, while the reference TT showed a value of 1.8×10^5. The SD values were detected by chemical analysis of the antigen according to the stechiometry of the molecule, based on the content of sialic acid [56] and protein [38], respectively equal to 0.04 (SD = 4) and 0.1 (SD = 10) w/w, as well as to the average MW determined for the oligosaccharide hapten.

Immunochemical analysis of the two glycoproteins

The specificity of polyclonal anti-TT antibodies for the glycosylated carrier protein was analysed by rocket immunoelectrophoresis [60]. The specificity of burro polyclonal anti-Group B capsular polysaccharide antibodies (Office of Biologics, Food and Drug Administration, Bethesda, MD, USA) for the derived oligosaccharide hapten before and after its chemical activation, was tested by differential immunoelectrophresis, under conditions similar to those reported [48].

Immunization of animals and immunological analysis

For each model of artificial glycoprotein synthesized, two animal models were used in order to test their immunological characteristics: guinea-pig and rabbit. The guinea-pig because it is a significant animal model able to predict the immunogenic potential of diphtheria and tetanus vaccines in humans [62]; the rabbit because it is well known that this model is unresponsive to highly purified bacterial capsular polysaccharides [33]. Thus, these two animal models would bc helpful in understanding the immunological characteristics of the protein carrier as well as the acquired antigenicity of the carried oligosaccharide haptens. The schedule of immunization and the immunological characteristics of the glycoproteins CRM197–oligo 6A as well as CRM197–oligo 6A,–oligo MenC, have been previously reported [48, 50]. The schedule of immunization for the glycoproteins CRM197–oligo Hib and TT–$(NANA)_6$ (SD4 and SD10) was identical to the one above mentioned and briefly involved: one group of ten guinea-pigs (average weight = 350 g) and one group of ten albino rabbits (average weight = 2 kg) were s.c.

injected with three doses of each of the artificial glycoproteins described, absorbed to the mineral adjuvant $AlPO_4$ (1.5 mg/dose) [48, 50]. The first booster dose was injected 28 days after the basal immunization and the second booster dose 11 days after the first one. Bleedings were performed either before the basal immunization of the booster dose were given and 11 days after the second booster dose.

Each dose of CRM197–oligo Hib contained 12.5 Lf of CRM197 [46, 48] corresponding to 31.2 μg of protein and 5.3 μg of oligosaccharide hapten. The amount of CRM197 was chosen on the basis of the considerations previously reported [46] and corresponding to the average amount of diphtheria toxoid present in the vaccine for human use. The amount of carbohydrate derived from the selected dose of the carrier protein CRM197, in consideration of the stechiometry of the glycoprotein.

Each dose of TT–$(NANA)_6$ contained 10 Lf of TT (the average amount present in the vaccine for human use) corresponding to 31.2 μg of protein and respectively 1.23 μg of carbohydrate in the case of the glycoprotein with SD = 4, or 3.1 μg of carbohydrate in the case of the glycoprotein with SD = 10. Control immunization was performed using TT alone with the same dose and schedule as described above. Control immunization by the purified oligosaccharide haptens used in the synthesis of either CRM–oligo Hib or TT–oligo MenB were omitted, based on the wide knowledge of the absence of significant immunogenicity in rabbits of highly purified bacterial oligo and polysaccharides.

Rabbit sera collected before and after immunization were analysed respectively for content of IgG isotype antibodies to the purified capsular polysaccharides of *H. influenzae* type b or *N. meningitidis* Group B, by ELISA using the procedure basically described previously [48].

In vitro bactericidal analysis of rabbit antisera for Group B meningococci and *H. influenzae* type b was performed basically according to the method reported by Wong [64], using the pre-immune rabbit sera as control.

Guinea-pig antisera were titred for neutralizing antibody to diphtheria toxin or tetanus toxin, according to the assay required by the US Pharmacopeia for these antigens when present in vaccines for human use. All the immunized animals were observed for adverse reactions at the site of injection.

Molecular mapping of neodeterminants potentially present in the synthesized artificial glycoproteins

In order to investigate the presence of IgG isotype antibody possibly induced for targets other than the capsular polysaccharide(s) and the carrier protein(s), the antisera of three rabbits belonging to each group immunized by three doses of each of the glycoproteins described were analysed by ELISA. In particular, the induction of boostable IgG isotype antibody specific for a potential neodeterminant involving the adipic acid spacer linked to the lysine residues of the selected carrier protein, was tested for all the glycoproteins injected. Furthermore, since a glycopeptide epitope has been reported to be present in a TT–meningococcal Group B oligosaccharide conjugate [31], the presence of such a hybrid determinant in TT–$(NANA)_6$ (SD10) was also investigated by inhibition-ELISA technique, using characterized molecules as inhibitors of specific immunochemical reactions. The list of these molecules included: bovine serum albumin (BSA); lysine; polylysine; adipic acid-activated BSA (BSA–AD); purified capsular polysaccharide of *N. meningitidis* Group B (Ps MenB); amino-activated oligosaccharide hapten $(NANA)_6$–NH_2; adipic acid (AD)-derived oligosaccharide hapten $(NANA)_6$–AD; $(NANA)_6$ conjugated to BSA [BSA–$(NANA)_6$]; $(NANA)_6$ conjugated to polylysine [polylysine $(NANA)_6$]. The chemically derived molecules as well as the BSA end polylysine conjugates were prepared according to the reported schedule of synthesis for the artificial glycoproteins described. BSA and polylysine replaced TT as carrier proteins in ELISA because the rabbit antiserum contained antibodies specifically induced towards TT (toxin). The ELISA technique was developed basically in the same conditions reported [48] using BSA–AD, BSA–$(NANA)_6$ and polylysine–$(NANA)_6$ as coating agents for the plastic plate supports (see Tables VII and VIII for their respective coating concentrations). The antiserum of one rabbit receiving three injections of TT–$(NANA)_6$ (SD10) was analysed by inhibition-ELISA after its pre-incubation at 37 °C × 30 minutes with increasing amount of the molecules listed as inhibitors (see Tables VII and VIII for the 'range' concentration of inhibitors used).

RESULTS

Physico-chemical characteristics of the synthesized glycoproteins

In Table I are reported the characteristics of the molecules used for this study. SDS–PAGE of glycosylated TT is shown in Figure 1.

Immunochemical characteristics of the oligosaccharide haptens

The specificity of polyclonal antibodies for their respective bacterial capsular polysaccharides, as well as for the homologous derived oligosaccharide haptens in unconjugated and conjugated form, is shown in Table II. The

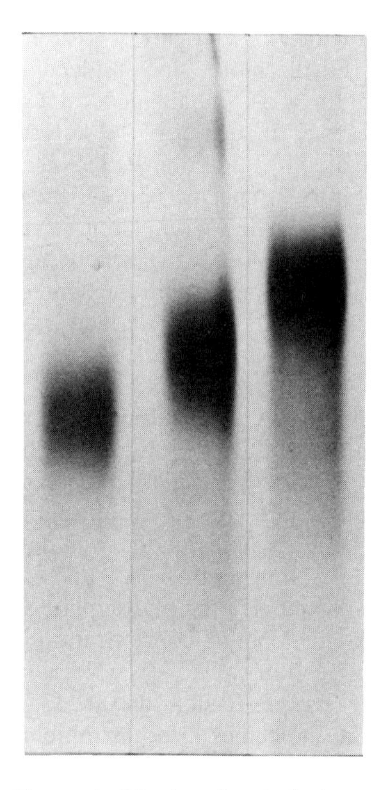

Figure 1. Physico-chemical characterization of the artificial glycoprotein TT–$(NANA)_6$ as detected by SDS–PAGE, in reducing conditions, using a 3–9% w/v gradient of acrylamide. (A) Reference tetanus toxoid; (B) TT–$(NANA)_6$ (SD = 4); (C) TT–$(NANA)_6$ (SD = 10). In all cases, the loaded protein concentration was 100 μg/ml. The average molecular weights were calculated based on the relative mobility of the reference proteins (not shown) ferritin (half unit = 2.2×10^5), albumin (6.7×10^4), catalase (6×10^4), lactate dehydrogenase (3.6×10^4) provided by Pharmacia (Uppsala, Sweden). Gel was silver stained [48]

Table I. Physico-chemical Characteristics of the Synthesized Glycoproteins

Artificial glycoprotein	MW ($\times 10^3$) carrier protein	MW ($\times 10^3$) glycoprotein (SD)	Hapten/ protein ratio (w/w)	Reference
CRM197–oligo 6A	62	75 (8)	0.18	[48]
oligo 6A		(4)	0.092	
CRM197	62	75		[50]
oligo MenC		(2)	0.057	
CRM197–oligo Hib	62	73 (6)	0.17	This work
TT–$(NANA)_6$(SD4)	180	190 (4)	0.04	This work
TT–$(NANA)_6$(SD10)	180	210 (10)	0.10	This work

specificity [8] increased for the oligosaccharide haptens in conjugated form, with respect to their homologous in unconjugated form, depending upon the SD of the synthesized glycoprotein. This observation indicated the exposure of the oligosaccharide haptens on the surface of the carrier protein, and the increase of specificity is explained by a higher amount of antibodies recognizing the carbohydrate in conjugated form, since for carbohydrate antigens, this amount has been related to the molecular weight of the antigen [11, 47]. In the case of a given glycoprotein, synthesized according to the model described, the carrier protein plays a role of spatial support for several oligosaccharide haptens, mimicking for the carbohydrate moiety a higher MW than that evidenced for the unconjugated oligosaccharide. Also shown, in Table III, is the unchanged specificity of meningococcal Group B antiserum for the $(NANA)_6$ oligosaccharide hapten before and after the chemical activation by introduction of a primary amino group at the hemiketal group of the end-reducing sialic acid residue.

Immunochemical characteristics of the carrier proteins

Molecular mapping of the main epitopes present in the carrier protein CRM197 after its chemical glycosylation by different oligosaccharide haptens, is shown In Table IV. In all cases reported, CRM197 retained the reactivity of the epitope located in the 8000-dalton carboxy-terminal region of the protein (approximately aa sequence 465–535) when analysed by specific monoclonal antibody.

Table II. Immunochemical specificity of reference polyclonal antibodies for their respective homologous capsular polysaccharides compared to that observed for the derived haptens in unconjugated or conjugated form with the carrier protein CRM197

Artificial glycoprotein	Reference antiserum	Native polysaccharide	Derived hapten	Immunodominant sugar	Conjugated hapten (SD)	Reference
CRM197–oligo 6A	Rabbit	1	10^{-3} (1800)	4×10^{-5} (Gal)	10^{-1} (8)	[48]
CRM197 oligo 6A	Rabbit	1	1.08×10^{-3} (1800)	4.2×10^{-5} (Gal)	1.09×10^{-2} (4)	[50]
CRM197 oligo MenC	Horse	1	1.06×10^{-3} (2100)	1.18×10^{-5} (NANA)	1.09×10^{-2} (2)	[50]
CRM197–oligo Hib	Rabbit	1	1.1×10^{-3} (1800)	1.05×10^{-5} (Rib)	10^{-1} (6)	This work

Note: The values were detected by differential immunoelectrophoresis under conditions described earlier [48], using the oligosaccharide haptens or the artificial glycoproteins as inhibitors of the respective homologous polysaccharide–antibody immunoprecipitates. Specificity expresses the ratio between the minimal inhibitory concentration experimentally observed for the native polysaccharides and that observed for their homologous oligosaccharide haptens, as well as for the identified immunodominant sugar in the type 6A polysaccharide of *S. pneumoniae* (galactose (Gal)), in that of Group C *N. meningitidis* (*N*-acetylneuraminic acid (NANA) and in that of type b *H. influenzae* (ribose (Rib)).

Table III. Specificity of horse meningococcal antiserum for the $(NANA)_6$ oligosaccharide hapten of *N. meningitidis* Group B. The values were detected by inhibition of immunoprecipitation in differential immunoelectrophoresis [48] with the $(NANA)_6$ oligosaccharide hapten and its chemically activated derivative used in the coupling procedure, as inhibitors of the homologous polysaccharide–antibody immunoprecipitation reaction

Specificity of meningococcal Group B antiserum		
Purified capsular polysaccaride	Derived hapten $(NANA)_6$	Amino-activated hapten $(NANA)_6$–NH_2
1	2.1×10^{-4}	2.08×10^{-4}

The specificity of horse polyclonal antibodies to tetanus toxin (Sclavo SpA, Siena, Italy) for the glycosylated carrier TT, as estimated by rocket immunoelectrophoresis, is shown in Figure 2. As one can see, the higher the glycosylation of the protein the lower appears the specificity of the antibodies for the carrier protein (detectable as minor definition of the corresponding 'rocket' immunoprecipitate) giving evidence for the lack of epitopes in its structure.

Immunological characteristics of the synthesized glycoproteins

The geometric mean ($\bar{x}g$) of IgG isotype antibody specifically induced in rabbits towards the native capsular polysaccharides of *S. pneumoniae* type 6A, *N. meningitidis* Groups B and C and *H. influenzae* type b are reported in Table V, also including the immunological properties of those antisera in terms of bactericidal activity for meningococci and *H. influenzae* and recognition of the bacterial capsule ('Quellung' reaction) for streptococci [5].

The titres of guinea-pig antisera neutralizing the activity of diphtheria toxin or tetanus toxin *in vivo* are shown respectively in Table VI and Figure 3.

No adverse reactions were observed at the site of injection in the treated animals.

Molecular mapping of neodeterminants present in the artificial glycoproteins

The ELISA technique, performed using BSA–AD as coating antigen (300 μg/ml) and three sera of rabbits immunized by three doses of the artificial glycoproteins described, gave a negative reaction when tested for the presence of IgG isotype antibodies. Because the theoretical structural similarity between the synthesized glycoproteins and BSA–AD involved only the region

Table IV. Immunochemical specificity of monoclonal antibodies to diphtheria toxin [65] for different epitopes of the protein CRM197 involved as carrier for oligosaccharide haptens

Artificial glycoprotein	Monoclonal antibody	Epitope recognized (approx. aa sequence in CRM197)	Specificity (%) for		Reference
			CRM197	Artificial glycoprotein	
CRM197–oligo 6A	Group I (clone 6B12)	1–156	100	82	This work
	Group II (clone 2A5)	157–193	100	80	
	Group IIIa (clone 2A7)	293–345	100	74	
	Group IV cl (clone 2E10)	465–535	100	97	
oligo 6A	Group I	1–156	100	31	[50]
CRM197	Group IIb	157–193	100	10	
oligo MenC	Group IIIa	293–345	100	21	
	Group IV cl	465–535	100	95	
CRM197–oligo Hib	Group I	1–156	100	76	This work
	Group IIb	157–193	100	10	
	Group IIIa	293–345	100	75	
	Group IV cl	465–535	100	100	

Note: The values were obtained by ELISA [50]. The percentage specificity was calculated assuming as 100 the specificity observed by measuring the absorbance values in the ELISA assay for CRM197.

Table V. Immunogenicity of the synthesized glycoproteins in groups of ten rabbits each by evaluation of the antibody response specific for the native homologous capsular polysaccharide of *S. pneumoniae* type 6A, *N. meningitidis* Groups B and C and *H. influenzae* type b

Artificial glycoprotein	$\bar{x}g$ of IgG isotype Ab (Abs–ELISA units)			$\bar{x}g$ of bactericidal titres (dil^{-1})			'Quellung' reaction (qualitative test)	Reference
	Basal immunization	First booster	Second booster	Basal immunization	First booster	Second booster		
CRM197–oligo 6A	0.18	1.00	2.93				Positive	[48]
Post/pre	5.6	2.9						
oligo 6A	0.04	3.39	n.d.				Positive	
CRM197	82.3							[50]
oligo MenC	0.33	2.94	n.d.	20	160	n.d.		
Post/pre	9.0			8.0				
CRM197–oligo Hib	0.1	0.36	0.74	5[a]	20[a]	80[a]		This work
Post/pre	3.6	2.2		4	4			
TT–$(NANA)_6$(SD4)	None detected			None detected				This work
TT–$(NANA)_6$(SD10)	None detected			None detected				This work

n.d. = not done.
[a] $\bar{x}g$ of three rabbit antisera randomly chosen.

Figure 2. Rocket immunoelectrophoresis of reference tetanus toxoid (A), as compared to TT–$(NANA)_6$ with SD = 4 (B) and TT–$(NANA)_6$ with SD = 10 (C). In all cases the loaded protein concentration was 110 μg/ml. Horse antiserum to tetanus toxoid was employed in 1% v/v in agarose gel 1% w/v (LKB, Bromma, Sweden). Electrophoretic run occurred at 70 V/cm for 60 minutes using a 0.02 M tris-barbiturate buffer (Gelman, Ann Arbor, MI, USA) pH = 8.8. The plate was stained by Coomassie Blue Brilliant R-250

encompassing the AD linked to the lysine residues of the carrier proteins, this result was interpreted in terms of absence of antigenically active neodeterminants in the structure of the artificial glycoproteins, at least so far as thymic-dependent neodeterminants able to induce boostable IgG isotype antibodies are concerned.

By contrast, in the serum of the rabbit receiving the TT–$(NANA)_6$ antigen, a hybrid immunodeterminant was detected and characterized as including the structure of the oligo $(NANA)_6$, the AD spacer and a lysine residue present in the structure of the carrier protein (Tables VII and VIII). In fact, ELISA reactions developed using either BSA–$(NANA)_6$ or

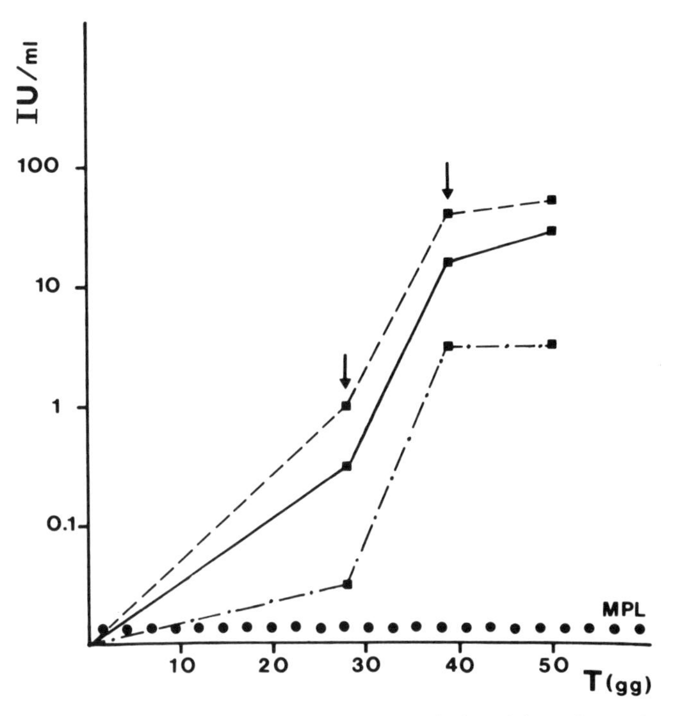

Figure 3. Antibodies to tetanus toxin induced in guinea-pigs by TT–(NANA)$_6$ with SD = 4 (———) or with SD = 10 (— · —), as compared to the reference tetanus toxoid (— — —). All the antigens were injected in absorbed form to the mineral adjuvant $AlPO_4$, as described in the Materials and Methods section. Arrows indicate the time when the first and the second booster dose were given. MPL indicates the minimum protective level estimated in humans [63]

polylysine–(NANA)$_6$ as 'coating' antigens and IgG rabbit antibodies induced by TT–(NANA)$_6$, were inhibited by 50% of their Abs value when BSA–(NANA)$_6$ was employed as inhibitor. Because the only structural similarity between TT, BSA and polylysine involves the aa lysine, this was localized as the residue included in the glycopeptide epitope able to induce IgG isotype antibodies. However, the IgG isotype antibodies specific for this neodeterminant were not specific either for the purified capsular polysaccharide of *N. meningitidis* Group B or for the capsule of group-specific living meningococci. A similar finding was reported by Jennings and Lugowski [31] using a model of artificial glycoprotein which did not involve the introduction of a chemical spacer in its structure, mirroring the observations reported above about the irrelevant role played by AD in introducing undesired neodeterminants in the structure of these synthetic molecules.

Table VI. *In vivo* diphtheria toxin neutralization test using the guinea-pig sera pool of each group of ten animals receiving the synthetic glycoproteins described, when CRM197 was the carrier protein for oligosaccharide haptens

Artificial glycoprotein	International units/ml serum of antidiphtheria toxin activity			Reference
	Basal immunization	First booster	Second booster	
CRM–oligo 6A	10^{-2}	1	5	[48]
CRM197 oligo 6A oligo MenC	$>10^{-2}$ $<10^{-1}$	>3 <6	>4 <6	[50]
CRM197–oligo Hib	$>2.5 \times 10^{-1}$ $<5 \times 10^{-1}$	>2 <3	>2 <3	This work

Table VII. Molecular mapping of the glycopeptide epitope present in the artificial glycoprotein TT–$(NANA)_6$, as estimated by inhibition of reaction in ELISA test[l]

Inhibitor[b]	Conc. NANA (μg/ml)	Conc. prot. (μg/ml)	% inhibition
BSA–$(NANA)_6$	0.0017	0.32	50
Purified Ps MenB[c]	0.0017–17		<10
$(NANA)_6$–NH_2[d]	0.0017–17		<10
$(NANA)_6$–AD[e]	0.0017–17		<10
Lysine		0.32	<10
Poly Lysine		0.32	<10
BSA		0.32	<10

[a] ELISA test performed with IgG rabbit antibodies induced by the glycoconjugate TT–$(NANA)_6$ (SD10).
[b] 'Coating' of the plates performed by BSA–$(NANA)_6$ (conc. NANA 17 μg/ml).
[c] Purified capsular polysaccharide of *N. meningitidis* Group B.
[d] Amino-activated oligosaccharide hapten.
[e] Amino-activated oligosaccharide hapten after chemical reaction with the spacer disuccinimidyl ester of AD used for the coupling procedure [48].

Table VIII. Molecular mapping of the glycopeptide epitope present in the artificial glycoprotein TT–$(NANA)_6$, as estimated by inhibition of reaction in ELISA test[a]

Inhibitor[b]	Conc. NANA (μg/ml)	% Inhibition
BSA–$(NANA)_6$	17	50
Purified Ps Men B	17	<10
$(NANA)_6$–NH_2	17	<10
$(NANA)_6$–AD	17	<10

[a] ELISA test performed with IgG rabbit antibodies induced by the glycoconjugate TT–$(NANA)_6$ (SD10).
[b] 'Coating' of the plates performed by polylysine–$(NANA)_6$ (conc. NANA 17 μg/ml).

DISCUSSION

The artificial glycoproteins described in this work were synthesized according to the same strategy of synthesis reported [48] in order to test the reliability of the model in object when different bacterial oligosaccharide haptens and different carrier proteins were involved in their preparation. The carrier proteins CRM197 and TT were chosen for this study because the immunization procedure for infants requires the inoculation of diphtheria and tetanus vaccines at an early stage of life. In particular, the non-toxic mutant protein CRM197 [57] was selected as a potential anti-diphtheria antigen [43, 46] since the aa sequence of this protein has been elucidated [19] and a collection of monoclonal antibodies specific for some important epitopes present in its structure became available [65]. Indeed, this protein represented a helpful model to study the immunochemical properties of a native antigen after its chemical glycosylation by oligosaccharide haptens.

The physico-chemical characteristics of the synthesized glycoproteins identified them as protein molecules, supporting on their surface covalently linked oligosaccharides. The immunochemical analysis indicated the availability of the oligosaccharide haptens to the recognition by polyclonal antibodies specific for the native homologous capsular polysaccharides, and unequivocally demonstrated that chemical glycosylation led to loss of epitopes in the structure of the carrier proteins.

The importance of the loss or retention of some of these epitopes was tested by monoclonal antibody reactivity in the case of the protein CRM197. One of the most important epitopes of CRM197, as well as of diphtheria toxin, was localized by Zucker and Murphy [65] in the 8000-dalton carboxy-terminal region of the protein. Some Group IV monoclonal antibodies specific for this epitope were proved almost as effective as a polyclonal antiserum in the neutralization of diphtheria toxin activity, either *in vitro* using sensitive cells or *in vivo* using the rabbit skin test. This neutralization activity was related to the inhibition binding of diphtheria toxin molecules to cell membrane. As a result, it would appear that it is extremely important that this region of the CRM197 antigen be retained after a given chemical manipulation of this protein. Following the glycosylation process by each of the three different oligosaccharide haptens, the 8000-dalton carboxy-terminal region of the protein CRM197 was still reactive when probed by the Group IV monoclonal antibody. By contrast, other epitopes were found to be unreactive, based on the reduction of specificity of monoclonal antibodies Groups I, II, and III by more than 50% when compared to their specificity for native CRM197. A theoretical explanation for this finding has been previously reported [50], based on the localization of the basic lysine residues (involved in the synthesis reaction) contained in the predicted most hydrophilic regions of the protein structure according to the Hopp and Woods analysis [26].

When the three artificial glycoproteins were injected into the animals, the amount of induced antibodies neutralizing the diphtheria toxin activity *in vivo* were detected at comparable levels. These levels largely exceeded the estimated minimum protective level (MPL) in humans for anti-diphtheria toxin activity [63]. A comparison with the antibody level induced by CRM197 in native form was not possible, because this protein is unable to induce significant levels of diphtheria toxin neutralizing antibodies without a chemical manipulation leading to improvement of its resistance towards proteolytic enzymes [43, 46]. These findings also prove that chemical glycosylation increases the immunogenicity of CRM197, although the basic reason for that has to be elucidated. However, the chemical glycosylation must not involve the 8000-dalton carboxy-terminal region of the protein if a significant amount of neutralizing antibodies has to be induced. In fact, when in another experiment the protein was overglycosylated by Hib oligosaccharide haptens (SD 10) the specificity of the Group IV monoclonal antibody was reduced by more than 90% with respect to that for native CRM197, and the level of neutralizing antibodies induced *in vivo* was not higher than 0.5 IU/ml after a booster dose of aluminium-absorbed artificial glycoprotein (personal observation). These results strongly support the role of the epitope localized approximately in the 70 aa of the carboxy-terminal sequence of CRM197 and suggest that predictions of the level of immunogenicity expressed by this protein could be carried out based on the specificity detected *in vitro* by the Group IV monoclonal antibody, when CRM197 is involved as carrier protein in a given glycoprotein synthesized according to the described procedure.

The *in vitro* specificity of polyclonal antibodies for the carrier protein TT, qualitatively determined by 'rocket' immunoelectrophoresis, evidenced that the higher the SD of the artificial glycoprotein TT–$(NANA)_6$ the lower was the antigenicity retained by the protein after the procedure of synthesis. Although monoclonal antibodies specific for the structure of tetanus toxin have been recently developed [59], the unknown aa sequence of this protein did not permit the precise localization of lysine residues in the main epitopes of the structure recognized by neutralizing monoclonal antibodies. In addition, the formalin treatment of the protein which leads to its detoxification, involves some lysine residues of the structure [12] making them unavailable to chemical glycosylation by oligosaccharide haptens using the procedure reported. Thus, at present it would be very difficult to apply for TT the same procedure used to map the glycosylated regions of CRM197 in order to explain the immunological properties of glycosylated TT in terms of induction of neutralizing antibodies. However, the polyclonal antibody analysis indicated a loss of epitopes in the structure of glycosylated TT, and these epitopes appeared to be important for induction of *in vivo* neutralizing antibodies, since the immunological data obtained by TT–(NANA) (SD4) and TT–$(NANA)_6$ (SD10) clearly mirrored the *in vitro* gradual loss of antigenicity in respect to TT. In any case the *in vivo* neutralizing antibody titres, largely exceeded the estimated MPL in humans for anti-TT activity [63].

The acquired T-helper dependency of carried oligosaccharide haptens, derived from the homologous high MW capsular polysaccharides of *S. pneumoniae* type 6A, *N. meningitidis* Group C and *H. influenzae* type b, was indirectly demonstrated by induction in rabbits of boostable IgG isotype antibodies specific for the purified homologous polysaccharide, as well as for the capsule of living homologous bacterial cells. In particular, rabbit antisera showed complement-dependent bactericidal activity for Group C meningococci and *H. influenzae* bacterial cells, as well as recognition of the capsule of type 6A streptococci. In this case the antisera were also specific for the capsule of type 6B streptococci [48], according to the structural similarity documented for these two bacterial antigens [35, 51].

The employed oligosaccharides used showed dimensions compatible with the size generally reported for the minimal structure of an epitope, either for protein or carbohydrate antigens [34, 58] which is approximately encompassing six to eight monomeric residues (amino acids or monosaccharides). All the derived oligosaccharide haptens used in the synthesis of the glycoproteins tested were able to inhibit the homologous immunoprecipitation reaction between the high MW polysaccharide and specific polyclonal antibodies. They also were specifically recognized by antibodies after either the chemical activation or the synthesis procedure. The chemical spacer AD interposed between the oligosaccharide and the protein moieties was chosen for two main reasons: (1) The optimal distance between a given hapten and the carrier support, permitting the T–B co-operative cells to deliver the 'help' signal, has been reported in the range 7–70 Å [1]. The calculated length of the AD molecule is 10.4 Å. (2) Adipic acid is a natural component of human and animal organisms, so that its structure would not be recognized as foreign to the host's immune system. Accordingly, no neodeterminants involving AD were found in animal sera after immunization by the artificial glycoproteins.

Despite its antigenicity, the $(NANA)_6$ oligosaccharide hapten derived from the Group B capsular polysaccharide of *N. meningitidis* did not induce detectable IgG isotype antibodies specific for the native antigen, after the coupling with the carrier protein. In this case, however, IgG isotype antibodies specific for a glycopeptide epitope present in the structure of the artificial glycoprotein, were induced. This 'hybrid' epitope encompassed a lysine residue of the carrier protein structure in addition to the oligosaccharide–spacer structure. Parallel results have been obtained in mice by Jennings and Lugowski [31], using a hapten of higher MW conjugated to the same carrier protein by a different procedure of synthesis. It appears evident that, in the case of the conjugate Group B capsular polysaccharide or oligosaccharide, neither the size of the hapten chosen nor the stechiometry of the glycoprotein synthesized (SD) is important in inducing a specific immunological response to the polysaccharide capsule of the micro-organism. Reasons other than a critical MW of the hapten or the method of synthesis involved in the preparation of the glycoprotein have to be considered to explain these results.

Attempts to explain this lack of anti-hapten IgG antibody induction could be sought in two main properties of the immune system: activation of the suppression mechanism and/or immunological tolerance of the immune system for self-antigens. The activation of a suppression mechanism preventing the expression of anti-hapten memory cells has already been described for chemical haptens (e.g. DNP) carried by protein molecules, when the adopted immunization schedule was carrier/hapten–carrier [25]. In that study, the authors reported the induction in mice of normal anti-hapten memory population cells following the injection of hapten–carrier conjugate in carrier-primed animals. However, they also reported the concomitant induction of a T cell-dependent suppression-effector mechanism that specifically prevented the expression of the activated memory cells. Suppression resulted, induced only when mice were primed with a carrier and then exposed to a hapten on the same carrier. This suppression prevented the IgG isotype anti-hapten response but did not interfere with the anti-carrier response. Similar observations have also been recently reported for synthetic peptide haptens in terms of carrier-induced epitopic suppression when high levels of anti-carrier antibodies were induced before the injection of the carried hapten [29, 53]. Although these findings seem very similar to the results reported here, they were obtained with a different schedule of immunization (carrier/hapten–carrier *versus* hapten–carrier/hapten–carrier) and using chemical haptens unrelated to molecules as the bacterial oligosaccharides. Furthermore, by immunization of the animal models with the glycoproteins described here, the anamnestic induction of IgG isotype antibodies specific for the native antigens by which the haptens were derived was always detected.

The immunological tolerance of the immune system for self-antigens could be explained in this case by the observation that the chemical structure of the meningococcal Group B capsular polysaccharide (2,8-α-D-*N*-acetylneuraminic acid)$_n$ is identical to the structure of the carbohydrate moiety present in human gangliosides [18] and to polysialosyl glycopeptides found in rat brain [16]. In particular, it has been reported that horse polyclonal anti-Group B meningoccoccal polysaccharide antibodies cross-reacted *in vitro* with these glycopeptide structures and the purified Group B capsular polysaccharide could specifically inhibit such a reaction [17]. Also, past clinical experience has shown the absence of significant immunogenicity in adult humans of the purified Group B capsular polysaccharide as compared with the high immunogenicity of the Group C capsular polysaccharide of *N.*

meningitidis [21, 22] which is composed of (2,9-α-D-*N*-acetylneuraminic acid)$_n$ [10, 30]. These clinical results were supported by the finding that, in human convalescent or post-vaccination sera, anti-Group B capsular polysaccharide antibody showed a binding constant value 10–28 times lower than anti-group C capsular polysaccharide antibody [41]. Comparable data were reported by the same authors, in the same work, using mouse monoclonal antibodies directed towards the two carbohydrate antigens. Thus, the lack of significant anti-hapten IgG isotype amplification using artificial glycoproteins could involve, in the case of the carried Group B meningococcal oligosaccharides or polysaccharide, a mechanism of self-defence for the organism receiving the antigen in order to prevent hazardous immunological reactions directed against self-targets. However, hazardous immunological reactions have still to be documented in patients recovered from the Group B meningococcal disease in which significant titres of anti-capsular polysaccharide antibodies have been detected [41].

The results achieved with the model of glycoprotein, when different bacterial haptens and antigens were involved in the procedure of synthesis, permit the following conclusions to be drawn.

1. Oligosaccharide haptens with a molecular size approximately comparable to the minimal structure able to be recognized by antibodies as an epitope [34, 58], may also have the immunogenic potential of a complete polysaccharide antigen when covalently bound to protein supports working as immunogenic carriers.
2. The carried oligosaccharide haptens do acquire the thymic-dependent immunogenic characteristics typical of a carrier protein, at least for the induction of boostable specific IgG isotype antibodies. These antibodies, induced either by the primary immunization or by the booster doses, were specific for the purified capsular polysaccharides homologous to the derived haptens, as well as for the native capsule of living bacteria to whom the polysaccharides belonged. Exception to this behaviour was shown by the carried Group B meningococcal oligosaccharide. In this case, however, reasons other than those regarding the model of glycoprotein used have to be considered.
3. Neodeterminants introduced in the linking region of the glycoproteins and able to induce IgG isotype antibodies were not detected, but an immunogenically active glycopeptide epitope was found in the structure of the glycoprotein TT–(NANA)$_6$.
4. The strategy of synthesis and the stechiometry involved in the preparation of the model of artificial glycoprotein reported, permitted the physiocochemical and immunochemical definition of the antigens in order to achieve the reproducibility needed understand to their antigenic characteristics. In particular, the exposure of the oligosaccharide haptens on the surface of the protein carriers was obtained using the model reported,

in order to predetermine the antigenicity of the glycoproteins used as antigens.

5. The carrier effect of a given protein antigen can be used for immunochemically different oligosaccharide haptens simultaneously carried by the same protein. The multivalent antigen is able to prime and boost an immunological response with specific characteristics required for a gram-positive and gram-negative capsular polysaccharide. The SD of a given hapten does not appear to be important for the quantitative level of boosted IgG isotype antibodies specific for the native homologous polysaccharide, but indeed appeared important for the expression of immunogenicity of the carrier protein.
6. The chemical glycosylation of a given protein carrier can lead to a decrease of its immunogenicity if the most important epitopes present in the structure are involved in the glycosylation process. When monoclonal antibodies specific for these epitopes are available, molecular mapping of their specificity for the synthesized glycoprotein can be helpful in predicting the immunogenic potential of the carrier protein.
7. The laboratory controls of these artificial antigens should include: (a) SDS–PAGE behaviour to control the average MW of the glycoprotein and to give evidence for covalent linkage of the oligosaccharide haptens; (b) chemical determination of the SD of the oligosaccharide haptens, based on the stechiometry of the glycoprotein, as well as on the physicochemical characteristics of the oligosaccharides involved; (c) detection of the specificity of monoclonal and/or polyclonal antibodies for the carrier protein as well as for the carried oligosaccharide haptens; (d) estimation of the quantitative levels of serum antibodies (in particular IgG isotype antibody) induced in animal models by a given glycoprotein towards the carrier protein and the native capsular polysaccharide by which the oligosaccharide hapten was derived.
8. Although in the case of diphtheria and tetanus antigens the guinea-pig model can be predictive for the immunogenicity of these proteins in humans, because of the past standardization of this model [62], the immunogenicity of the carried oligosaccharide haptens in animal models cannot be fully evaluated or standardized until extensive clinical trials demonstrate the levels of immunogenicity and protection attainable by the use of these artificial antigens in the infant population.

REFERENCES

1. Alkan, S. S., Bush, M. E., Nitecki, D. E., and Goodman, J. W. Antigen recognition and the immune system: structural requirements in the side chain of tyrosine for immunogenicity of L-tyrosine-azobenzenarsonate. *J. Exp.*, **136**, 387–91 (1972).

2. Anderson, P. Antibody responses to *H. influenzae* type b and diphtheria toxin induced by conjugates of oligosaccharides of the type b capsule with the non-toxin protein CRM197. *Infect. Immun.*, **39**, 233–8 (1983).
3. Anderson, P., Pichichero, M. E., and Insel, R. Immunogens consisting of oligosaccharides from the capsule of *Haemophilus influenzae* type b coupled to diphtheria toxoid or the toxin protein CRM197. *J. Clin. Invest.*, **76**, 52–9 (1985).
4. Anderson, P. W., Pichichero, M. E., Insel, R. A., Betts, R., Eby, R., and Smith, D. H. Vaccines consisting of periodate–cleaved oligosaccharides from the capsule of *Haemophilus influenzae* type b coupled to a protein: structural and temporal requirements for priming in the human infant. *J. Immunol.*, **137**, 1181–6 (1986).
5. Austrian, R. The Quellung reaction, a neglected microbiology technique. *Mt Sinai J. Med.*, **43**, 699–709 (1976).
6. Austrian, R. Pneumococcal vaccine: development and prospects. *Am. J. Med.*, **67**, 547–9 (1979).
7. Avery, O. T., and Goebel, W. F. Chemoimmunological studies on conjugated carbohydrate proteins. II. Immunological specificity of synthetic sugar-protein antigens. *J. Exp. Med.*, **50**, 533–50 (1929).
8. Berzofsky, J. A., and Schechter, A. N. The concepts of cross-reactivity and specificity in immunology. *Molec. Immun.*, **18**, 751–63 (1981).
9. Beuvery, E. C., Rossum, F. V., and Nagel, J. Comparison of the induction of immunoglobulin M and G antibodies in mice with purified penumococcal type 3 and meningococcal Group C polysaccharides and their protein conjugates. *Infect. Immun.*, **37**, 15–22 (1982).
10. Bhattacherjee, A. R., Jennings, H. J., Kenny, C. P., Martin, A., and Smith, I. C. P. Structural determination of the sialic acid polysaccharide antigens of *N. meningitidis* serogroup B and C with carbon 13 nuclear magnetic resonance. *J. Biol. Chem.*, **250**, 1926 (1975).
11. Bishop, C. T., and Jennings, H. J. Immunology of polysaccharides. In *The Polysaccharide* (ed. G. O. Aspinal), Vol. 1, Academic Press, New York, 1982, pp. 292–330.
12. Blass, J., Bitten, B., and Raymond, M. Etudes sur le mécanisme de la détoxification des toxines protéiques par le formol. *Bull. Soc. Chim. France*, 3957–65 (1967).
13. Crisel, R. M., Baker, R. S., and Dorman, D. E. Capsular polymer of *Haemophilus influenzae* type b. I. Structural characterization of the capsular polymer of strain eagan. *J. Biol. Chem.*, **250**, 4926 (1975).
14. Douglas, R. M., Paton, J. C., Duncan, S. J., and Hausman, D. J. Antibody response to pneumococcal vaccination in children younger than five years of age. *J. Infec. Dis.*, **148**, 131–7 (1983).
15. Douglas, R. M., and Miles, H. B. Vaccination against *Streptococcus pneumoniae* in childhood: lack of demonstrable benefit in young Australian children, *J. Infec. Dis.*, **149**, 861–9 (1984).
16. Finne, J. Occurrence of unique polysaccharide carbohydrate units in glycoproteins of developing brain. *J. Biol. Chem.*, **257**, 11966–70 (1982).
17. Finne, J., Leinonen, M., and Makela, P. H. Antigen similarities between brain components and bacteria causing meningitis. Implications for vaccine development and pathogens. *Lancet*, **8346**, 355–7 (1983).
18. Fredman, P., Manson, J. E., Svennrholm, L., and Samuelson, B. E. The structure of the tetrasiologanglioside from human brain. *FEBS Lett.*, **110**, 80 (1980).
19. Giannini, G., Rappuoli, R., and Ratti, G. The amino acid sequence of two non-

toxic mutants of diphtheria toxin: CRM45 and CRM197. *Nucleic Acid Res.*, **12**, 4063–9 (1984).
20. Goebel, W. F. Chemo-immunological studies on conjugated carbohydrate proteins. IV. The immunological properties of an artificial antigen containing cellobiuromic acid. *J. Exp. Med.*, **68**, 469–84 (1938).
21. Gotschlich, E. C., Goldschneider, I., and Artenstein, M. S. Human immunity to the meningococcus. IV. Immunogenicity of Group A and Group C meningococcal polysaccharides in human volunteers. *J. Exp. Med.*, **129**, 1367–84 (1969).
22. Gotschlich, E. C. Development of polysaccharide vaccines for the prevention of meningococcal diseases. *Allergy*, **9**, 245–58 (1975).
23. Granoff, D. M., and Cates, K. L. *Haemophilus influenzae* type by polysaccharide vaccines (medical progress). *J. Pediatrics*, **107**, 330–6 (1985).
24. Granoff, D. M., and Munson, R. S. Prospects for prevention of *Haemophilus influenzae* type b disease by immunization. *J. Infect. Dis.*, **153**, 448–61 (1986).
25. Herzenberg, L. A., Tokuisa, T., and Herzenberg, L. A. Carrier priming leads to hapten specific suppression. *Nature*, **285**, 665 (1980).
26. Hopp, T. P., and Woods, K. A. Prediction of protein antigenic determinants from amino acid sequences. *Proc. Natn. Acad. Sci. USA*, **78**, 3824–8 (1981).
27. Insel, R. A., Anderson, P., Pichichero, M. E., Amstey, M. S., Ekborg, G., and Smith, D. H. Anticapsular antibody to *Haemophilus influenzae* type b. In *Haemophilus influenzae: Epidemiology, Immunology and Prevention of the Disease* (ed. S. H. Sell and P. F. Wright), Elsevier Biomedical, New York, 1982, pp. 155–68.
28. Insel, R. A., and Anderson, P. W. Oligosaccharide-protein conjugate vaccines induce and prime for oligoclonal IgG antibody responses to the *Haemophilus influenzae* b capsular polysaccharide in human infants. *J. Exp. Med.*, **163**, 262–9 (1986).
29. Jacob, C. O., Arnon, R., and Sela, M. Effect of carrier on the immunogenic capacity of synthetic cholera vaccine. *Molec. Immunol.*, **22**, 1333–9 (1985).
30. Jennings, H. J., Bhattacharjee, A. K., Bundle, D. R., Kenny, C. P., Martin, A., and Smith, I. C. P. Structures of the capsular polysaccharides of *N. meningitidis* as determined by ^{13}C NMR spectroscopy. *J. Infect. Dis.*, **136**, 578–83 (1977).
31. Jennings, H. J., and Lugowski, C. Immunochemistry of Groups A, B and C meningococcal polysaccharide-tetanus toxoid conjugates. *J. Immunol.*, **127**, 104–8 (1981).
32. Johnston, R. B., Anderson, P., Rosen, F. S., and Smith, D. H. Characterization of human antibody to polyribophophate, the capsular antigen of *Haemophilus influenzae* type b. *Clin. Immunol. Immunopathol.*, **1**, 234–40 (1973).
33. Kabat, E. A. Methylpentose determination In *Experimental Immunochemistry* (ed. E. A. Kabat and M. Mayer), Thomas, Springfield, Illinois, 1964, pp. 538–41.
34. Kabat, E. A. The nature of an antigenic determinant. *J. Immunol.*, **97**, 1–11 (1966).
35. Kenne, L., Lindberg, B., and Madden, J. K. Structural studies of the capsular antigen from *Streptococcus pneumoniae* type 26. *Carbohydr. Res.*, **73**, 175–82 (1979).
36. Kimball, J. W. Maturation of the immune response to type III pneumococcal polysaccharide. *Immunochemistry*, **9**, 1169–84 (1972).
37. Laemmli, U. K. Cleavage of structural proteins during the assembly of the head of bacteriophage T4. *Nature, Lond.*, **227**, 680–5 (1970).
38. Lowry, O. H., Rosebrough, N. J., Farr, L., and Randall, R. J. Protein measurement with the Folin phenol reagent. *J. Biol. Chem.*, **193**, 265–73 (1951).

39. Makela, P. H., Peltola, H., Kayhty, H., Jousimies, H., Rusolahti, E., Sivonen, A., and Renkonen, O. V. Polysaccharide vaccines of Group A *Neisseria meningitidis* and *Haemophilus influenzae* type b: a field trial in Finland. *J. Infect. Dis.*, **136**, 243–50 (1977).
40. Makela, P. H., Leinonen, M., Pukander, J., and Karma, P. A study of the pnemococcal vaccine in prevention of clinical acute attacks of recurrent otitis media. *Rev. Infect. Dis.*, **3**, S124–30 (1981).
41. Mandrell, R. E., and Zollinger, W. D. Measurement of antibodies to meningococcal group B polysaccharide; low activity binding and equilibrium binding constants. *J. Immunol.*, **129**, 2172–8 (1982).
42. Mond, J. J., Monglin, P. K. A., Siekman, D., and Paul, W. E. Role of T lymphocites in the response to TNP–AECM ficoll. *J. Immunol.*, **125**, 1066 (1980).
43. Pappenheimer, A. M. Jr, Uchida, T., and Harper, A. A. An immunological study of the diphtheria toxin molecule. *Immunochemistry*, **9**, 891–906 (1972).
44. Paul, W. E., Katz, D. H., and Benacerraff, B. Augmented anti-SIII antibody responses to an SIII-protein conjugate. *J. Immunol.*, **107**, 685–8 (1971).
45. Peltola, H. Meningococcal disease: still with us. *Rev. Infect. Dis.*, **5**, 71–91 (1983).
46. Porro, M., Saletti, M., Nencioni, L., Tagliaferri, L., and Marsili, I. Immunogenic correlation between cross-reacting material (CRM197) produced by a mutant of *C. diphtheriae* and diphtheria toxoid. *J. Infect. Dis.*, **143**, 716–24 (1980).
47. Porro, M., Fabbiani, S., Marsili, I., Viti, S., and Saletti, M. Immunoelectrophoretic characterization of the molecular weight polydispersion of polysaccharides in multivalent bacterial capsular polysaccharide vaccines. *J. Biol. Stand.*, **11**, 65–74 (1983).
48. Porro, M., Costantino, P., Viti, S., Vannozzi, F., Naggi, A., and Torri, G. Specific antibodies to diphtheria toxin and type 6A pneumococcal capsular polysaccharide induced by a model of semi-synthetic glycoconjugate antigen. *Molec. Immun.*, **22**, 907–19 (1985).
49. Porro, M., Costantino, P., Fabbiani, S., Pellegrini, V., and Viti, S. A semisynthetic glyconjugate antigen prepared by chemical glycosylation of pertussis toxin by a meningococcal group C oligosaccharide hapten. In *Proc. Fourth Intl. Symp. on Pertussis, Develop. Biol. Stand.* (S. Karger, Basle) **61**, 525–30 (1985).
50. Porro, M., Costantino, P., Giovannoni, F., Pellegrini, V., Tagliaferri, L., Vannozzi, F., and Viti, S. A molecular model of artificial glycoprotein with predetermined multiple immunodeterminants for Gram-positive and Gram negative encapsulated bacteria. *Molec. Immunol.*, **23**, 385–91 (1986).
51. Rebers, P. A., and Heidelberger, M. The specific polysaccharide of type VI pneumococcus. II. The repeating unit. *J. Am. Chem.*, **83**, 3056–9 (1961).
52. Rijkers, G. T., and Mosier, D. E. Pneumococcal polysaccharides induce antibody formation by human B lymphocytes in vitro. *J. Immunol.*, **135**, 1–4 (1985).
53. Schutze, M. P., Ledere, C., Tolvert, M., Audibert, F., and Chedid, L. Carrier-induced epitopic suppression, a major issue for future synthetic vaccines. *J. Immunol.*, **135**, 2319–22 (1985).
54. Schneerson, R., Barrera, O., Sutton, A., and Robbins, J. B. Preparation, characterization and immunogenicity of *Haemophilus influenzae* type b polysaccharide-protein conjugates. *J. Exp. Med.*, **152**, 361–76 (1980).
55. Schneerson, R., Robbins, J. B., Parke, J. C., Bell, C., Schlesselman, J. J., Sutton, A., Wang, Z., Schiffman, G., Karpas, A., and Shiloach, J. Quantitative and qualitative analyses of serum antibodies elicited in adults by *Haemophilus influenzae* type b and pneumococcus type 6A capsular polysaccharide–tetanus toxoid conjugates. *Infec. Immun.*, **52**, 519–28 (1986).

56. Svennerholm, L. Quantitative estimation of sialic acids. II. A colormetric resorcinol–hydrochloric acid method. *Biochem. Biophys. Acta.*, **24**, 604–11 (1957).
57. Uchida, T., Pappenheimer, A. M. Jr, and Greany, R. Diphtheria toxin and related proteins. I. Isolation and properties of mutant proteins and serologically related to diphtheria toxin. *J. Biol. Chem.*, **248**, 3838–44 (1973).
58. Van Vunakis, H., Kaplan, H., and Levin, L. Immunogenicity of polylisine and polyornithine when complexed to phosphorylated bovine serum albumin. *Immunochemistry*, **3**, 393–402 (1966).
59. Volk, W. A., Bizzini, B., Snyder, R. M., Bernhard, F., and Wagner, R. R. Neutralization of tetanus toxin by distinct monoclonal antibodies binding to multiple epitopes on the toxin molecule. *Infec. Immun.*, **45**, 604–9 (1984).
60. Weeke, B. Rocket immunoelectrophoresis. In *A Manual for Quantitative Immunoelectrophoresis* (ed. N. H. Axelson, J. Kroll and B. Weeke); *Scand. J. Immun.*, **2** S37–46 (1973).
61. WHO Expert Committee on Biological Standardization. Requirements for menigococcal polysaccharide vaccine. *Technical Report Series*, **594**, 50–75 (1976).
62. WHO Expert Committee on Biological Standardization. Requirements for diphtheria toxoid, Pertussis vaccine, tetanus toxoid and combined vaccines. *Technical Report Series*, **638**, 37–115 (1979).
63. Wilson, G. S., and Miles, A. Diphtheria and other diseases due to corynebacteriae. In *Topley and Wilson's Principles of Bacteriology, Virology and Immunity* (ed. E. Arnold), Arnold, London, 1975, pp. 1800–42.
64. Wong, K. H., Barrera, O., Sutton, A., May, J., Hochstein, D., Robbins, J. D., Robbins, J. B., and Parkman, P. O. Jr Standardization and control of meningococcal vaccines group A and group C polysaccharides. *J. Biol. Stand.*, **5**, 197–215 (1977).
65. Zucker, D., and Murphy, J. R. Monoclonal antibody analysis of diphtheria toxin. I. Localization of epitopes and neutralization of cytoxicity. *Molec. Immun.*, **21**, 785–93 (1984).

As Dr Porro was unable to attend the meeting the contents of his paper were summarized by Dr Jennings.

There was no discussion.

Towards Better Carbohydrate Vaccines
Edited by R. Bell and G. Torrigiani

Published by John Wiley & Sons Ltd

21

Vaccines composed of polysaccharide–protein conjugates: current status, unanswered questions, and prospects for the future

RACHEL SCHNEERSON, JOHN B. ROBBINS, SHOUSUN CHEN SZU AND YONGHONG YANG
National Institute of Child Health and Human Development, National Institutes of Health, Bethesda, MD 20892, USA

INTRODUCTION

It is probable that vaccines composed of polysaccharides (PS) covalently bound to proteins (conjugates) will be certified by national authorities and in widespread use in the next several years. Conjugates designed to prevent meningitis and other invasive diseases due to *Haemophilus influenzae* type b (Hib) are being extensively studied and will probably be the first of these semi-synthetic vaccines to be licensed [1–4, 8, 9, 13, 16, 22, 24–26, 40, 41, 43, 57, 60–64]. The principles underlying this approach to Hib vaccines have been extended to other bacterial PS and to peptides of bacterial, viral and parasitic origin.

Our experience with developing synthetic schemes, standardization methods and clinical evaluation of the safety and immunological properties of bacterial PS–protein conjugates is reviewed. We have been concerned with Hib and pneumococci (Pn) as causes of invasive diseases in infants and children. A list is appended. (Table I), describing the synthesis and evaluation of PS–protein conjugates intended for or that could be considered for human use.

Table I. Polysaccharide–protein conjugates considered for human diseases

Haemophilus influenzae type b
Capsular polysaccharide–tetanus toxoid [9, 60–64]
Oligosaccharide–CRM_{197} [1–4, 24–26]
Capsular polysaccharide–diphtheria toxoid [8, 22, 40, 41]
Capsular polysaccharide–Group B meningococcal outer membrane proteins [13, 43]
Pneumococcus
Type 6A and type 6B-capsular polysaccharide–tetanus toxoid [60–64]
Type 6A oligosaccharide–CRM_{197} [53, 54]
Type 3 capsular polysaccharide–tetanus toxoid [7]
Type 3 hexasaccharide–BSA [69]
Phosphocholine–BSA [77]
Meningococci
Groups A, B, C oligosaccharide–tetanus toxoid [27]
Group B *N*-propionyl capsular oligosaccharide derivative–tetanus toxoid [29]
Group C capsular polysaccharide–tetanus toxoid [7]
R-type LPS oligosaccharide–tetanus toxoid [28, 39]
Pseudomonas aeruginosa
LPS immunotype 1-pili [66]
LPS immunotype 5-exotoxin A [11]
LPS immunotype 1-BSA [76]
Escherichia coli
K13 capsular polysaccharide–BSA [33, 63]
K100 capsular polysaccharide–tetanus toxoid [64]
Salmonella typhimurium
LPS disaccharide–BSA [31]
LPS oligosaccharides–BSA [14, 15, 30, 42, 58, 71–74]
Klebsiella pneumoniae
Type 2 oligosaccharide–BSA [18]
Type 11 oligosaccharide–BSA [83]

HIB CAPSULAR POLYSACCHARIDE–PROTEIN CONJUGATES

We were prompted to synthesize and characterize the immunological properties of Hib–capsular polysaccharide (CPS) conjugates for several reasons. Hib, a gram-negative bacterium, is pathogenic for humans only [57]. It is found almost exclusively in the upper respiratory tract of infants and children. In non-immune individuals, Hib may invade the blood and multiply. If its concentration in the blood reaches 10^3 per ml or greater, Hib may penetrate several tissues, most notably the meninges (meningitis), pericardium (pericarditis), periosteum (osteomyelitis) or the periarticular tissues (septic arthritis) [46]. About one in 250 infants and children contracts meningitis due to this organism in the USA (the incidence is higher in selected populations, such as native Americans, and in patients with splenic dysfunction, such as sickle-cell anaemia and hereditary spherocytosis) [10, 48, 57, 79]. Despite effective antibiotics and supportive therapy, 5–10% of patients succumb and 30–50% of those who recover endure permanent central nervous system damage [57, 65). Hib is also the leading cause of septic arthritis and osteomyelitis in infants and children. Epiglottitis, a serious and potentially fatal upper respiratory infection, is also caused by Hib. In summary, Hib causes several serious diseases with a significant frequency, morbidity and mortality [57].

The type b CPS is an essential virulence-promoting and a protective antigen for Hib [56, 70]. The CPS confers the property of invasiveness by 'shielding' Hib organisms from the protective actions of complement [5, 21, 57]. Antibodies, therefore, are required to activate the protective actions of complement; anti-CPS antibodies are especially efficient in affording such protection [55]. The Hib CPS was purified and standardized according to methods established for meningococal and Pn CPS vaccines [5, 21, 57]. Clinical studies established its safety, effectiveness and its potential for routine immunization of children 2 years or older [50, 57]. Hib CPS failed, however, to induce protective levels of serum antibodies in infants and children, that age-group with the highest attack rate of Hib meningitis [50, 55]. In addition to its age-related immunogenicity, reinjection of Hib failed to induce a booster response: a single injection yielded the maximum antibody response characteristic for the age of the vaccinate (this latter immunological property is conveniently termed T-independence) [35]. To overcome these limitations, the approach of covalently binding PS to proteins, as first suggested by Landsteiner for haptens and then by Avery and Goebel for Pn type 3 and its disaccharide repeat unit, was used [6, 19, 20].

SYNTHESIS OF Hib CPS-TETANUS TOXOID CONJUGATE (Hib-TT)

After we experimented with several proteins, tetanus toxoid (TT) was chosen for the carrier protein because of its medical usefulness and long history as an effective vaccine component. Tetanus toxoid was passed through Sephacryl S-300 and the fractions corresponding to a molecular weight of about 1.4×10^5 daltons were used. Hib CPS does not contain active groups, such as uronic acid or a sufficient concentration of reducing end groups, which could bind to proteins [85]. Accordingly, an active group must be introduced by clinically acceptable methods that do not depolymerize or chemically alter the CPS. Our current scheme is as follows:

1. Hib CPS is activated with cyanogen bromide to form the isocyanate intermediate [80].
2. The Hib CPS cyanate intermediate is reacted with the bifunctional nucleophile, adipic acid dihydrazide, to form the adipic hydrazide derivative of Hib CPS. This adipic hydrazide derivative facilitated the coupling reaction between Hib CPS and proteins both by providing a 'spacer' between the two macromolecules and by providing active nucleophilic hydrazide groups.
3. The Hib CPS adipic hydrazide and TT are coupled by carbodiimide-mediated condensation. The reaction mixture is passed through a CL-4B Sepharose column and the void volume material, containing only the conjugate, is used, Yields of about 70%, based upon the weights of the Hib CPS and TT, have been obtained with this synthetic scheme. The ratio of Hib CPS to TT (w/w%) can be varied according to the concentration of the two components in the reaction mixture. The ratio of protein to PS in most of the conjugates was about 2 : 1.

This synthetic scheme has been used with Pn type 6A and type 6B, and *Escherichia coli* K13 and K100 CPS [9, 63]. The conjugates satisfy the FDA requirements for safety of CPS and TT vaccines.

Hib–TT lots have been evaluated in both inbred and outbred laboratory mice and in juvenile and infant rhesus monkeys [9, 60, 62]. They have been injected alone or concurrently with two other conjugates (Pn type 6A CPS or *E. coli* K100 CPS bound to TT), with TT (fluid), or with DTP (adsorbed). The results of these studies may be summarized as follows:

1. Hib CPS was non-immunogenic in most mice and in juvenile and infant rhesus monkeys: CPS are more immunogenic in humans than in other species. Hib–TT, in contrast, elicited protective levels of Hib CPS antibodies in inbred and outbred mice and in juvenile and infant rhesus monkeys. Antibody responses were dose-dependent, increased with carrier priming or with incorporation into complete Freud's adjuvant, and could be boosted with second and third injections. Hib CPS therefore, has both increased immunogenicity and T-dependent properties as a conjugate with TT.
2. Concurrent injection of Hib–TT and the cross-reacting Pn type 6A–TT enhanced the Hib CPS antibody response. No effect (enhancement or depression) was observed on the Pn 6A antibody response in animals injected with the two conjugates. It follows that two conjugates can be injected in the same formulation [68].
3. Concurrent injection of TT along with Hib–TT accelerated the Hib antibody responses in both adult and infant rhesus monkeys ('carrier' effect). Hib–TT and Pn6A–TT could be incorporated in DTP formulation as part of routine infant immunization.
4. Passive immunization of juvenile rhesus monkeys with an adult human

dose of tetanus immune globulin did not affect the serum Hib antibody response elicited by the Hib–TT. We were particularly interested in this because of the potential for maternally derived TT antibodies to inhibit the immunogenicity of Hib–TT in infants [47].

6. Following three injections of Hib–TT to juvenile and infant rhesus monkeys, spaced 3 weeks apart, TT was injected about 1 month later. No effect upon the levels of conjugate-induced Hib CPS antibodies was observed after this immunization. Thus, reinjection of the carrier protein alone, such as would be expected to occur with TT in children and adults, did not affect the level of Hib CPS antibodies.
7. The carrier protein was immunogenic; increases in TT antibodies were observed after each injection of the Hib–TT conjugate.
8. The anti-CPS and carrier protein antibodies had biological activities which correlated with protection (bactericidal and mouse-protective activity for Hib CPS antibodies, mouse protection for Pn6A antibodies and neutralizing antibodies for TT).
9. The nature of the carrier protein affected the immunogenicity of the Hib CPS in the resultant conjugate: the immunogenicity of the Hib CPS in mice was increased with conjugates prepared with cholera toxin, pseudomonas exotoxin A or meningococcal Group B outer membrane protein. Hib conjugates, prepared with horseshoe crab haemocyanin (HCH), were more immunogenic in mice than in rhesus monkeys. This unexpected finding was in accordance with the lesser immunogenicity of this carrier protein in rhesus than in mice.

Clinical evaluation of our Hib CPS and other CPS conjugates

Following experiments with mice, rabbits and primates, we conducted a clinical evaluation of our conjugates [64]. Hib–TT, Pn6A–TT or cross-reacting *E. coli* K100 covalently bound to TT, were injected into young adult volunteers, singly or in combination, randomly assigned to groups of about 20 each. Local reactions were common and were probably due to Arthus reactivity mediated by pre-existing TT antibodies. Fever occurred in about 10% of the volunteers after the first injection; none had fever after the second injection. Similar levels of Hib or Pn6A CPS antibodies were elicited by either 50 μg or 100 μg doses or following concurrent injection of two different conjugates (Hib–TT and Pn6A–TT or Hib–TT and K100—TT). The Hib–TT elicited about a 180-fold increase in Hib antibodies and the Pn6A–TT conjugate elicited about a eight-fold increase in Pn6A CPS antibodies after one injection. Booster reactions were not elicited in adults; similar levels of post-immunization antibodies in the five groups suggested that the response elicited by the conjugates were maximal. A one-way cross-reaction was noted as Pn6A conjugates elicited two-fold or greater increases in the levels of Hib CPS antibodies in 13/20 of the volunteers; only 4/59 immunized with Hib–TT had an increase in Pn6A antibodies. Pre-immunization Hib antibodies were composed of IgM, IgA and IgG immunoglobulins. Post-immunization sera showed increases in all three isotypes; elevation of IgG was the highest of the three isotypes. Conjugate-induced antibodies to both the PS and TT exerted secondary biological activities that have been correlated with immunity. The cross-reactive Hib CPS antibodies, observed in 13/20 volunteers that received Pn6A–TT, also had bactericidal activity against Hib organisms.

All 73 volunteers examined maintained a four-fold or greater elevation of Hib CPS antibodies over their pre-immunization levels 6 months after their second immunization. The post-immunization levels declined in 6 months to about 50% of the maximum attained by immunization. The fold increases and post-immunization geometric mean antibody levels elicited by the conjugates, used in our experiments and those synthesized by other methods, were about five times higher than those elicited by the Hib CPS at the same dose, confirming the increased immunogenicity of the Hib–TT (Table II). The lack of a booster response in the adults was likely due to the high levels of antibodies to both the protein and CPS components elicited by the conjugates (probably the maximal attainable by subcutaneously injected saline solutions). Both Hib CPS and Hib conjugates induced an increase in IgM, IgA and IgG isotypes; IgG was the predominate isotype induced by both, and the level of this isotype declined the most after 6 months. Preliminary experiments indicate that the IgG subclasses and the 'clonotype', as revealed by isoelectric focusing, are similar in recipients of either the Hib CPS or the conjugate. The relative homogeneity of CPS antibodies compared to the heterogeneity of anti-protein antibodies, reported by Yount *et al.* [82], is observed in antibodies elicited by CPS as well as by CPS-protein conjugates: the difference between the serum antibodies elicited by the two immunogens seems to be quantitative not qualitative. Accordingly, it appears that both the Hib CPS and Hib–TT are stimulating lymphoid cells previously differentiated to synthesize antibodies of a single specificity.

CURRENT STATUS OF EXPERIMENTATION WITH BACTERIAL POLYSACCHARIDE–PROTEIN CONJUGATES UNDER CLINICAL INVESTIGATION

Most activity in this field has been directed towards conjugates composed of Hib CPS and carrier proteins. Conjugates prepared by Connaught Ltd, have been studied for their safety and immunogenicity in adults through infants [8, 22, 40, 41]. This firm has employed a Hib CPS–diphtheria toxoid (DT)

Table II. Comparison of the serum antibody responses elicted by *Haemophilus influenzae* type b (Hib)[a] and pneumococcus (Pn) type (Pn6A)[b] capsular polysaccharides (CPS) alone or as conjugates with tetanus (TT) or diphtheria toxoid in adult volunteers.

Vaccine	Geometric mean of anibodies			Reference
	Pre-immunization	Post-immunization	Fold increase	
Hib CPS	1.99	29.5	14.8	[22]
Hib CPS	0.56	15.9	28.4	[55]
Hib-TT	1.12	202.2	180.5	[64]
Hib-DT	3.03	248.0	75.3	[22]
Hib-DT	0.56	89.0	158.9	[3]
Pn6A CPS	220	686	3.1	[64]
Pn6A CPS	117	686	5.3	[64]
Pn6A CPS	167	1385	8.2	[64]

[a] Micrograms of antibody protein per ml.
[b] Nanograms of antibody nitrogen per ml.

conjugate, prepared by the original method of Schneerson *et al.* [60] with a modification: the Hib CPS was heated in order to reduce its molecular weight prior to activation by cyanogen bromide. No serious adverse reactions were observed in adults, children and infants injected with wt μg of the vaccine (calculated on the basis of the Hib CPS content of the vaccine). Hib CPS antibodies elicited by the Hib CPS–DT had similar bactericidal and opsonic activities to antibodies elicited by the Hib CPS. Vaccinates injected with the conjugate responded with IgG Hib CPS antibodies and there was a booster response observed in children. The immunogenicity of the Hib CPS–DT in infants, however, was disappointing; only one-half of vaccinates in this age-group responded with protective levels of Hib CPS antibodies [13]. Currently, an effectiveness trial of this conjugate in Alaskan Eskimo infants is going on [79, 80] (it should be noted that the attack rate is considerably higher and age-distribution of Hib meningitis in this selected population is lower than in most infants and children in the USA, with about 50% of the cases occurring in infants of 6 months or less). Our original scheme was modified to make adipic hydrazide derivatives of the Hib CPS, rather than the carrier protein, and coupling this intermediate to carrier proteins by carbodiimide condensation [9]. Comparison of these two synthetic schemes indicated that conjugates made by the latter procedure elicit more Hib CPS and carrier protein antibodies [13].

Another method for synthesizing Hib CPS conjugates, using a spacer and forming a lattice, has been proposed by Marburg *et al.*, at Merck, Sharp & Dohme [43]. These workers replaced the metallic cation of the Hib CPS (usually sodium or calcium depending upon the purification process) with *t*-

butyl ammoniun ions [12, 85]. The resultant Hib CPS compound was soluble in organic solvents. Hydroxyls were activated with *N,N'*-carbonyldiimidazole and a propylamino moiety was added as a spacer to bind the Hib CPS to Group B meningococcal outer membrane proteins (OMP) via a sulphhydryl bond. The Hib CPS–Group B meningococcal OMP elicited antibodies in adults, children and infants [13]. The Hib CPS–OMP conjugate elicited protective levels of Hib CPS antibodies in 10/10 infants after three injections. The choice of Group B meningococcal OMP may require further investigation by these workers; their preparation contained higher levels of lipopolysaccharide (LPS or endoxtoxin) than have been tolerated for vaccines composed of Group A, C, Y and W135 CPS. The conjugate had to be adsorbed to aluminium hydroxide in order to avoid systemic reactions, including fever, in the infants. Further improvement in the purity of the carrier protein for this conjugate is required if it is to be incorporated into the formulation of infant immunizations. The levels and secondary biological activities of, antibodies elicited by the OPM preparation towards Group B meningococci were not cited.

Anderson reported the synthesis of conjugates composed of oligosaccharides of Hib CPS bound to the non-toxic CRM_{197} protein of *Corynebacteria diphtheria* [1, 2, 4]. The concentration of terminal reducing groups in the Hib CPS was increased by controlled acid hydrolysis. The aldehyde groups of the oligosaccharides were bound to the protein by reductive amination. This type of conjugate contained about one to three oligosaccharides per protein molecule. Recently, Anderson has reported an improvement in this synthesis which increased the amount of oligosaccharides bound to the carrier protein [3]. Hib CPS was subjected to limited periodate oxidation. This reaction requires the presence of vicinal hydroxyls which are confined to the ribitol moieties of the Hib CPS [85]. Theoretically, oligosaccharides are created by this reaction which have aldehydes at both ends. The periodate-treated Hib CPS was subjected to gel filtration and oligosaccharides, with about 8 and about 20 repeating units, were isolated. These two preparations of oligosaccharides, presumably differing only in their molecular weights, were then individually bound to DT by reductive amination. Analysis of these conjugates by gel filtration showed a small proportion that was of high molecular weight, presumed by these investigators to be composed of a lattice formed by the bifunctional oligosaccharides cross-linking the carrier protein. The two conjugates, formed with the oligosaccharides of 8 or 20 repeating units, elicited similar levels of Hib CPS antibodies in adults (interpretation of these data is difficult since only three subjects were in each experimental group). Both increased immunogenicity and T-dependence were demonstrated in adults and children with both conjugates. Interestingly, only the conjugate prepared with the oligosaccharides composed of 20 repeating units induced protective levels of Hib CPs antibodies consistently in infants. Antibodies to both Hib CPS and DT elicited by this conjugate had secondary biological properties correlated with immunity. A more detailed analysis of the Hib CPS antibodies elicited in infants by the conjugates has been reported by these workers [25]. Using the technique of isoelectric focusing and radioautography with ^{125}I-labelled Hib CPS, the authors have demonstrated that serum Hib CPS antibodies elicited by the conjugate and the Hib CPS alone had similar oligoclonal properties. We have confirmed their results identifying this oligoclonal property of the Hib CPS antibodies in adult subjects.

CONJUGATES FOR THE PREVENTION AND TREATMENT OF HOSPITAL-ACQUIRED INFECTIONS

The diverse aetiologies, frequency, morbidity and mortality of hospital-acquired infections continue to pose serious problems. Active immunization is not a realistic possibility for prevention of these infections because most of these patients have depressed antibody synthesis or acquire their disease soon after their hospital admission. A leading cause of serious infections among hospitalized patients with decreased resistance is *Pseudomonas aeruginosa*. Pre-existing serum antibodies to the LPS and exotoxin A of this organism have been shown to confer protection against invasive infection with this organism [11, 49]. Cryz *et al.* [11] have approached the problem of hospital-acquired infections due to *P. aeruginosa* by preparing a conjugate composed of the *O*-specific side-chain of LPS bound to exotoxin A. An aldehyde derivative of the LPS, created by limited periodate oxidation, was bound to the adipic hydrazide derivative of the exotoxin A by reductive amination. The conjugate was separated from the unreacted exotoxin A and the LPS by gel filtration. The LPS used for synthesis of the conjugate had a molecular weight of about 50 000 and should have had multipoint attachment to the exotoxin A. The nature of the conjugate, i.e. its molecular weight and whether or not a lattice was formed, was not discussed. Rabbits immunized with this conjugate responded with both LPS and exotoxin A antibodies; the post-immunization sera had both anti-bacterial and anti-toxin activities. Preliminary studies in adult volunteers showed no serious local or systemic adverse reactions. Vaccinates responded with both LPS-specific and exotoxin A antibodies that had protective secondary biological activities (personal communication from Dr Cryz). It is planned to evaluate such vaccine-induced antibodies in healthy adults as passive immunization reagents in patients at risk for invasive diseases due to *P. aeruginosa*.

Variables affecting the immunogenicity of conjugates

Molecular weight of the polysaccharide

In their original experiments, Avery and Goebel reported that Pn type 3 CPS formed a more immunogenic conjugate than its disaccharide repeating unit [6, 19, 20]. Since then, many investigators, including us, have confirmed the increased immunogenicity of conjugates made with higher molecular weight PS [4, 72]. Seppela *et al.* [67] suggested that there is an optimal immunogenic size of the PS component of a conjugate. The immunogenicity of albumin–dextran conjugates, prepared with dextrans of high, intermediate and low molecular weights, was compared [67]. The highest levels of anti-dextran antibodies were elicited by conjugates with dextran of intermediate size (*circa* 40 000). Interpretation of these data must take into consideration the difficulties in preparing conjugates with dextrans of varying sizes as their only variable. The extent of derivatization of the dextran with adipic acid dihydrazide, the ratio of protein to carbohydrate and the molecular weights of these conjugates, prepared with dextrans of varying sizes, were different. We have not explored this approach extensively. Our preliminary results show that conjugates composed of CPS of higher molecular weight are better immunogens; a decrease in immunogenicity with our highest molecular weight Hib CPS, Pn6A CPS and the Vi CPS of *Salmonella typhi* was not observed.

Spatial relation between the polysaccharide and the protein ('spacer' effect)

The binding of some ligands to their parent molecule is reduced when they are directly attached to a macromolecule such as an insoluble PS [32, 37, 81]. This reduced binding may be restored if the ligand is bound to the PS via a 'spacer'. The explanation for this has been that steric hindrance, due to the proximity of the ligand to the support, interferes with its binding to the parent molecule. Similar phenomena have been demonstrated for hapten–protein conjugates [17, 75]. The immunogenicity of DNP and arsenilic acid were related to the length of the spacer between them and their site of attachment to the protein. These findings may offer another explanation for Svenson's findings that a single repeat unit of *S. typhimurium O*-specific side-chain bound to a protein was not immunogenic despite its ability to bind to antibodies [74]. Oligosaccharides of two or more repeat units were required for conjugates to elicit antibodies specific for the PS. The explanation for this, and other similar findings, has been that the disaccharide is too small to interact with the combining site of the *O*-specific antibodies and trigger B-cell differentiation and antibody formation. Another possibility however, is that the first repeat unit of the more immunogenic octasaccharide could have served as a 'spacer'. This possibility could be experimentally tested. Stearyl derivatives of trisaccharides, however, elicited anti-dextran antibodies [38], suggesting that the hindrance of the antigenic determinant caused by the carrier protein resulted in the lack of immunogenicity of the disaccharide–protein conjugate. We also observed this 'spacer' effect in our early attempts to synthesize Hib CPS conjugates in high yields. By themselves, only about 3% of the reactants formed a conjugate. A slightly higher yield of conjugate was achieved by treatment of BSA with the *N*-carboxanhydride (Leuch's anhydride) of L-alanine. This reaction results in the formation of multiple short chains of D-alanine to emanate from the surface of the protein ending in an alpha amino acid. This resultant poly-L-ala-BSA, when reacted with cyanogen bromide-activated Hib CPS formed a conjugate in slightly higher yield than the previous reaction. Low yields of conjugates were also obtained with protein derivatives of diaminohexane (this compound is similar to adipic acid dihydrazide except that the latter has more nucleophilic end groups). In contrast, adipic hydrazide derivatives with the same 6-carbon spacer but with more active nucleophilic end groups combined readily with the activated Hib CPS to form conjugates in high yields [9].

Configuration of polysaccharide–protein conjugates

Conjugates synthesized to date for clinical evaluation may be divided into two types, based upon their supposed overall configuration. The first approach, uses multiple attachments of both components to form a lattice (see Table I). Spacers, such as adipic acid or diaminopropyl, have been used to facilitate the binding of the PS to the protein [8, 9, 11, 13, 22, 33, 40, 41, 43, 60–64, 66]. The molecular weight of such conjugates may be very high. The second approach to synthesizing conjugates uses oligosaccharides. The naturally occurring aldehyde moiety at the reducing end, or a derivative created either at the reducing or non-reducing end, is bound to the carrier protein: the configuration of the resultant conjugate may be described as a sun (protein) with rays (oligosaccharides). Several techniques have been used to bind these oligosaccharides covalently to the protein carrier; reductive amination facilitated by cyanoborohydride, perhaps modified by new findings, has been used [59]. There may be a limit to the molecular weight of the PS, especially those with a negatively charged moiety in their repeat unit, that could be bound by their reducing end to the carrier protein. Comparative studies of conjugates composed of the same CPS and carrier protein, prepared by the two different methods, have not been reported.

Carrier protein

It is probable that much of the information gained by the study of haptens is applicable to the understanding of the immunological properties of PS–protein conjugates. The covalent binding to a protein imparts new immunological properties to a hapten (PS). The immunogenicity of the carrier protein is an important factor in determining the amount of antibody directed towards the hapten or PS. For example, little or no anti-hapten antibody is elicited by conjugates prepared with homologous serum proteins. The results obtained with Hib CPS conjugate prepared with HCH-injected into mice and rhesus monkeys provide further evidence. High levels of specific antibodies in mice were elicited by HCH [9]. Juvenile rhesus monkeys, unexpectedly, responded poorly to this protein antigen. Correspondingly, Hib–HCH elicited high levels of Hib CPS antibodies in mice and low levels in the rhesus monkeys [62]. No increase in the immunogenicity of Hib CPS was observed when it was bound to Pn type 3 CPS [60], another T-independent antigen (there are numerous other examples in the literature). A T-independent response to the DNP hapten was elicited by DNP conjugated to Pn type 3 CPS [44]. Guinea-pigs, unresponsive to DNP when presented as a conjugate of poly-L-lysine, responded with antibody formation when this hapten-cationic polymer was complexed to the polyanionic carrier methylated bovine serum albumin [23]. Similar results were obtained with the non-immunogenic DNA and DNA-methylated bovine albumin complexes. The immune response to the hapten (PS) elicited by conjugates does not take on all of the characteristics of the protein carrier: the restricted nature of the anti-PS antibodies elicited is preserved even when induced by PS–protein conjugates. The antibodies elicted by conjugates are qualitatively similar but quantitatively higher than those elicted by the CPS. The subclass homogeneity of the CPS antibodies elicited by the conjugates are unaffected by the heterogeneity of the antibodies specific to the protein [24]. In our clinical study in adults pre- and post-immunization levels of TT and Hib CPS antibodies were unrelated, indicating that the pre-immune status was unrelated to the magnitude of the immune response elicited by the conjugate to either of its components.

What is the mechanism (or mechanisms) by which conjugates impart increased immunogenicity and T-dependence to PS?

An enormous literature followed Mitchison's article describing the carrier effect [34, 45]. Yet, to our minds, there is no satisfying explanation for the differences in the serum antibodies elicited by a subcutaneous injection of a saline solution of the Hib CPS contrasted to that elicited by Hib–TT. The applicability of data from studies of both hapten and PS protein conjugates to the problem of inducing immunity in infants to invasive bacterial infections must take into account the restrictions imposed on delivering vaccines to humans, e.g. data from experiments using the intravenous, intraperitoneal routes of immunization of incorporation of the immunogen into Freund's adjuvant have a limited value in considering the problem of vaccinating healthy infants.

What qualities confer both an increased immunogenicity and T-dependence to Hib CPS (and to other PS) when injected in a clinically acceptable fashion? A review of our and others' failure to increase the immunogenicity of PS in infants by modifications of the PS, or by synthetic schemes other than the formation of conjugates, provides some insight into this problem. These unsuccessful attempts to increase the immunogenicity of Hib CPS and other PS are listed.

1. Use of established adjuvants: adsorption on to aluminium hydroxide or incorporation with complete Freund's adjuvant [55, 60].
2. Mix Hib CPS with DTP in order to exploit the adjuvant effect of *Bordetella pertussis* [16, 36].
3. Randomly acylate Hib CPS with fatty acid derivatives [Schneerson, Liu, unpublished].
4. Form multivalent electrostatic charge complexes with methylated proteins [61].
5. Incorporation of fatty acid derivatives of Hib PS into liposomes [Schneerson, Lieve, unpublished].
6. Formation of multivalent electrostatic charge complexes of Hib CPS with positively charged synthetic peptides [61].
7. Polymerization of Hib CPS to a higher molecular weight by creating additional PO_4 [Schneerson, Liu, unpublished] bonds or by covalently binding it to Pn type 3 CPS (61).
8. Non-covalent complexes formed with outer membrane proteins of Hib CPS and Group B meningococcal CPS [2, 78, 84].
9. Formation of Hib CPS–antibody complexes in antibody or antigen excess or at equivalence [Schneerson, Robbins, Barrera, unpublished].
10. Covalent addition of muramic acid dipeptide or its derivatives to meningococcal Group C CPS [51, 52] or admixture with Hib CPS [Schneerson, Robbins *et al.*, unpublished

To date, only conjugates composed of CPS of sufficient size, covalently attached to an immunogenic and T-dependent carrier confer increased immunogenicity and T-dependence to the CPS when prepared in a clinically acceptable fashion (only protein carriers have been found to confer these properties though Ficoll, a polymer of polymerized fructose, has been shown to serve as an immunogenic and T-independent carrier for haptens) [75]. 'Complexes' formed by non-covalent forces, such as those formed between outer membrane proteins of gram-negative bacteria, polycations such as methylated albumins and synthetic polypeptides or Hib CPS-antibody precipitates, elicited anti-PS antibodies when injected either intravenously or intraperitoneally into mice or rabbits. Yet, these 'complexes' did not elicit increased levels of CPS antibodies when injected subcutaneously [2]. Similar findings have been reported for 'complexes' of outer membrane proteins of Group B meningococci with its CPS [78, 85]. Repeated intravenous injections of capsulated bacteria into laboratory animals elicited levels of Hib CPS and other CPS antibodies that are among the highest achieved by any immunization scheme. These bacteria elicit lower levels of Hib CPS antibodies than our Hib–TT when injected subcutaneously. It is probable that intravenous injection avoids a cellular or metabolic step encountered by immunogens injected subcutaneously, which permits a direct interaction with T cells in the spleen.

What can we deduce from the observation that the bond with the protein must be covalent in order to impart the properties of increased immunogenicity and T-dependence to the PS when the conjugate is injected subcutaneously? First, it is likely that the conjugate is transported to lymphoid tissue adjacent to the injection site. There, the conjugate is subjected to physicochemical modification that does not disturb the proximity of the protein and the PS (presumably 'complexes' would be disrupted by this process). Second, the protein component of the 'processed' conjugate interacts with and stimulates a T-cell response that results in the differentiation and secretion of both anti-protein and anti-PS antibodies. The B cells that respond to this signal and synthesize anti-PS antibodies are 'qualitatively' the same as those elicited by the PS alone. This is deduced from the observations that the isotype, IgG subclass, 'clonotype' and biological activities of the Hib CPS and conjugate-induced antibodies are qualitatively indistinguishable from those elicited by the CPS alone (the authors point out that only incomplete information for one CPS is available at this time). Do these B cells respond to signals (presumably lymphokines) synthesized by carrier-specific T cells or to T cells stimulated by the conjugate but that are specific for the PS? The experiments with haptens suggest that the latter possibility is not the case; the secondary response to the hapten is induced by the original carrier protein only. Insel *et al.* have suggested that the Hib CPS conjugates may directly stimulate B cells. According to their hypothesis, T cells may act as helper cells only after they have recognized a surface membrane complex formed by class II histocompatibility antigen and the 'processed' carrier protein on the B cell [24]. The proposed carrier-induced T-cell signal for PS synthesis is antigen-specific; there is no detectable change in the levels of other PS antibodies [60, 62, 64]. Another possibility is that the conjugate induces a T cell–macrophage interaction, that is, an antigen-specific B-cell stimulant. We plan to test this hypothesis further. Knowledge of both the structural and the immunological properties of conjugates will be essential for predicting their *in vivo* actions (standardization).

SUMMARY

Polysaccharide–protein conjugates, acceptable for clinical use, provide immunologists with compounds similar to the hapten and PS conjugates used to explore lymphoid structure and function in animals. There is reason to expect that clinical and *in vitro* studies of conjugates will provide new and important information about the human immune response. We are excited by the observations that conjugates elicit more CPS antibodies in animals than Hib organisms as well as in patients (especially infants) that have recovered from systemic infection or asymptomatic colonization with Hib. These semi-synthetic vaccines seem to be better immunogens for Hib CPS antibodies than the homologous bacteria or other stimuli encountered in nature. There is reason to expect that a similar increase in immunogenicity can be achieved for CPS conjugates of other encapsulated bacterial pathogens. Conjugates for infants will have to be compatible with DPT vaccines in order not to exceed our public health resources. Our information about the 'priming' effect of tetanus and diphtheria toxoids on conjugates prepared with these carrier proteins as well as the enhanced CPS and protein antibody responses in animals injected with TT and Hib CPS–TT concurrently suggest that this will be feasible. Polysaccharide–protein conjugates may be able to immunize patients with certain immunodeficiencies and to protect patients from hospital-acquired infections by passive immunization with immune sera from recipients of these new semi-synthetic vaccines.

REFERENCES

1. Anderson, P. Antibody responses to *Haemophilus influenzae* type b and diphtheria toxin induced by conjugates of oligosaccharides of the type b capsule with the nontoxic protein CRM 197. *Infect. Immun.*, **39**, 233–8 (1983).
2. Anderson, P., Insel, R. A., Farsad, P., Smith, D. H., and Petrusick, T. Immunogenicity of 'aggregated PRP', 'PRP complex' and covalent conjugates of PRP with a diphtheria toxin. In *Haemophilus influenzae. Epidemiology, Immunology and Prevention of Disease.* (ed. S. H. Sell and P. Wright), Elsevier Science Publishing Co., Inc. New York, 1982, pp. 275–83.
3. Anderson, P. W., Pichichero, M. E., Insel, R. A., Betts, R., Eby, R., and Smith, D. H. Vaccines consisting of periodate-cleaved oligosaccharides from the capsule of *Haemophilus influenzae* type b coupled to a protein carrier: structural and temporal requirements for priming in the human infant. *J. Immunol.*, **137**, 1181–6 (1986).
4. Anderson, P., Pichichero, M., Insel, R., Farsad, P., and Santosham, M. Capsular antigens noncovalently or covalently associated with protein as vaccines to *Haemophilus influenzae* type b: comparison in two-year-old children. *J. Infect. Dis.*, **152**, 634–6 (1985).
5. Austrian, R. Pneumococcal infections. In *Bacterial Vaccines* (ed. R. Germanier), Academic Press, New York, 1984, pp. 257–88.

6. Avery, O. T., and Goebel, W. F. Chemo-immunological studies on conjugated carbohydrate-proteins. II. Immunological specificity of synthetic sugar-proteins. *J. Exp. Med.*, **50**, 521–33 (1929).
7. Beuvery, E. C., van Rossum, F., and Nagle, J. Comparison of the induction of immunoglobulin M and G antibodies in mice with purified pneumococcal type 3 and meningococcal group C polysaccharides and their protein conjugates. *Infect. Immun.*, **37**, 15–22 (1982).
8. Cates, K. L., Marsh, K. H., and Granoff, D. M. Serum opsonic activity after immunization of adults with *Haemophilus influenzae* type b-diphtheria toxoid conjugate vaccine. *Infect. Immun.*, **48**, 183–9 (1985).
9. Chu, CY., Schneerson, R., Robbins, J. B., and Rastogi, S. C. Further studies on the immunogenicity of *Haemophilus influenzae* type b and pneumococcal type 6A polysaccharide protein conjugates. *Infect. Immun.*, **50**, 245–56 (1983).
10. Cochi, S. L., Broome, C. V., and Hightower, A. W. Immunization of US children with *Hemophilus influenzae* type b polysaccharide vaccine. *J. Amer. Med. Assoc.*, **253**, 521–9 (1985).
11. Cryz, S. J. Jr, Furer, E., Sadoff, J. C., and Germanier, R. *Pseudomonas aeruginosa* immunotype 5 polysaccharide-toxin A conjugate vaccine. *Infect. Immun.*, **52**, 161–5 (1986).
12. Egan, W., Schneerson, R., Werner, K. E., and Zon, G. Structural studies and chemistry of bacterial capsular polysaccharides. Investigations of phosphodiester-linked capsular polysaccharides isolated from *Haemophilus influenzae* types 1, b, c, and f: NMR spectroscopic identification and chemical modification of endgroups and the nature of base-catalyzed hydrolytic depolymerization. *J. Amer. Chem. Soc.*, **104**, 2898–910 (1982).
13. Einhorn, M. S., Weinberg, G. A., Anderson, E. L., Granoff, P. D., and Granoff, D. M. Immunogenicity in infants of *Haemophilus influenzae* type B polysaccharide in a conjugate vaccine with *Neisseria meningitidis* outer-membrane protein. *Lancet*, **ii**, 299–302 (1986).
14. Ekborg, G. K., Elkind, P. J., Garegg, P. J., Gotthammar, B., Carlsson, H. E., Lindberg, A. A., and Svenungsson, B. Artificial dissaccharide protein conjugates as immunogens for the preparation of specific anti-*Salmonella* O-antisera. *Immunochem.*, **14**, 153–7 (1977).
15. Ekborg, G. K., Elkind, P. J., Garegg, P. J., Gotthammar, B., Carlsson, H. E., Svenson, S. B., and Lindberg, A. A. Artificial salmonella vaccines: *Salmonella typhimurium* O-antigen-specific oligosaccharide–protein conjugates elicit protective antibodies in rabbits and mice. *Infect. Immun.*, **32**, 490–6 (1981).
16. Eskola, J., Peltola, H., Makela, P. H., Kayhty, H., Karanko, V., Samuelson, J., and Gordon, L. K. Antibody levels achieved in infants by course of *Haemophilus influenzae* type b polysaccharide/diphtheria toxoid conjugate vaccine. *Lancet*, **i**, 1184–6 (1985).
17. Fong, S., Nitecki, D. E., Cook, R. M., and Goodman, J. W. Spatial requirements between haptenic and carrier determinants for T-dependent antibody responses. *J. Exp. Med.*, **148**, 817–22 (1978).
18. Geyer, H., Stirm, S., and Himmelspach, K. Immunochemical properties of oligosaccharide protein conjugate with *Klebsiella*-K2 specificity. I. Specificity and cross-reactivity of anti-conjugate versus anti-bacterial antibodies. *Med. Microbiol. Immunol.*, **165**, 271–88 (1979).
19. Goebel, W. F. Chemo-immunological studies on conjugated carbohydrate-proteins. XII. The immunological properties of an artificial antigen containing cellobiuronic acid. *J. Exp. Med.*, **50**, 469–520 (1929).

20. Goebel, W. F., and Avery, O. T. Chemo-immunological studies on conjugated carbohydrate protein. I. The synthesis of p-aminophenol β-glucoside, p-aminophenol β-galactoside and their coupling with serum globulin. *J. Exp. Med.*, **50**, 521–32 (1929).
21. Gotschlich, E. C. Meningococcal meningitis. In *Bacterial Vaccines* (ed. R. Germanier), Academic Press, New York, 1984, pp. 237–52.
22. Granoff, D. M., Boies, E. G., and Munson, R. S. Immunogenicity of *Haemophilus influenzae* type b polysaccharide-diphtheria toxoid conjugate vaccine in adults. *J. Pediat.*, **105**, 22–7 (1984).
23. Green, I., Vassallii, P., and Benacerraf, B. Cellular location of anti-DNP-PLL and anti-conveyer albumin antibody in genetically non-responder guinea pig with DNP-PLL albumin complexes. *J. Exp. Med.*, **125**, 527–36 (1967).
24. Insel, R. A., and Anderson, P. W. Oligosaccharide-protein conjugate vaccines induce and prime for oligoclonal IgG antibody response to the *Haemophilus influenzae* type b capsular polysaccharide in human infants. *J. Exp. Med.*, **163**, 262–9 (1985).
25. Insel, R. A., and Anderson, P. W. Response to oligosaccharide-protein conjugate vaccine against *Haemophilus influenzae* type b in two patients with IgG2 deficiency response to capsular polysaccharide vaccine. *New Eng. J. Med.*, **315**, 499–501 (1986).
26. Insel, R. A., Kittelberger, A., and Anderson, P. Isoelectric focusing of human antibody to the *Haemophilus influenzae* type b capsular polysaccharide: restricted and identical spectrotypes in adults. *J. Immunol.*, **135**, 2810/15 (1985).
27. Jennings, H., and Lugowski, C. Immunochemistry of Groups A, B and C meningococcal polysaccharide tetanus toxoid conjugates. *J. Immunol.*, **127**, 104–8 (1981).
28. Jennings, H. J., Lugowski, C., and Ashton, F. E. Conjugation of meningococcal lipopolysaccharide R-type oligosaccharides to tetanus toxoid as route to a potential vaccine against Group B *Neisseria meningitidis. Infect. Immun.*, **43**, 407–12 (1984).
29. Jennings, H. J., Roy, R., and Gamian, A. Induction of meningococcal Group B polysaccharide-specific IgG antibodies in mice by using an *N*-propionylated B polysaccharide-tetanus toxoid conjugate vaccine. *J. Immunol.*, **137**, 1708–13 (1986).
30. Jorbeck, H. J. A., Svenson, S. B., and Lindberg, A. A. Artificial *Salmonella typhimurium* O-antigen-specific oligosaccharide–protein conjugates elicit opsoninizing antibodies that enhance phagocytosis. *Infect. Immun.*, **32**, 497–502 (1981).
31. Jenkin, C. R., Karnovsky, M., and Rowley, D. Preparation of an artificial antigen and immunity to mouse typhoid. *Immunol.*, **13**, 361–8 (1967).
32. Jost, R., Miron, T., and Wilchek, M. The mode of absorption of proteins to aliphatic and aromatic amines coupled to cyanogen bromide activated agarose. *Biochim. Biophys. Acta*, **362**, 75–81 (1974).
33. Kaijser, B., Larsson, P., Olling, S., and Schneerson, R. Protection against acute ascending pyelonephritis caused by *Escherichia coli* in rats using isolated capsular antigen conjugated to bovine serum albumin. *Infect. Immun.*, **39**, 142–9 (1983).
34. Katz, D., Paul, W. E., Goidl, E., and Benacerraf, B. Carrier function in anti-hapten immune responses. I. Enhancement of primary and secondary anti-hapten responses by carrier preimmunization. *J. Exp. Med.*, **132**, 261–74 (1970).
35. Kayhty, H., Karanko, V., Peltola, H., and Makela, P. H. Serum antibodies after vaccination with *Haemophilus influenzae* type b capsular polysaccharide and

responses to reimmunization: no evidence of immunological tolerance or memory. *Pediatrics*, **74**, 857–65 (1984).
36. King, S. D., Wynter, H., Ramlal, A., Moodie, K., Castle, D., Kuo, J. S. C., Barnes, L., and Williams, C. L. Safety and immunogenicity of a new *Haemophilus influenzae* type b vaccine in infants under one year of age. *Lancet*, **ii**, 705/708 (1981).
37. Kohn, J., and Wilchek, M. Activation of polysaccharide resins by CnBr. In *Solid Phase Biochemistry* (ed. W. H. Scouten), John Wiley & Sons, 1983, pp. 599–629.
38. Lai, E., and Kabat, E. A. Immunochemicsl studies of conjugates of isomaltosyl oligosaccharides to lipid. Production and characterization of mouse hybridomas specific for stearyl-isomaltosyl oligosaccharides. *Molec. Immunol.*, **22**, 1021–37 (1985).
39. Lambden, P. R., and Heckels, J. E. Synthesis of immunogenic oligosaccharide-protein conjugates from the lipopolysaccharide of *Neisseria gonorrhoeae* P9. *J. Immunol. Methods*, **48**, 233–40 (1982).
40. Lepow, M., Randolph, M., Cimma, R., Larsen, D., Ragon, M., Schumacher, J., Lent, B., Gaintner, S., Samuelson, J., and Gordon, L. Persistence of antibody and response to booster dose of *Haemophilus influenzae* type b polysaccharide diphtheria toxoid conjugate vaccine in infants immunized at 9 to 15 months of age. *J. Pediat.*, **108**, 882–6 (1986).
41. Lepow, M. L., Samuelson, J. S., and Gordon, L. K. Safety and immunogenicity of *Haemophilus influenzae* type b polysaccharide-diphtheria toxoid vaccine in infants 9 to 15 months of age. *J. Pediat.*, **106**, 185–90 (1985).
42. Lindberg, A. A., Rosenberg, L. T., Ljunggren, A., Haregg, P. J., and Wallin, N.-H. Effect of synthetic dissacharide–protein conjugate as an immunogen in *Salmonella* in mice. *Infect. Immun.*, **10**, 541–50 (1974).
43. Marburg, S., Jorn, D., Tolman, L., Arison, B., McCauley, J., Kniskern, P. J., Hagopian, A., and Vella, P. P. Bimolecular chemistry of macromolecules: synthesis of bacterial polysaccharide conjugates with *N. meningitidis* membrane protein. *J. Amer. Chem. Soc.*, **108**, 5282–7 (1986).
44. Mitchell, G. F., Humphrey, J. H., and Williamson, A. R. Inhibition of secondary anti-hapten responses with the hapten coupled to type 3 pneumococcal polysaccharide. *Eur. J. Immunol.*, **2**, 460–4 (1972).
45. Mitchison, N. A. The carrier effect in the secondary response to hapten-protein conjugates. II. Cellular cooperation. *Eur. J. Immunol.*, **1**, 18–30 (1971).
46. Moxon, R., and Murphy, P. A. *Haemophilus influenzae* bacteremia and meningitis resulting from the survival of a single organism. *Proc. Natl. Acad. Sci. USA*, **75**, 153–6 (1978).
47. Osborn, J. J., Dancis, J., and Julia, J. F. Studies on the immunology of the newborn infant. II. Interference with active immunization by passive transplacental circulating antibody. *Pediat.*, **10**, 328–33 (1952).
48. Parke, J. C. Jr, Schneerson, R., and Robbins, J. B. The attack rate, *influenzae* type b meningitis in Mecklenburg County, North Carolina. *J. Pediat*,, **81**, 765–9 (1972).
49. Pollack, M., and Young, L. S. Protective activity of antibodies to exotoxin A and lipopolysaccharide at the onset of *Pseudomonas aeruginosa* septicemia in man. *J. Clin. Invest.*, **63**, 276–86 (1979).
50. Peltola, H., Käyhty, H., Virtanen, M., and Mäkelä, P. H. Prevention of *Haemophilus influenzae* type b bacteremic infections with the capsular polysaccharide vaccine. *New. Eng. J. Med.*, **310**, 1561–6 (1984).
51. Ponpipom, M. M., and Rupprecht, K. M. Methyl b-glycosides of *N*-acetyl-6-0(*w*-

aminoacyl)muramyl-L-alanyl-D-isoglutamines, and their conjugates with meningococcal Group C polysaccharide. *Carb. Res.*, **113**, 45–56 (1983).
52. Ponpipom, M. M., and Rupprecht, K. M. *w*-aminoalkyl *b*-glycosides of *N*-acetylmuramyl-L-alanyl-D-isoglutamine, and their conjugates with meningococcal Group C polysaccharide. *Carb. Res.*, **113**, 57–62 (1983).
53. Porro, M., Costantino, S., Viti, S., Vannozzi, F., Naggi, A., and Torri, G. Specific antibodies to diphtheria toxin and type 6A pneumococcal capsular polysaccharide induced by a model of semi-synthetic glycoconjugate antigen. *Mol. Immunol.*, **22**, 907–19 (1985).
54. Porro, M., Constantino, P., Giovannoni, F., Pellegrini, V., Tagliaferri, L., Vannozzi, F., and Viti, S. A molecular model of artificial glycoprotein with predetermined multiple immunodeterminants for Gram-negative and Gram-positive encapsulated bacteria. *Mol. Immunol.*, **23**, 385–91 (1986).
55. Robbins, J. B., Parke, J. C., Schneerson, R., and Whisnant, J. K. Quantitative measurement of 'natural' and immunization-induced *Haemophilus influenzae* type b capsular polysaccharide antibodies. *Pediat. Res.*, **7**, 103–10 (1973).
56. Robbins, J. B., Schneerson, R., Egan, W. B., Vann, W., and Liu, D. T. Virulence properties of bacterial capsular polysaccharides – unanswered questions. In *The Molecular Basis of Microbial Pathogenicity* (ed.) H. Smith, J. J. Skehel and M. J. Turner), Dahlem Konferenzen, 22–26 October 1980, Verlag Chemie GmbH, Weinheim, 1980, pp. 115–32.
57. Robbins, J. B., Schneerson, R., and Pittman, M. *Haemophilus influenzae* type b infections. In *Bacterial Vaccines* (ed. R. Germanier), Academic Press, New York, 1984, pp. 289–316.
58. Robertsson, J. A., Svenson, S. B., and Lindberg, A. A. *Salmonella typhimurium* infection in calves: delayed specific skin reactions directed against the O-antigenic polysaccharide chain. *Infect. Immun.*, **34**, 328–32 (1982).
59. Roy, R., Katzenellenbogen, E., and Jennings, H. J. Improved procedures for the conjugation of oligosaccharides to protein by reductive amination. *Canad. J. Biochem. Cell Biol.*, **62**, 270–80 (1984).
60. Schneerson, R., Barrera, O., Sutton, A., and Robbins, J. B. Preparation, characterization and immunogenicity of *Haemophilus influenzae* type b polysaccharide-protein conjugates. *J. Exper. Med.*, **152**, 361–76 (1980).
61. Schneerson, R., Robbins, J. B., Barrera, O., Sutton, A., Habig, W. B., Hardegree, M. C., and Chaimovich, J. *Haemophilus influenzae* type b polysaccharide-protein conjugates: model for a new generation of capsular polysaccharide vaccines. In *New Developments with Human and Veterinary Vaccines* (ed. A. Mizrahi, I. Hertman, M. A. Klingberg and A. Kohn), Alan R. Liss, New York, 1980, pp. 77–94.
62. Schneerson, R., Robbins, J. B., Chu, C.-Y., Sutton, A., Vann, W., Vickers, J. C., London, W. T., Curfman, B., Hardegree, M. C., Shiloach, J., and Rastogi, S. C. Serum antibody responses of juvenile and infant rhesus monkeys injected with *Haemophilus influenzae* type b and pneumococcus type 6A polysaccharide-protein conjugates. *Infect. Immun.*, **45**, 582–91 (1984).
63. Schneerson, R., Robbins, J. B., Egan, W., Zon, G., Sutton, A., Vann, W. F., Kaijser, B., Hanson, L. A., and Alhstedt, S. Bacterial capsular polysaccharide conjugates. In Seminars in Infectious Disease, Vol. 4, (ed. L. Weinstein and B. N. Fields) *Bacterial Vaccines*, (ed J. B. Robbins, J. L. Hill and J. C. Sadoff, Thieme-Stratton, New York, 1982, pp. 311–21.
64. Schneerson, R., Robbins, J. B., Parke, J. C. Jr, Sutton, A., Wang, Z., Schlesselman, J. J., Schiffman, G., Bell, C., Karpas, A., and Hardegree, M. C.

Quantitative and qualitative analyses of serum *Haemophilus influenzae* type b, pneumococcus type 6A and tetanus toxin antibodies elicited by polysaccharide--protein conjugates in adult volunteers. *Infect. Immun.*, **52**, 501–18 (1986).
65. Sell, H. W., Merrill, R. E., Doyne, E. O., and Zimsky, E. P. Long-term sequelae of *Hemophilus influenzae* meningitis. *Pediat.*, **49**, 206–11 (1972).
66. Seid, R. C., and Sadoff, J. C. Preparation and characterization of detoxified lipolysaccharide–protein conjugates. *J. Biol. Chem.*, **256**, 7305–10 (1981).
67. Seppela, I., Pelkonen, J., and Makela, O. Isotypes of antibodies induced by plain dextran or a dextra-protein conjugate. *Eur. J. Immunol.*, **15**, 827–33 (1985).
68. Siber, G. R., Weitzman, S. A., Aisenberg, A. C., Weinstein, H. J., and Schiffman, G. Impaired antibody response to pneumococcal vaccine after treatment for Hodgkin's disease. *New Engl. J. Med.*, **299**, 442–8 (1978).
69. Snippe, H., Van Houte, A.-J., Van Dam, J. E. G., DeReuver, M. J., Jansze, M., and Millers, J. M. N. Immunogenic properties in mice of hexasaccharide from the capsular polysaccharide of *Streptococcus pneumoniae* type 3. *Infect. Immun.*, **40**, 856–61 (1983).
70. Sutton, A., Schneerson, R., Kendall-Morris, S., and Robbins, J. B. Differential complement resistance mediates virulence of *Haemophilus influenzae* type b. *Infect. Immun.*, **35**, 94–104 (1982).
71. Svenson, S. B., and Lindberg, A. A. Oligosaccharides-protein conjugate: a novel approach for making *Salmonella* O antigen immunogens. *FEMS Microbiol. Lett.*, **1**, 145–8 (1977).
72. Svenson, S. B., and Lindberg, A. A. Immunochemistry of Salmonella O antigens: preparation of an octasaccharide-bovine serum albumin immunogen representative of *Salmonella* serogroup O antigen and characterization of the antibody response. *J. Immunol.*, **120**, 1750–7 (1978).
73. Svenson, S. B., and Lindberg, A. A. Coupling of acid labile *Salmonella* specific oligosaccharides to macromolecular carriers. *J. Immunol. Methods*, **25**, 323–35 (1979).
74. Svenson, S. B., Nurminen, M., and Lindberg, A. A. Artificial *Salmonella* Vaccines: O-antigen oligosaccharide–protein conjugates induce protection against infection with *Salmonella typhimurium. Infect. Immun.*, **25**, 863–70 (1979).
75. Toshinori, K., Lawn, C.-Y., Amsden, A., and Leskowitz, S. Hapten-specific T cell response to azobenezenearsonate-*N*-acetyl-L-tyrosine in the Lewis rat. III. Effects of peptide-spacer structure on eliciting ASA-specific helper activity with TNP-haptened ABA–peptide–Ficoll. *J. Immunol.*, **130**, 586–9 (1983).
76. Tsay, G. C., and Collins, M. S. Preparation and characterization of a nontoxic polysaccharide-protein conjugate that induces active immunity and passively protective antibody against *Pseudomonas aeruginosa* immunotype 1 in mice. *Infect. Immun.*, **45**, 217–21 (1984).
77. Wallick, S., Claflin, J. L., and Briles, D. E. Resistance to *Streptococcus pneumoniae* is induced by a phosphocholine–protein conjugate. *J. Immunol.*, **130**, 2871–5 (1983).
78. Wang, L. Y., and Frasch, C. E. Development of a *Neisseria meningitidis* Group B serotype 2b protein vaccine and evaluation in a mouse model. *Infect. Immun.*, **46**, 408–14 (1984).
79. Ward, J. J., Lum, M. K. W., and Margolis, H. S. *Haemophilus influenzae* in Alaskan eskimos: characteristics of a population with an unusual incidence of invasive disease. *Lancet*, **1**, 121–5 (1981).
80. Ward, J. I., Lum, K. W., Hallo, D. B., Silimperi, D. R., and Bender, T. R.

Invasive *Haemophilus influenzae* type b disease in Alaska: background epidemiology for a vaccine efficacy trial. *J. Infect. Dis.*, **153**, 17–26 (1986).
81. Wilchek, M., and Lamed, R. Immobilized nucleotides for affinity chromatography. *Methods Enzymol.*, **50**, 475–7 (1974).
82. Yount, W. J., Dorner, M., Kunkel, H., and Kabat, E. A. Studies on human antibodies. VI. Selective variation in subgroup composition and genetic markers, *J. Exp. Med.*, **127**, 633–46 (1968).
83. Zigterman, J. W. J., van Dam, J. E. G., Snippe, H., Rotteveel, F. T. M., Jansze, M., Willers, J. M. M., Kammerling, J. P., and Vliegenthart, J. F. G. Immunogenic properties of octosaccharide-protein conjugates derived from *Klebsiella* serotype 11 capsular polysaccharide. *Infect. Immun.*, **47**, 421–8 (1985).
84. Zollinger, W. D., Mandrell, R. E., and Griffiss, J. M. Enhancement of immunological activity by noncovalent complexing of meningococcal Group B polysaccharide and outer membrane proteins. In *Seminars in Infectious Diseases* (ed. J. B. Robbins, J. C. Hill and J. C. Sadoff), Thieme Stratton, New York, 1982, pp. 254–62.
85. Zon, G., and Robbins, J. D. ^{31}P- and ^{13}C-NMR-spectral and chemical characterization of the end-group and repeating-unit components of oligosaccharides derived by acid hydrolysis of *Haemophilus influenzae* type b capsular polysaccharide. *Carb. Res.*, **114**, 103–21 (1983).

DISCUSSION – Chaired by Professor G. L. Ada

ADA: Can we start off with clarification about this, then perhaps some might want to discuss a more general question: what is the best sort of carrier – should it be the homologous carrier, i.e. from the same organism, or should it be a heterologous carrier, such as has been used here?

MOSIER: Dr Robbins, I was very intrigued by the last point you made. Actually, the last two points: that you need a good spacer molecule and you need apparently very high epitope density to prime neonatal cells. I think these are important features to keep in mind in designing potential vaccines. It is certainly true in neonatal mice that, if one makes hapten conjugates of polyacrylamide beads, the density of conjugation must be much higher to stimulate neonatal B cells than it is to stimulate mature B cells. I think the logical inference of those kinds of experiments is that practically every immunoglobulin receptor on an immature B cell needs to be engaged before that cell can be triggered, whereas only partial binding to immunoglobulins on mature B cells seems to suffice for B-cell triggering. It also seems to be the case that putting on these longer spacers increases the possibility of multivalent binding. So I think the two features that you emphasized are very important in designing potential vaccines, making sure that you do have very high conjugation ratios and that there is a long spacer. In mice, there is an absolute threshold effect on conjugation ratio of acrylamide beads that are about a half-micron in diameter and below a certain conjugation ratio hapten one obtains no response at all.

ADA: Is this simply a reflection of the density of Ig molecules on the surface of the cell?

MOSIER: One wouldn't think so, because on neonatal B cells the absolute density of Ig molecules is actually somewhat higher than it is in mature B cells.

MORENO: Another factor that could be important here is the ratio between IgD and IgM on the surface, because the flexibility of those molecules to accommodate to different types of epitopes is different, one is far more flexible than the other.

MOSIER: Sorting B cells on the basis of sIgM : sIgD ratios makes no difference for antipolysaccharide responses. There was a lot of speculation about IgM : IgD delta ratios on neonatal B cells, and the fact that the low level of IgD expression might preclude antipolysaccharide responses. The direct experiment suggests that that is probably not the case.

JENNINGS: I would just like to point out one thing, that I am not sure the spacer *per se* is necessary, provided the oligosaccharide is long enough, because it functions as its own spacer.

ADA: How long does the antibody persist?

ROBBINS: We have checked only 6 months later, it falls to about one-half to two-thirds levels.

ADA: So you might expect it to retain high enough levels of antibody for several years in order to prevent subsequent infection by a challenge organism? Is that a fair assumption?

ROBBINS: That's right. That's what it looks like. And with these type of diseases, that's all you need to do.

ADA: That's the critical point. We now come to the second part of the discussion, either you are going to use the heterologous or the homologous carrier. The only benefit of using the homologous carrier is that if you don't have persisting antibody and you want to have a very quick response, this would be facilitated by the memory-T cells to the homologous carrier. However, if you have persistence of the antibody which would prevent infection, the use of the homologous carrier becomes less important.

ROBBINS: I would like to make a point here. There is the notion in the literature that vaccines serve to activate the immune response so that, when the host encounters the pathogen later, he will respond quickly enough to it not to have disease. That may be true, but I think the overwhelming evidence favours that the most prudent way to achieve immunity is to have in place a protective level of serum antibody to the diseases that need serum antibody and not a 'sensitized' state that *may* be sufficiently responsive to prevent disease.

ADA: I am not going to dispute that at all. The only case where it falls down is when you have antigenic variation at the B-cell level. Here, antibody produced to a previous infection is not much help against a subsequent one and one needs a rapid response in which cell-mediated immunity might be critical.

ROBBINS: I would like to make one another point about these conjugates that is interesting to me. When we first thought of this approach, many people said, 'Well you can't prevent *Haemophilus meningitis* because, when the infants get disease, they don't make antibodies so if the disease can't do it, how are you going to do it?' But tetanus does not usually confer immunity to second cases of tetanus and diphtheria did not universally confer immunity to diphtheria, and vaccinia did not universally confirm immunity to further infection with vaccinia, at least immunity usually did not last after 5–7 years. But these conjugates make antibody at an age when disease does not do it, so that we have achieved something with a semi-synthetic product that is better than the disease itself.

ADA: But have you done sufficient to show that you do not have a proportion of poor responders?

ROBBINS: The work is only beginning in infants. But it is interesting that these conjugates produce responses in animal species that do not respond to the polysaccharide itself, and if you inject mice with bacteria the conjugates make more antibody than the bacteria themselves.

SÖDERSTRÖM: I am intrigued by the parallel in time with the development of IgG_2 and IgG_4 in the infants and the capacity to respond to carbohydrate antigens. I would like to ask Dr Mosier, are there any experimental data at all to suggest that IgG_2-, and in mice, IgG_3-producing cells would require a higher epitope density?

MOSIER: I do not think there is any direct evidence, very few people have looked directly at Ig_3 responses very early in ontogeny and, certainly, there is no clear relationship between the ability to make IgG_3 and the surface Ig density, or the multivalency of antigen binding.

ROBBINS: If we could move on to the carrier protein, that is not an easy problem. We only inject two or three proteins into humans whose efficacy and usefulness has been verified. So that when one would go to another carrier protein, one would be using a material that would not, of necessity, be of use to the host, that is why we chose tetanus and diptheria, but I think the technique of using a CRM 1 is a terrific idea. We hope to be using tetanus toxid preparations from the Institut Mérieux that have been purified by affinity chromatography. It looks to me as though there is not very much difference between diphtheria and tetanus. We chose the tetanus because it was of higher molecular weight and, in general, it is a better immunogen. Concurrent injection of the carrier protein seems to have a beneficial effect, which has now been verified in preliminary clinical experiments. But those are not the best carrier proteins you can use. I think that among the many carrier proteins we have tried, probably the outer membrane proteins of Group B meningococcus and pseudomonas exotoxin A and cholera toxin have been much better than tetanus toxoid. Cholera-toxin induced serum antibodies, however, have never been shown to confer any protection against cholera. Whether cross immunity could occur to heat-labile toxins of *E. coli* we do not know. The outer membrane proteins of Group B, theoretically, should be protective but, as you know, that has not been verified by clinical study. We recently have made a conjugate of *H. influenzae* type b and a major outer-membrane protein for *H. influenzae* type b. It was something that Dr Schneerson and Dr Munson worked very hard with. We are going to verify whether or not the protective activity of that conjugate may exceed the level of polysaccharide antibodies induced by it. Our preliminary experiments show that it is a good carrier for *Haemophilus*, certainly better than tetanus, but whether or not this is an advantage of working with outer membrane protein for *Haemophilus* has to be verified. It is not easy to work with and probably will need a lot of chemical engineering to make it commercially feasible. But it can be done.

KABAT: It seems to me that some of the findings on the synthetic glycolipids suggest that these should be explored as potential antigens.

ADA: Carriers or antigens?

KABAT: The lipid is a carrier for carbohydrate antigens.

ROBBINS: Dr Kabat, we made stearic acid derivatives of the polysaccharide. Not as elegantly used as you did, these were randomly acylated. In addition to those alone, Dr Schneerson and Dr Loretta Levy collaborated to incorporate them in liposomes. In mice, they did not induce antibodies, that is not to say that it would not occur in humans, but the dextran seems to be a better immunogen in mice than are polysaccharides.

KABAT: I do not think that the stearyl group will be good enough to hold a very, very large molecule. I think you have got to work with a determinant, coupled with the stearyl moiety so that you get something where the material is on the surface of your cells.

ROBBINS: So you think that something like a 20 mer, or an 18 mer, plus the lipid and not the entire polysaccharide?

KABAT: I am not sure about a 20 mer, or an 8 mer, we have not worked with anything beyond 7, but these are all quite good. We were astounded to get the kinds of precipitating antibody that we got with dextran. I do not think that the polysaccharide has much to do with it. I think it is the size of the lipid group *versus* the size of the oligosaccharide group which we put on. Now one could consider using a branched chain fatty acid, amine, to couple, where you would have tighter binding on the cell surface.

ROBBINS: I think it is a good idea. It is a little difficult with *Haemophilus* because there is the phosphate in the repeating group, so that you have to go a couple of repeat units on either side of it to get the entire determinant.

KABAT: I think there is room for exploration of this glycolipid story.

FEIZI: Yes, I agree with Dr Kabat's comments. In fact, we are now comparing the antigenicities of neoglycolipids constructed using a variety of lipids as 'carriers'.

GRIFFISS: *Haemophilus* and *Neisseria* have outer-membrane glycolipids that bear oligosaccharides of roughly 8–12 glycoses. These are quite immunogenic during disease in infancy. The most bactericidal antibody that we have detected in the serum of children recovering from meningococcal disease has been directed at a very short oligosaccharide, probably about 5 mer. That antibody is and quite cross-reactive, and would appear to be protective. Now we would not want to use endotoxin as a vaccine *per se*. When we purify the oligosaccharide, it loses 10^2 of affinity for the antibody. But if we steriolate the oligosaccharide we recover antigenicity and recover the affinity binding. The point I want to make is that most of this conference, and indeed, most of our thoughts, have been structured around how to make the immune system of the infant respond to the antigens we wish it to respond to, namely, the capsular polysaccharide. But there is an alternative set of glycose antigens on the surface of, at least, *Meningococcus* and *Haemophilus*, to which the infant is fully capable of responding. An alternative approach would be to take advantage of the natural responsiveness of the infant and work with it.

JENNINGS: There are a couple of points I would like to make. As this technology develops, it is obvious that we will need a greater repertoire of proteins. It seems that the outer membrane proteins are probably the most obvious candidates. But, there was a point made yesterday, I think by Dr Mosier, where he said that you may be able to use proteins that might be more mitogenic or something like that, which would also be an advantage in preparing these conjugate vaccines.

ADA: I think that that comes back to the question that we raised earlier. Theoretically, the proteins from the same organism should be better carriers. If you wish to stimulate the immune response quickly when you get infection by the pathogenic organism. If you can get persisting antibody production so that antibody is present when the organism comes and so will prevent infection, then the carrier becomes a less critical point. Is my interpretation correct Dr Robbins?

ROBBINS: I am sure that is your interpretation. Whether it is right we will have to find out! Outer membrane proteins are very difficult to work with, they aggregate, they are the dickens to work with.

ADA: If I interpret correctly what you said this morning, adults naturally become immune to these organisms. Is that so?

ROBBINS: Older children do.

ADA: Right, older children do. Then your real requirement is to get a system which causes antibody production to persist for a certain number of years. What is that number?

ROBBINS: It is to erase that period when maternally derived antibodies have disappeared and the natural immunity hasn't . . ., it is about 5 years.
ADA: Five years. So you need a system using any conjugate basically, which causes antibody production for that period of time. That seems to be the answer.
ROBBINS: What is nice about this, too, is the following. We have had so much experience now with polysaccharide antibodies that, when we measure them, we can predict immunity. So that, whatever system induces the most antibodies the quickest and lasts the longest, will be the best. We do not have to conduct extensive trials. Once we know that, these conjugates can prevent disease in infants. The immunochemical analysis of these polysaccharide antibodies is going along very well. These have been very useful probes for understanding development of immunity. It is the first time that immunologists can work with humans, with materials that have been available since the turn of the century. I think that we are going to learn a lot about human immunology and the things it has to teach us in general, in addition to developing useful prophylactic methods.

Part V: General Discussion

Towards Better Carbohydrate Vaccines
Edited by R. Bell and G. Torrigiani

Published by John Wiley & Sons Ltd

General discussion – Chaired by Professor G. L. Ada

A. HOW DOES THE IMMUNE SYSTEM HANDLE ANTIGEN PROTEINS VERSUS CARBOHYDRATE?

ADA: I thought it may be useful if, at the start of our general discussion, we try to pinpoint differences between the handling of polypeptides and carbohydrates by the immune system. Now we are not all immunologists, so I have tried to simplify my description of the immune system.

In the simplest terms, there are three crucial points about the immune system. One is, as Don Mosier showed a number of years ago, antigen must be presented to the immune system in a special way. The second point is that T cells and B cells differ in their recognition mechanisms in two critical ways. Gell and Benacerraf showed in the early 1960s that if the proteins were denatured, B cells would no longer recognize the denatured protein in the same way as the original protein was recognized, but you would still get a T-cell response, such as a delayed-type hypersensitivity response. And the third point about presentation is that, whereas a B cell can recognize antigen *per se*, a T cell can only recognize antigen in association with a major histocompatibility complex antigen of which there are two classes, I and II. In the following description, I will not talk about suppressor-T cells very much as that is a very complex story and may not be very relevant to the present discussion.

Until about 10 years ago we thought that the main antigen-presenting cells were macrophages. Two things have happened since then: the first is that there are other forms of antigen-presenting cells, dendritic cells and Langerhans cells which are potentially very important. Cell for cell, it is claimed that a dendritic cell is 100 times more efficient at presenting antigen to T cells than is a macrophage. I don't know how to compare these cells one to the other, because dendritic cells don't have the same properties as macrophages. They don't, as far as we know, phagocytose antigens at all and they don't have Fc receptors on their surface, and yet they seem to be remarkably efficient at presenting antigens to T cells. It has been proposed that there may be collaboration between a macrophage and a dendritic cell in the presentation of antigen. It seems certain when you are dealing with things as complex as whole bacteria that they may have to be degraded in some particular way and that the degradation products may be passed on to the dendritic cell.

The other point is that it became clear, about 10 years ago, that the B cell itself might be efficient at presenting antigen, and this has been stimulated very much by recent work by Lanzavecchia and others in the last few years. If the antigen is a complex particle, not a simple protein but, say, a virus particle with repeating units, two things and happen. It can go to an antigen-presenting cell, such as a macrophage, and be processed in that cell. Processing can mean at least one of two things. A protein may simply have a conformational change, so that hydrophobic groups are exposed, because Berzofsky and others have shown in recent years that perhaps the critical thing about recognition by T cells is that the antigen should have what is called an amphipathic structure, that is, it has a component which is hydrophilic and a component which is hydrophobic, and this can be achieved simply by changing the conformation of a protein so that hydrophobic groups are exposed. Or it may be achieved by degradation of the protein so that a particular peptide with this physical characteristic is produced in the macrophage. The other mechanism is that the virus can bind directly to the B cell, be adsorbed to the immunoglobulin receptors on the B cell and taken into that B cell and processed within the B cell.

The main evidence, to my way of thinking, which supports this type of presentation is work done with viruses. Let me just quote one example. We know with the influenza virus that the haemagglutinin molecule is the main protein involved in neutralization of infectivity, and there are four sites on that protein molecule which are important. The haemagglutinin exists on the virus particle as a trimer, not as a monomer, and many monoclonals have been made to the virus particles which recognize the haemagglutinin molecule and one group has selected four monoclonals reacting with each of these sites, that is, a total of 16 monoclonals. Most efficiently neutralize infectivity of the virus. So they have examined the ability of those monoclonals to bind to the trimeric protein, the monomeric protein or the denatured protein, which would still have the primary amino-acid structure. They find that monoclonals against three of the sites virtually bind only to the trimer and not to the monomer, or to the denatured protein. For the other site, the monoclonals bind both to the trimer and to the monomer but, again, not to the denatured protein. So, obviously, these monoclonals recognize conformational structures which are best expressed by the trimeric protein. It is difficult to see how the trimeric structure could survive in a macrophage stage and so the concept is that the virus particle *selects* the B cell which recognizes this conformational structure. It is taken into that B cell, processed and expresses fragments of that antigen on the surface of the B cell associated with a class II MHC antigen. The important thing to realize is that the specificity of the fragments expressed on the surface of the B cell is entirely different from the specificity of the immunoglobulin which that B cell produces. The second thing is that, while that B cell has one Ig specificity on its surface, the expressed fragments will vary in their specificity. Some of the fragments produced in this way, will have the same specificity of fragments produced by degradation in the macrophage. So you will get activation of a MHC class II-restricted T cell by macrophage-processed antigen. The T cell so activated recognizes similar fragments on the surface of the B cell and this results in the liberation of factors which cause differentiation and replication of the B cell, so that it turns into a plasma cell and produces that antibody with the original specificity.

ROBBINS: That's the best explanation I have heard, and also provides a method for understanding how the help conferred to the polysaccharide, which I think is a non-degradable or poorly degradable component, is mediated by the carrier, that is, the T cells recognize the carrier protein on the surface of the B cell and the help is mediated by the carrier protein, and not by the polysaccharide.

ADA: Just let me expand that point. The concept now prevailing is quite different from the Mitchisonian concept of a hapten–carrier complex, in that the antigenic epitope is recognized by the Ig on the surface of the B cell and is probably protected by that globulin inside the B cell so that it is not expressed on the B-cell surface. The 'carrier' epitope is expressed on the surface of the B cell, rather than the original epitope recognized by that immunoglobulin. Now the question is, how are carbohydrates different from polypeptides? My guess is, if we 'put aside' aspects that Don Mosier talked about yesterday of different subtypes of B cells, that the polysaccharide can, generally speaking, react directly with an appropriate B cell, it may not be degraded in the B cell. The difference may be in what happens in the cell presenting the antigen to the T cell.

Now let us look at the potential steps where 'blocking' might occur. One is that the carbohydrate cannot be processed by the antigen-presenting cell – whatever processing might be, such as a change in conformation or degradation to an appropriate size. A second possible blocking step might be that it may not be able to associate with MHC antigen, and we don't know very much about this except the need for an amphipathic structure. The amphipathic structure is thought to be involved in one of two ways. First of all, the hydrophilic portion of the epitope is recognized by the T-cell receptor, and the hydrophobic portion of the molecule is either to associate with the MHC antigen or to be incorporated into the membrane, or both, so it becomes mobile and can contact the MHC antigen. That has not been resolved yet, as far as I know. There are differing experimental results, one of which says that the T-cell receptor sees the epitope associated with the MHC antigen, the other one says that the T-cell receptor brings the other two together effectively. It holds them in association with each other. We don't know which is the correct interpretation. So a second point is, can a carbohydrate antigen become associated with a class II MHC antigen? Dr Lemieux said the other day that tetrasaccharides can have amphipathic structures. So maybe that's not the blockage. Another possible restriction is the size of the repertoire of the T-cell receptors. Do T-cell receptors have a repertoire which includes recognition of carbohydrates? I don't know. All I have done now is to suggest a general scheme, which it might be useful to consider for 5 or 10 more minutes and see if the blocking step can be pinpointed. This is now open to discussion. Don Mosier, any comments?

MOSIER: I would just like to comment on one point and that is the evidence for different methods of antigen presentation of carbohydrates. It has been appreciated, since John Humphrey first demonstrated it, that polysaccharide antigens have different initial sites of localization in lymphoid organs from polypeptide antigens. But the absolute importance of that has been somewhat difficult to discern. I would like to call your attention to a very recent paper by Eric Claassen (*European Journal of Immunology*, **16,** 492 (1980)). That study demonstrated that a small cytotoxic specifically eliminated dendritic cells in the marginal zone of the spleen. Animals treated with this compound could no longer respond to polysaccharide antigens, such as TNP–Ficoll, but made perfectly normal responses to protein antigens such as haptenated KLH and, in fact, had little-diminished responses to antigens like TNP–lipopolysaccharide and TNP–*Brucella abortus*, antigens that addressed other subsets of B cells. So, I think this is one of the first experiments that directly suggest that the initial site of antigen presentation of polysaccharide antigen is quite distinct. The further point of this paper, and actually several of the papers about antigen presentation of polysaccharides to B cells, is that the actual frequency of cells which can perform this antigen-presenting function is quite small. We have estimated in limiting dilution experiments that only about one out of 20 000 cells in the spleen seems to be capable of presenting TNP–Ficoll. This immediately eliminates the possibility that conventional macrophages are good at presenting polysaccharide antigens to B cells, since the frequency of macrophages is very much higher. So I still think we have a lot to learn about the rules for antigen presentation of carbohydrates, but it is very safe to say at this point that the rules are quite different than they are for presentation of polypeptide antigens.

GEYSEN: I would like to make a comment. Again, I have really got no experience in looking at responses to carbohydrate antigens, but I would like to make a comment with respect to protein antigens. As to antigen processing, what I find very difficult to come to grips with is, if there is in actual fact significant antigen processing by either of the two methods, i.e. conformational change in the antigen or actual physical processing of the antigen, then it is very difficult to understand how the eventual products of the immune response bear very well-defined relationships to intrinsic properties of the native antigen. Because, if there were processing, one wouldn't expect that correlation to be maintained in the products produced after processing. That must have been lost, and, in actual fact, there is very good correlation between the intrinsic properties of the native antigen and the final observable products of the humoral side of the immune response, and that would argue against antigen processing.

ADA: My understanding is that that explains it essentially. That is what has been difficult to explain until relatively recently.

ROBBINS: Capsular polysaccharide antibodies are comparatively restricted. I think we can say that, if you inject a polysaccharide or a protein polysaccharide conjugate, the composition of the polysaccharide antibodies is similar. To me, that would say that the polysaccharide is doing the cell selection and that the cell selection does not change, even though the material is altered. I interpret these findings by thinking that antigen processing by another cell type *per se* doesn't satisfy me as an explanation for what happens. The problem in dealing with experiments such as that of Humphrey is that there may be many methods by which foreign molecules are treated. The question that we have to ask is, which is the process which directly involves antibody synthesis? They may not be directly related.

MOSIER: I totally agree with that, which is why I cited the study of Claassen which is the first evidence that abolishing this form of antigen localization abolishes immune responsiveness. I think that, with that additional information, the findings of Humphrey are much more important.

MORENO: To me the main point made by Lanzavecchia was that there was an alternative to the original scheme for presentation of antigen. Now, the fact that antigen processing does take place in the macrophage does not rule out the possibility that some of the antigen presented on the surface of the macrophage is not processed, because both things could happen simultaneously. Some of the antigen is predigested and presented in the context of Ia antigens. Another fraction of that antigen could be partially, or completely unprocessed and still be available for combination with antibody, without undergoing degradation. I think the fact that there is an alternative of presenting antigen in the context Ia on the surface of B cells, does not to rule out that the same phenomenon is happening in the macrophage.

ADA: I think you are saying is that there can be a mechanism inside the body for holding the antigen in a relatively undegraded form, so that the B cell to be selected can come along and meet it. This role, of course, can be played by the dendritic follicular cell, although most of the evidence suggests that it is very important for the generation of a B-memory response. But, the antigen might also be held on the surface of macrophages. In fact, if you present a labelled antigen to a macrophage, you can find for some considerable time the label still present on the surface of that macrophage. So I am not ruling out this possibility at all.

MÄKELÄ: At great risk of being wrong, I suggest that, for processing purposes, an antigen should have two characteristics that proteins do have, and polysaccharides may not have. The full T-helper cell antigen on the macrophage surface or on the B-cell surface consist of the MHC class I molecule, and the external half-antigen. The two must stick together. This can conceivably be achieved so that they have a high affinity for each other. The problem is that one type of MHC class II molecule should have high affinity for many structures. Alternatively, if not only the MHC class II molecule but also the external antigen is anchored to the membrane, the affinity requirement between these two is reduced. Therefore, I propose that an ideal half-antigen has a hydrophobic moiety which can anchor it to the membrane.

On the other hand, a successful external half-antigen cannot be very large in size. If it is large, it will interfere with the interaction between the T-cell receptor and the MHC half.

Native polysaccharides do not meet these two requirements. They are not easily broken down in cells and they have only tiny hydrophobic moieties. Proteins are probably broken down in cells and some breakdown products may have lipophilic sequences which reside in the interior of the native protein. Breakdown products of polysaccharide protein conjugates can also have both of the required characteristics if the polysaccharide moiety is not too big.

HANDMAN: I just have a comment in support of this hypothesis. I read a very recent paper from Benacerraf's lab showing that antigen processing may involve, or does involve, fatty-acid acylation of the peptide, and the antigen-presenting cell, as well as many other cells in the body, do have already a mechanism for fatty-acid acylation of various internal proteins. It is possible to understand that they do this to external protein antigen as well, whereas they may not have this mechanism for acylation of carbohydrate antigens.

ADA: It is a question of whether the protein is a fragment or not. There is increasing evidence to show that, as far as T-cell recognition is concerned, peptides may be important rather than intact proteins. We can go through this evidence if necessary, but I do not want to because it would take some time.

SUTHERLAND: I think there is one point that we tend to forget about as far as polysaccharides are concerned, and yet we have been hearing all the time about the need for a certain size of molecule, and Dr Mäkelä has just pointed out to us the problem of the very large molecule.

In terms of a protein, the linkages are relatively non-specific in that they are broken down by very many enzymes. In terms of the polysaccharides, we have unique situations in almost all polysaccharides, and enzymes breaking down such unique linkages simply do not exist. There are exceptions – dextrans are relatively easily broken down. There are a small number of polysaccharides broken by phosphodiesterases, but the great majority of polysaccharides are molecules which, as far as we know, are totally recalcitrant to enzymes. The only enzymes known to break these down are often of very localized occurrence in, for example, bacteriophages infecting the capsulate bacteria. No other sources of enzymes which will break down these polysaccharides are known.

ADA: So the message you have is that the blockage is at the processing step, if that involves a degree of degradation.

SUTHERLAND: Yes.

SÖDERSTRÖM: I am missing one thing in the scheme, it should be about a 1000-fold higher chance for the antigen to encounter circulating antibodies linked on the cells, or the antigen receptors on the cells. Therefore, I think one may have to add immune complexes instead of antigens there somewhere.

ADA: In a secondary situation?

SÖDERSTRÖM: Yes, but perhaps there are not so many primary situations. Unless there is a skewed repertoire, you should have approximately the same antibodies represented in the circulation as you have on the cell surfaces.

ADA: You can have many primary situations. There is no evidence that influenza, for example, is a native pathogen of mice. There is no anti-influenza naturally occurring antibody detectable which limits infectious cases. So that you do have many primary situations.

SÖDERSTRÖM: So, what about the secondary?

ADA: What you propose is more likely for a secondary situation. But not infrequently, the does of antigen necessary to induce a secondary response needs to be quite larger.

ROBBINS: We have shown that antigen–antibody complexes, either in antigen excess, or antibody excess do not immunize. *Haemophilus* polysaccharide bound to pneumococcus type 3, which is in general a good polysaccharide, does not immunize. Electrostatic, not covalent, complexes of the two do not work when they are injected subcutaneously. Another, epidemiological note: *H. influenzae* type b, and many of these other pathogens, including meningococcus, are habitants of humans only. I do not think that it is impossible to start thinking here today that, if we had effective vaccines, even if we do not get a few cases for 2 or 3 months, if we achieve epidemiological control in a population we might be able to do the same as was done with smallpox – eliminate these species from the earth. That would not surprise me at all.

GRIFFISS: It would surprise me enormously. These vaccines do not prevent pharyngeal colonization. The study that purported to show that the vaccine does, was improperly analysed statistically. It would be an absolute shock if we were able to eradicate the meningococcus from the face of the earth by providing everyone with circulating antibodies. That would turn my world upside-down. But that was not the comment I wanted to make.

The comment I wanted to make was that antigen processing of at least two polysaccharides, those from *Pseudomonas* and from one of the Group B streptococci, has been shown in the mouse to depend upon binding of complement. When an animal is decomplemented, there is no response. That can be understood in terms of the complement receptors on antigen-processing cells, including splenic dendritic cells. It would also suggest that the complement system acts as a recognition system for these molecules, and that it is precisely that characteristic of the molecules that allows them to confer pathogenic potential to a bacterium, namely their down-regulation of complement, that makes them not recognized, taken up or processed appropriately by antigen-presenting cells. For instance, properdin serves as a recognition molecule for some, but not all, meningococcal polysaccharides, and for the lipooligosaccharides of the meningococcus and gonococcus.

ADA: Do we have any evidence that, when you present a complex polysaccharide to a macrophage, that it is taken up quite adequately and the macrophage suffers from indigestion? Because that would point to the stage being where antigen presentation fails to occur.

FEIZI: Coming back to lypophilicity. If lypophilicity is really important for an immune response, then glycolipids are the ideal saccharide antigens and we come back to the point that Dr Kabat made earlier, that perhaps we should study in detail the immune response to oligosaccharides derived from bacterial polysaccharides and conjugated to lipids.

ADA: I can make perhaps one more comment. My understanding is that it will not be long before we will have x-ray structures of some of the MHC antigens. Once these are available we will have a better appreciation of the property required of a T-cell epitope in order for it to become associated with the MHC antigen.

ROBBINS: Am I mistaken that two patients with C3 deficiency have been immunized and made antibodies for the polysaccharides?

GRIFFISS: I do not know that particular work. For the meningococcus the alternative pathway is more important than the classical pathway, and so the fact that someone is C3 deficient might not be as important as properdin deficiency, although I would assume that the receptor on the antigen-presenting cell is a C3 NC3g receptor, that is, the CR2.

ROBBINS: An investigator at the University of Connecticut and, I think, someone in South Africa have been immunized and have made antibodies to meningococcus A and C and pneumococcus, so that, at least in those situations, the C3 component is not obligatory for producing antibody.

GRIFFISS: But if they were older children or adults, they might have antibody induced by enteric organisms and they could use the Fc receptor independent of the complement receptor and, in fact, without any antibody to the polysaccharide would be dependent on the complement receptor.

ADA: Any more discussions on this? I think the feeling now is that one of the major blocks is the ability of this cell to process the complex polysaccharide. It may be that some experiments should be done, as has been done with peptides, to see whether, in liposomes containing MHC antigens, a tetrasaccharide would associate with MHC antigens. I think there are experiments that can be done to look at this particular blockage further. Last question on this point.

GRIFFISS: It raises another quite different point. If you swallow a bacterium, as we all do, that has a meningococcal polysaccharide on its surface, the bacterium can be found deep within Peyer's patch after a few days and in association with macrophage-like cells. Some time later the animal, either a mouse or man, will have antibody to that polysaccharide in their bloodstream. So there must be something going on in Peyer's patch that relates to antigen processing and that might be quite different from subcutaneous antigen processing. It is a system that can be studied quite readily using cross-reacting bacteria.

ADA: Yes, but if you try hard enough, you can make antibody to almost any structure. While the usual procedure may be to make antibody predominantly to conformational structures, such as tertiary or quaternary structures, it is amazing what can serve as an antigen. So some of the products of digestion of, say, a whole bacterium in a macrophage could well escape from that cell and be presented to a B cell. I do not have too much trouble with that possibility.

GRIFFISS: But the question is, what happens if you immunize an individual subcutaneously after they have been primed at Peyer's patch? Does the processing of the bacterium through Peyer's patch permit the individual to now respond to the polysaccharide?

MORENO: One aspect in relation to simplicity of the structure and virulence could be related to the fact that the more complex the polysaccharide, the greater the variety of antibody responses that can be made against it. The heterogeneity of the response is going to increase enormously every time you introduce a new monosaccharide along the chain. Now, the restrictive element operating here makes the genetic vulnerability in the capacity of the individuals to respond play a more and more relevant role, because they do not have an arsenal of antibodies to respond in terms of variable chains that would be specific against it. Also, the level of antibodies that you are going to produce is going to be inferior because the number of B-cell clones in the repertoire is going to be lower.

The other point that could be related – and it is not necessarily an immunological one – is that many of these polysaccharides are considerably less stable than others and they degrade discontinuously, so they do not trigger the immune system very effectively. Isn't it so that the rate of degradation *in vivo* could differ considerably?

ROBBINS: Dr Moreno, I think your first point is well taken, although you would not predict that something that is ribose ribitol phosphate would not differ so much from glucose ribitol phosphate with respect to the number of potential epitopes that there might be. The other point, about *in vivo* degradation – I do not think that that is an explanation, because phosphorylated polysaccharides can be degraded by mammalian alkaline phosphatases and something like pneumococcus type 3 must persist in our tissues for life. I do not think there is terribly much difference in the virulence of the organism. I do not think that biodegradability is likely.

MORENO: All I am saying is that it could be an additional factor, not necessarily the most important.

ROBBINS: I think we are looking for phenomena to give us an explanation which, I am sure, is physico-chemical.

MORENO: If our strategy to produce vaccines is going to reduce the number of potential clones to respond, rather than increase it as you do, for instance, when you go for idiotype-specific responses, then the capacity to use the whole potential of the organism to produce a diversity of antibodies is also narrowed down if it is not utilized.

ROBBINS: If you feed an organism to rats and immunize with the polysaccharide later, compared to the rats which were not fed with the organism the differences between the two groups is not great, but feeding does prime for an immune response.

ADA: But do you have proteins associated with the breakdown product?

MÄKELÄ: The fact that the bacteria are found inside phagocytes or phagocyte-like cells does not say that structures of this bacterium will be processed towards the T-cell antigen.

ADA: No, but it may liberate some products, that could subsequently come into contact with an appropriate B cell. That was the point being made.

MÄKELÄ: It may, but it may not.

ADA: Oh, but it may.

SÖDERSTRÖM: We have also done experiments feeding rats live or killed bacteria and, and I think one has to be a bit cautious not to generalize, since there may be differences with different capsules, also when it comes to processing in the Peyer's patches. Generally, feeding killed bacteria repeatedly induced the most efficient priming for an anti-polysaccharide response upon later encounter with polysaccharide or conjugate.

ADA: Let me make a final comment in this respect. Nossal and I did some experiments over 20 years ago in which we labelled the flagella proteins of *Salmonella*, and injected this into rats. The labelled material stayed in macrophages for as long as we cared to look, and yet we got a continuous antibody response. So you could take the point of view that it wasn't being degraded because it was still there, but it is just as likely that some pieces were being cleaved from it all the time, but it persisted sufficient to continuously stimulate an antibody response.

Let us now get on to the next topic.

B. WHAT HAPPENS WHEN AN OLIGOSACCHARIDE IS BOUND BY A LECTIN OR ANTIBODY?

LEMIEUX: Mr Chairman, as you have noticed, I have been sitting there in the corner very quietly for the last 2 days, not feeling very competent to get engaged in much of the discussion that is going on here. But I did feel that perhaps I should talk about some work we have done recently because I have seen a decided interest in things like molecular recognition – memory. The major effort we have made in recent years is to try and understand how antibodies and lectins recognize oligosaccharides. It is going to be very hard for me to try and condense about 20 person-years' work into 5 minutes, but I hope I can give you the gist of what we are finding and what appears to be the picture that is developing.

I think the first thing to recognize regarding these associations is that there exists in the several cases we have so far measured a rather regular pattern for the kinds of surfaces that are specifically bound by the protein. I should mention that all our thermodynamic studies have been with lectins. However, the kind of recognition patterns we find for lectins and for antibodies are so similar that I expect that similar information will be found for antibodies. We tried to examine antibodies, but these bound our haptens too strongly for the physical methods that we have for measuring association constants.

These binding reactions are all accompanied by very important decreases in entropy. Thus, a great deal of organization occurs – as is expected for these complexation reactions. Interestingly enough, the binding of the Lewis b tetrasaccharide (α LFuc(1 → 2) β DGal(1 → 3)[α LFuc(→ 4)] β DGlcNAc—) by a lectin, the so-called lectin IV of *Griffonia simplicifolia*, was near equal in strength to the binding by the so-called Y determinant, which is a closely related structure (α LFuc(1 → 2) β DGal(1 → 4)[α LFuc(1 → 3)] β DGlcNAc—) but of the so-called type 2 core structure.

In fact these have ends for which the topographies are essentially the same. On the other hand, the other parts of these molecules have surfaces that are completely different. So, it was most probable that the lectin is looking at the topography that is common to both structures and this was proved to be the case. Molecular models will show that this surface is an amphiphilic-type structure and we believe that these oligosaccharides maintain these conformations in aqueous solution. For example, in the case of the B human blood group determinant (α LFuc(1 → 2)[α DGal(1 → 3)] β DGal—) we do know, by nuclear magnetic resonance, what the conformation is in water and we find exactly the same conformation in the x-ray structure, including some compressions between atoms in different sugar units which are very powerful. We often find this kind of van der Waals' conflict in branched oligosaccharides and this suggests that these oligosaccharides sit in rather deep and narrow energy wells and will not move away much from this conformation in order to form a complex with a protein.

In each case, for the seven proteins that we have so far studied, monoclonal antibodies and lectins, the binding involves the interaction of a polar grouping that is adjacent to an extensive rather non-polar surface. Briefly, what we did was to synthesize a wide variety of slightly modified forms of these oligosaccharides. Then, using a radioimmunoassay, we determined the effects of the structural changes on the 50% inhibitions. It was discovered that, for each of the proteins studied, a cluster of certain hydroxyl groups is essential to the binding. This appears to be so, since replacement of any one of the two or three hydroxyl groups in the cluster by hydrogen provides an essentially inactive compound. In other situations, replacement of an hydroxyl by hydrogen actually provides a better inhibitor. In certain cases the effect was truly remarkable; for example, the replacement by hydrogen of the 6^b-hydroxyl group of the Lewis b tetrasaccharide gave a structure that was 18 times more potent as an inhibitor of the binding by a monoclonal anti-Lewis b antibody. We have noticed this kind of phenomenon often and, in every case, such a hydroxyl group is one that is well situated for intramolecular hydrogen bonding. I don't have the time to go into this today, but I wish to assure you that the evidence seems to be quite compelling that certain hydroxyl groups may be forced to leave water and become intramolecularly hydrogen bonded in order to be accepted into the complex. Now this is something rather phenomenal if you think about it, because this process must be importantly demanding in energy. The question then arises as to why the binding reaction involves stripping of at least part of the water away from the hydroxyl group and then the organization of the hydroxyl group in order to form an intramolecular hydrogen bond, so that it can then be accepted by the protein. Surely, if so, this involves acceptance of the hydroxyl group into a non-polar region of the combining site.

As you well know, there exist polar interactions which are directional in character, and may be repulsive if the orientations are not correct. On the other hand, London–van der Waals' dispersion forces are distant dependent only, and occur between any two atoms whether or not these are engaged in polar or non-polar covalent bonds.

In the case of an oligosaccharide, we have termed the cluster of hydroxyl groups essential to binding as the 'key polar grouping'. Of course, in water it is strongly hydrated. The hydration, of course, involves polar interactions which are highly directional and should tend to orient the water molecules in certain ways. Now the energetically most favourable orientations of these water molecules need not be such that they will come close to the adjacent non-polar surface. Therefore, it is reasonable to expect that some sort of void will exist, on the average, between the water molecules and the non-polar surface. Similarly for the protein. Now, if the two surfaces are complementary, then of course these will tend to form a complex in order to fill the voids along the two amphiphilic surfaces and thereby maximize the dispersion forces of attraction. This is, I think, how hydrogen bonding is most importantly involved in the driving of these molecular associations. The complex will form, however, only when the requirements of the polar interaction (involving the key polar grouping) are well met and, thereby, provide an important source of the specificity of the interaction. To prove that this is in fact the case will be difficult, but I believe that it will be found to be so. At this time, we are doing some theoretical calculations trying to support this idea. Using an energy minimization programme, developed by Dr Fraga of our department, we attempt to simulate the minimum energy conglomerate of α-methyl fucopyranosides and a sufficient number of water molecules to completely cover its surface. The calculation is highly demanding in computer time since the placing of near 500 water molecules was required. After the fucoside was completely covered with water, we stripped away the water molecules, except those that formed the first layer and, as was expected, there was a substantial cavity next to the hydrophobic side of the glycoside.

GEYSEN: At the beginning you showed the relationship with ΔH and ΔS, and it was a linear relationship and that was consistent with one of the later slides that you showed in which the ΔG, that was measured on the interaction, was very, very constant. It didn't vary by very much at all and, of course, if I remember my thermodynamics correctly, ΔG is equal to ΔH minus $T\,\Delta S$. Now I assume you did most of the measurements at the same temperature, let's say room temperature . . .

LEMIEUX: Ten to 45 degrees but best in the range 15–35 °C.

GEYSEN: In fact, you would expect that, if the ΔG were constant, that that relationship exists. But I think the interesting thing is that the fact that your ΔG remained constant suggests that it hadn't interfered with the bit that was doing the binding, and that the fact that you changed you ΔG and ΔS

terms suggests that those modifications which you had made in the molecule affected things like the solvation of the molecule which just partitioned out the ΔH with respect to the ΔS, but you still hadn't affected the actual entity that was binding, the binding entity between the two.

LEMIEUX: Well I think you are part right, and probably in part . . . we also have affected parts of the molecule that are involved intimately in the binding.

GEYSEN: It is very difficult to see how you get a constant ΔG then.

LEMIEUX: Well, it is not constant.

GEYSEN: It is very, very close.

LEMIEUX: Well, I wished only to indicate the trend.

GEYSON: I think that one of your early and one of your last slides showed a very narrow range of ΔG, there was only one slide in which the ΔG differed . . .

LEMIEUX: It may be of interest to note that, if you take the literature data for other lectins and other structures, you obtain a similar trend.

GEYSEN: Again, I think it is consistent with the fact that you can make a lot of changes which don't affect the binding entity. It is just changing the relationship between the . . .

LEMIEUX: I see what you mean, and certainly we wondered about this. The simplest interpretation is that we are introducing hydrophobic effects, which are compensating a bit for what you are losing in entropy and that is why the ΔG stays about constant. But both the ΔH and ΔS have changed.

ADA: I suggest we move to the third topic.

C. ALL POLYSACCHARIDES ARE NOT CREATED EQUAL, ONLY SOME ARE ASSOCIATED WITH VIRULENCE AND THEIR IMMUNOGENICITY IS UNEQUAL. WHY? HOW CAN IT BE MEASURED BY PHYSICO-CHEMICAL ASSAY?

ROBBINS: I think one of the levels of understanding that would help us in making better vaccines is to understand why bacteria cause invasive disease in humans. We need to know more about the physico-chemistry of the polysaccharides themselves. I don't know if it's appreciated but, for each bacterial species, there are many more capsular polysaccharides of the organism than those that are associated with disease. With *Pneumococcus* there are 84 capsular polysaccharides and almost all the infections are caused by 24 or 25. With *Haemophilus influenzae* there are six. Some of them, like type c and type d and type f, are very encapsulated, have much more capsule than the type b. Why does only the type b polysaccharide cause invasive disease? I don't know how many capsules of meningococcus have been discovered now, Dr Jennings?

JENNINGS: I think there are eleven.
ROBBINS: But most diseases are caused by three, and almost all are caused by five. I don't think that is an accident. There is something in the tertiary structure of those capsules that determines whether or not those organisms are going to cause disease. In addition to that, there is a relation between the immunogenicity of these organisms and the propensity to cause disease. Those seem to be related. The more immunogenic ones seem to be less virulent and yet one can't take a polysaccharide in a test-tube or look at the structure on a blackboard and say 'this is going to be a poor immunogen' or 'this is one that is going to be associated with disease'. I think that level of understanding, if we could achieve it, would be very important to understanding the nature of these diseases. I think it's built into the structure, the composition may give us a clue but I don't know how to study it. I think it is an important question.
ADA: Is it related to the presence or absence of receptors on cells for those organisms, or those particular capsular materials? There are receptors for viruses on certain cells which determine the tropism of the virus. What do we know about receptors on cells for the tropism of the bacteria?
ROBBINS: I can only give you the most indirect information on that and I don't think its good information. I don't know the answer to that question.
ADA: If you have monoclonal antibodies against these different capsular polysaccharides that might give you a tool to look at that question.
ROBBINS: There were some suggestions, that is, it seems that the polysaccharides that are comparatively simple, composed of monosaccharides, tended to be associated with more virulent bacteria and less immunogenic polysaccharides. For the *Meningococcus* that seems to hold, that is, A, B and C are monosaccharides and are the most virulent of all of them, the rest of the capsules of meningococous are all disaccharides in a repeat unit, and aside from Y and W and 35, the others don't seem to cause any more disease than any other bacteria out in the open. Sialic acid is another important marker. How many capsules have sialic acid that don't cause disease?
JENNINGS: It is generally that the more simple the structure is the more likely it is to be involved in disease. Another important factor is that the presence of sialic acid in a capsular polysaccharide and the ability of the related organism to cause disease is 100%. It would certainly be nice to identify a structural feature common to the capsular polysaccharides of all pathogenic organisms, but so far this has eluded us. For instance, it is difficult to see a relationship between the structure of sialic acid and that of the capsular polysaccharide of the highly virulent type b *Haemophilus influenzae*. On this evidence one must assume that any relationship between the pathogenicity of an organism and the structure of its capsular polysaccharide must be fairly complex.
ROBBINS: Sialic acid may not be the only determinant that determines viru-

lence but, when it's there, it seems to be related to virulence and comparatively poor immunogenicity when it's in a monomeric unit. You know the *E. coli* K92 organism, the capsule of K92, the alternating 28 29 capsule, is very difficult to find in people. We searched and searched and found it very irregularly. In the infant rat model it is a pathogenic organism. It is not as pathogenic as the K1 strains, but it does induce bacteraemia in a small proportion of rats when it is fed. So at least it holds that, where there is sialic acid, and sialic acid is in a monomeric or simple fashion, the capsule is associated with virulence and, if you will, comparatively poor immunogenicity, although we haven't got good data to state that in unequivocal terms. With *Haemophilus*, our observations showed the following. If you take fully encapsulated type B organisms and put them into antibody-free complement, they survive. If you take *H. influenzae* type F, which is a heavily encapsulated strain, and put it in the same antibody-free complement, it disappears quickly. That is why we think that antibody is required for immunity to *H. influenzae*, that is required to induce protective complement reactions. There are just two corollaries to that: (1) if we induce antibody to *H. influenzae* type b in the population, the other types are not going to cause disease because we are resistant to them already. We are not going to have the emergence of other types as pathogen; (2) the next most common type to *Haemophilus* type b that causes invasive disease is type a. Compositionally they are similar, one is ribose ribitol phosphate, the other is glucose ribitol phosphate. Now I know I may be falling into a trap by saying that the composition may be related, but it is interesting that that's the organism that is next in its resistance to complement. So there is some structural basis for saying that the structure is important, at least in *Haemophilus*. With *Pneumococcus* it is harder because the structures are so diverse.

MORENO: One aspect in relation to simplicity of the structure and virulence could be related to the fact that, the more complex the polysaccharide, the greater the variety of antibody responses that can be made against it. The heterogeneity of the response is going to increase enormously every time you introduce a new monosaccharide along the chain. Now, the restrictive element operating here makes the genetic vulnerability in the capacity of the individuals to respond play a more and more relevant role, because they do not have an arsenal of antibodies to respond in terms of variable chains that would be specific against it. Also, the level of antibodies that you are going to produce is going to be inferior because the number of B-cell clones in the repertoire is going to be lower.

The other point that could be related, and that is not necessarily an immunological one, is that many of these polysaccharides are considerably less stable than others and they degrade discontinuously, so they do not trigger the immune system very effectively. Isn't it so that the rate of degradation *in vivo* could differ considerably?

ROBBINS: Dr Moreno, I think your first point is well taken, although you would not predict that something that is ribose ribitol phosphate, would not differ so much from glucose ribitol phosphate with respect to the number of potential epitopes that there might be. The other point, about *in vivo* degradation – I do not think that that is an explanation, because phosphorylated polysaccharides can be degraded by mammalian alkaline phosphatases and something like pneumococcus type 3 must persist in our tissues for life. I do not think there is terribly much difference in the virulence of the organism. I do not think that biodegradability is likely.

MORENO: All I am saying is that it could be an additional factor, not necessarily the most important.

ROBBINS: I think we are looking for phenomena to give us an explanation which, I am sure, is physico-chemical.

MORENO: If our strategy to produce vaccines is going to reduce the number of potential clones to respond, rather than increase it as you do, for instance, when you go for idiotype-specific responses, then the capacity to use the whole potential of the organism to produce a diversity of antibodies is also narrowed down, it is not utilized.

ROBBINS: I do not understand what you have just said.

ADA: Let's come back to this.

FEIZI: You have raised, Dr Ada, the question of other mechanisms for virulence or tropisms, rather, of bacteria apart from the polysaccharides, and I just wanted to comment on quite a large body of evidence that is accumulating now to show that bacteria contain adhesins, which are proteins which adhere to specific sugar residues on host-cell membranes. Of course these, being proteins on the bacteria, are likely to be immunogenic and good candidates for vaccines.

MÄKELÄ: I thought that one aim, when bacteria started to produce capsules, was to convert the non-capsulated surface, which is an activator of the alternative pathway of complement, into a surface that is not an activator of the alternative pathway of the complement. I thought that the K1 capsule is superior to the K2 capsule because K1 is not an activator and K2 is an activator of the alternative pathway. But from Dr Griffiss's talk, I understood that he is turning the picture the other way around, saying that perhaps one good, efficient capsule, the meningococcus B, is sufficient because it does activate the alternative pathway of complement. I am slightly confused what to think.

ADA: Dr Griffiss, could you clarify this confusion?

GRIFFISS: I doubt that I can clarify any confusion I create. The problem is distinguishing between complement molecules acting as recognition molecules for triggering effector mechanisms and the activation of complement as an effector mechanism. The recognition of a molecule, in physico-chemical terms, by another molecule does not mean that an effector mechanism has been activated. The α2-8 sialic acid capsule of K1 *E. coli* and Group B *N. meningitidis* binds the recognition component of the alternative complement pathway in such a way that effective complement activation does not occur on the cell surface and effector mechanisms are not triggered. It does this better than any other polysaccharide that we have studied. That is quite different from saying that it is not recognized by the ACP. Rather, it is recognised in a way that does not lead to activation of effector mechanisms – sort of a false recognition.

Let me also mention that whereas I agree with most of Dr Robbins's ruminations about these capsules and their physical and chemical structures, any unifying hypothesis must encompass all of the possibilities, and the Group X meningococcal capsule is as simple as the Group A, being glucosamine phosphate rather than mannosamine phosphate. It is very similar, structurally, to some of the newer capsules that Harry Jennings has studied. It is also reminiscent of the *E. coli* capsules that are cross-reactive with the Group A meningococcal capsule. Yet this group never causes diseases. So a hypothesis has to be a uniform one that takes into account all these capsules; it does not seem to me that we are there yet.

ROTTA: Well, just listening to the discussion, it may seem that one is inclined to simplify a little the virulence of a bacterium by identifying one or two factors decisive for the initial stage of the infection. I am wondering whether some other factor(s) in addition to the capsular polysaccharides of the bacteria discussed at this meeting are considered to play a contributory role in virulence, as they do in the Group A streptococci. The receptor for fibrinogen located on the surface of the Group A streptococcus and the hyaluronic acid in the capsule clearly enhance the virulence of this bacterium.

ROBBINS: I assume that we all realize that if you took a baseball and covered it with a capsule, it would not cause meningitis. The bacterium has to have something more than a capsule. The capsule exerts an essential, but not sufficient, role for the virulence of a bacteria. We try to understand one component at a time, to understand the composite. I think that the old experiments that say that encapsulated bacteria resist the protective actions of complement are critical. The ones that have capsules that do not cause disease are affected by complement; there is also a relation between those capsulated organisms that resist complement and their immunogenic properties. I think they are related but, as Dr Griffiss says, it is not a one-to-one relation and there is no obvious simple explanation. But it has to be physicochemical. A bacterium that is covered by some capsules lives in blood, multiplies and causes systemic infections. The quality and not the quantity determines this ability to survive in the blood. That, I think, is the essence of what it is. Now, certainly, the bacteria have to have other adaptive mechanisms to live in humans, but with the streptococcus, if they do not have an M protein they do not cause disease. But an M protein itself is not a disease-producing material.

I am a little concerned about some issues that Dr Griffiss brought up and I guess they have to be studied. One thing that always surprised me is that people and disease with encapsulated bacteria, in which there was an abscess, like an empyema, or pericarditis, can have circulating capsular antigen for months afterwards and in not insignificant amounts, hundreds of μg for 1 ml of blood, but they do not have any symptoms. That is, the capsule itself prepares a pure form as a vaccine and, as a component of the body, it is not reactive. It does not play a role in the pathogenisis of inflammation in the disease. It seems that its function to the bacteria is to protect the bacteria, but it does not make you sick. That is why I am surprised that you find so much complement activation. I was surprised, I would not have predicted it.

GRIFFISS: I am not finding complement activation, I am finding complement non-activation. The capsule variously binds whatever it is that activates complement in a way that does not lead to complement activation. It is the initiator molecule, not C3b, that is being bound and removed.

ADA: Can we now move on to the next topic?

D. DO PEPTIDES AND CARBOHYDRATES CROSS-REACT?

FEIZI: I just want to briefly comment on this rather provocative possibility. We have heard during this meeting some data that seem to suggest that there are antigenic cross-reactions between peptides and carbohydrates, and that they might be exploited in vaccination. I would like to bring up, once again, the question of what constitutes idiotypic determinants, or idiotopes. Are they peptide determinants or are they carbohydrate structures shared by immunoglobulins and the original glycosylated immunogens? I think it will be important to determine the biochemical basis of idiotypic reactions. The question of carbohydrate specificity can now be tackled using our neoglycolipid procedure. I certainly would be very pleased to collaborate with groups who have monoclonal anti-idiotypic antibodies, particularly antibodies that react with or mimic the original immunogens that are glycosylated. Dr Capron presented observations that schistosomal glycoproteins, snail-vector glycoproteins and KLH inhibit the reactivities of (AB_3) iodiotypic antibodies raised against (AB_2) antibodies which themselves were raised against AB_1 antibodies to schistosomal glycoproteins. Dr B. Fields, in Boston, has described idiotypic systems involving receptors for reovirus. I think these are tremendously interesting experimental systems. Then, Dr Söderström has a system where anti-idiotype induces production of antibodies to *E. coli* polysaccharides. Even more provocative is Dr Geysen's suggestion that anti-carbohydrate antibodies with blood-group A specificities bind to chemically synthesized peptides. I think that his system is eminently testable now, using his chemically synthesized peptides as inhibitors of well-characterized monoclonal anti-A antibodies that are specific for structural variants of blood group A. Both the 'idiotope' and the 'mimotope' systems are, I think, potentially important and they are very relevant to the subject-matter of this meeting. I think they are topics that might be the subject of WHO collaborative programmes involving laboratories that can work towards consolidating their biochemical basis, and considering their applications.

ADA: We thought they were important, that is why we put them in the programme. Would you like to make a comment, Dr Söderström?

SÖDERSTRÖM: We have already agreed on how to proceed in the K13 business. I have no difficulty, functionally, to envision protein carbohydrate complementarity. The mere fact that you can induce antibodies against carbohydrates, to me, suggests that you can have complementarity between proteins and carbohydrates.

MORENO: The diagram that I have made was designed to explain what Dr Robbins did not understand, probably because I did not explain it properly. If you think of one circle as the anti-epitope repertoire (Figure 1), in other words all those antibodies that recognize the antigen, and you have another universe overlapping, that is the idiotype repertoire and you challenge with an anti-idiotype, you will only have the overlapping section being used out of the total potential of that individual to respond to that particular antigen. This is what I meant when I said that there is a restriction of the total potential of that individual to respond, and it is very relevant in the context of this last point because, for many years, I thought it was unlikely that these cross-reactivities could emerge, but apparently I have been wrong all the time. However, probably the cross-reactivities are going to be tailor made and that would also reduce the potential for responses.

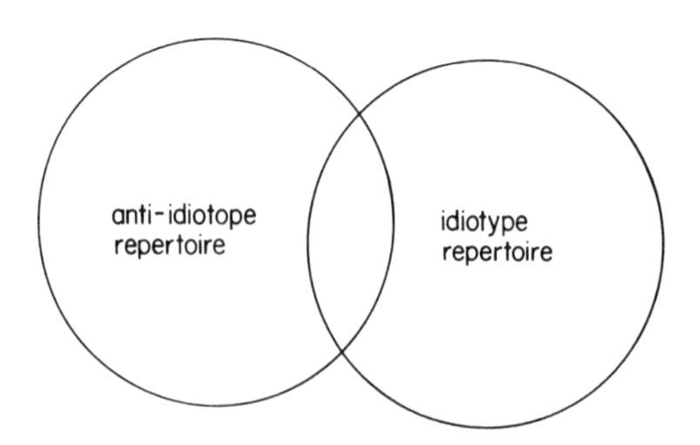

List of Contributors

G. L. ADA, Department of Microbiology, John Curtin School of Medical Research, Australian National University, Canberra, ACT 2601, Australia
F. E. ASHTON, Bureau of Microbiology, Laboratory Center for Disease Control, Ottawa, Ontario, Canada K1A 0L2
F. A. ASSAAD, Director, Division of Communicable Diseases, World Health Organization, 1211 Geneva 27, Switzerland
A. CAPRON, Centre d'Immunologie et de Biologie parasitaire, Unité mixte, Institut national de la Santé et de la Recherche médicale, Centre national de la Récherche scientifique, Institut Pasteur, 59019 Lille, France
M. CAPRON, Centre d'Immunologie et de Biologie parasitaire, Unité mixte, Institut national de la Santé et de la Recherche médicale, Centre national de la Récherche scientifique, Institut Pasteur, 59019 Lille, France
C. DISSOUS, Centre d'Immunologie et de Biologie parasitaire, Unité mixte, Institut national de la Santé et de la Recherche médicale, Centre national de la Récherche scientifique, Institut Pasteur, Lille, France
C. S. F. EASMON, Department of Medical Microbiology, Wright–Fleming Institute, St Mary's Hospital Medical School, London W2 1PG, UK
W. EGAN, Office of Biologics Research and Review, Food and Drug Administration, Bethesda, MD 20892, USA
J. ESKOLA, Department of Bacteriology and Immunology, University of Helsinki and the National Public Health Institute, Helsinki, Finland
A. J. FEENEY, Division of Immunology, Medical Biology Institute, La Jolla, CA 92037, USA
T. FEIZI, Immunochemistry Research Group, Medical Research Council Clinical Research Centre, Harrow, Middlesex MA1 3UJ, UK
A. GAMIAN, Division of Biological Sciences, National Research Council of Canada, Ottawa, Ontario, Canada K1A 0R6
H. M. GEYSEN, Department of Molecular Immunology, Commonwealth Serum Laboratories, Parkville, Victoria 3052, Australia
C. P. J. GLAUDEMANS, National Institutes of Health, Bethesda, MD 20892, USA
J. McL. GRIFFISS, The Centre for Immunochemistry and the Departments of Laboratory Medicine and Medicine, University of California, San Francisco, CA 94123, USA
J. M. GRZYCH, Centre l'Immunologie, et de Biologie parasitaire, Unité mixte, Institut national de la Santé et de la Recherche médicale, Centre national de la Récherche scientifique, Institut Pasteur, Lille, France

E. HANDMAN, The Walter and Eliza Hall Institute of Medical Research, Melbourne, Victoria 3050, Australia
J. G. HOWARD, The Wellcome Trust, 1 Park Square West, London NW1 4LJ, UK
P. M. JACQUINOT, Unité associée, Centre national de la Recherche scientifique 217, Université des Sciences et Techniques, 59655, Lille, France
H. J. JENNINGS, Division of Biological Sciences, National Research Council of Canada, Ottawa, Ontario, Canada K1A 0R6
E. A. KABAT, Departments of Microbiology, Genetics and Development and Neurology, Columbia University, New York, NY 10032, and the National Institute of Allergy and Infectious Diseases, Bethesda, MD 20892, USA
W. W. KARAKAWA, Department of Biochemistry, Pennsylvania State University, University Park, PA 20742, USA
H. KÄYHTY, Department of Bacteriology and Immunology, University of Helsinki and the National Public Health Institute, Helsinki, Finland
R. U. LEMIEUX, Department of Chemistry, University of Alberta, Edmonton, Alberta, Canada T6G 2G2
R. MACFARLAN, Department of Molecular Immunology, Commonwealth Serum Laboratories, Parkville, Victoria 3052, Australia
P. Helena MÄKELÄ, Department of Bacteriology, National Public Health Institute, Helsinki, Finland
O. MÄKELÄ, Department of Bacteriology and Immunology, University of Helsinki and the National Public Health Institute, Helsinki, Finland
T. J. MASON, Department of Molecular Immunology, Commonwealth Serum Laboratories, Parkville, Victoria 3052, Australia
M. J. McCONVILLE, The Walter and Eliza Hall Institute of Medical Research, Melbourne, Victoria 3050, Australia
F. MICHON, Division of Biological Sciences, National Research Council of Canada, Ottawa, Ontario, Canada K1A 0L2
G. F. MITCHELL, The Walter and Eliza Hall Institute of Medical Research, Melbourne, Victoria 3050, Australia
F. MODABBER, Parasitic Diseases Programme, World Health Organization, 1211 Geneva 27, Switzerland
H. MOLL, The Walter and Eliza Hall Institute of Medical Research, Melbourne, Victoria 3050, Australia
J. MONTREUIL, Unité associée, Centre national de Recherche scientifique, Université des Sciences et Techniques, 59655 Lille, France
C. MORENO, Medical Research Council Tuberculosis and Related Infections Unit, Hammersmith Hospital, London W12 0HS, UK
A. MORRIS HOOKE, The Department of Pediatrics and Microbiology, Georgetown University School of Medicine, Washington, DC 20007, USA
D. E. MOSIER, Division of Immunology, Medical Biology Institute, La Jolla, CA 92037, USA
M. PORRO, Sclavo SpA, Siena 53100, Italy
N. RAUTONEN, Department of Bacteriology and Immunology, University of Helsinki and the National Public Health Institute, Helsinki, Finland
J. B. ROBBINS, National Institute of Child Health and Human Development, National Institutes of Health, Bethesda, MD 20892, USA
S. J. RODDA, Department of Molecular Immunology, Commonwealth Serum Laboratories, Parkville, Victoria 3052, Australia
J. ROTTA, Institute of Hygiene and Epidemiology, 10042 Prague 10, Czechoslovakia

R. ROY, Division of Biological Sciences, National Research Council of Canada, Ottawa, Ontario, Canada K1A 0R6

P. SCHERLE, Immunology Graduate Program, University of Pennsylvania, Philadelphia, PA 19104, USA

R. SCHNEERSON, National Institute of Child Health and Human Development, National Institutes of Health, Bethesda, MD 20892, USA

P. SCHOOFS, Department of Molecular Immunology, Commonwealth Serum Laboratories, Parkville, Victoria 3052, Australia

I. SEPPÄLÄ, Department of Bacteriology and Immunology, University of Helsinki and the National Public Health Institute, Helsinki, Finland

G. SPIK, Unité associée, Centre National de la Recherche scientifique 217, Université des Sciences et Techniques, 59655 Lille, France

T. SÖDERSTRÖM, Department of Clinical Immunology, Sahlgrenska Hospital and the University of Göteborg, 41346 Göteborg, Sweden

I. W. SUTHERLAND, Department of Microbiology, Edinburgh University, Edinburgh, EH9 3JG, UK

S. C. SZU, National Institute of Child Health and Human Development, National Institutes of Health, Bethesda, MD, 20892 USA

G. TRIBBICK, Department of Molecular Immunology, Commonwealth Serum Laboratories, Parkville, Victoria 3052, Australia

W. F. VANN, Office of Biologics Research and Review, Food and Drug Administration, Bethesda, MD, USA

Y. YANG, National Institute of Child Health and Human Development, National Institutes of Health, Bethesda, MD 20892, USA

Index